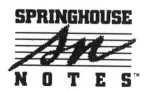

MEDICAL-SURGICAL NURSING

=== SECOND EDITION ===

Mildred Wernet Boyd, RN, MSN
Associate Professor of Nursing
Essex Community College
Baltimore

Barbara L. Tower, RN, MA, MSN, CCRN
Associate Dean of Instruction, Academic Programs
Essex Community College
Baltimore

Springhouse Corporation
Springhouse, Pennsylvania

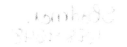

Staff

Executive Director, Editorial
Stanley Loeb

Director of Trade and Textbooks
Minnie B. Rose, RN, BSN, MEd

Art Director
John Hubbard

Clinical Consultant
Maryann Foley, RN, BSN

Editors
David Moreau, Carol Munson

Copy Editor
Pamela Wingrod

Designers
Stephanie Peters (associate art director),
Jacalyn Facciolo

Typography
David Kosten (director), Diane Paluba (manager),
Elizabeth Bergman, Joyce Rossi Biletz, Phyllis
Marron, Robin Mayer, Valerie L. Rosenberger

Manufacturing
Deborah Meiris (manager), T.A. Landis, Anna
Brindisi

SNMS-041294

A member of the Reed Elsevier plc group

Library of Congress Cataloging-in-Publication Data

Boyd, Mildred W.
  Medical-surgical nursing/Mildred Wernet
Boyd, Barbara L. Tower. — 2nd ed.
  p. cm. — (Springhouse notes)
  Includes bibliographical references and
index.
  1. Nursing. 2. Surgical nursing. I. Tower,
Barbara L. II. Title III. Series.
  [DNLM: 1. Nursing Care—outlines. 2.
Surgical Nursing—outlines. WY 18 B789m]
RT41.B64   1993
610.73'—dc20
DNLM/DLC   92-2254
ISBN 0-87434-483-2   CIP

Contents

Advisory Board and Reviewer

How to Use Springhouse Notes

Springhouse Notes is a multi-volume study guide series developed especially for nursing students. Each volume provides essential course material in an outline format, enabling the student to review the information efficiently.

Special features recur throughout the book to make the information accessible and easy to remember. *Learning objectives* begin each chapter, encouraging the student to evaluate knowledge before and after study. Next, within the outlined text, *key points* are highlighted in shaded blocks to facilitate a quick review of critical information. Key points may include cardinal signs and symptoms, current theories, important steps in a nursing procedure, critical assessment findings, crucial nursing interventions, or successful therapies and treatments. *Points to remember* summarize each chapter's major themes. *Study questions* then offer another opportunity to review material and assess knowledge gained before moving on to new information. Difficult, frequently used, or sometimes misunderstood terms (indicated by small capital letters in the outline) are gathered at the end of each chapter and defined in the *glossary*, Appendix A; answers to the study questions appear in Appendix B.

The Springhouse Notes volumes are designed as learning tools, not as primary information sources. When read conscientiously as a supplement to class attendance and textbook reading, Springhouse Notes can enhance understanding and help improve test scores and final grades.

CHAPTER 1

Cardiovascular System

Learning objectives

Check off the items below once you've mastered them:

☐ Describe the psychosocial impact of cardiovascular disorders.

☐ Differentiate between modifiable and nonmodifiable risk factors in the development of a cardiovascular disorder.

☐ List three probable and three possible nursing diagnoses for a patient with any of the cardiovascular disorders.

☐ Identify nursing interventions for a patient with any of the cardiovascular disorders.

☐ Write three teaching goals for a patient with any of the cardiovascular disorders.

I. Anatomy and physiology

A. Cardiac structures
1. The heart is a muscular organ composed of two atria and two ventricles
2. It is surrounded by a pericardial sac that consists of two layers
   a. Visceral (inner) layer
   b. Parietal (outer) layer
3. The heart wall has three layers
   a. Epicardium (visceral pericardium)
   b. Myocardium
   c. Endocardium
4. The heart has four valves
   a. Tricuspid
   b. Mitral
   c. Pulmonary
   d. Aortic

B. Myocardial blood supply
1. The left coronary artery (LCA) branches into the left anterior descending artery (LAD) and the circumflex artery
   a. The LAD artery supplies blood to the anterior wall of the left ventricle, the anterior ventricular septum, and the bundle branches
   b. The circumflex artery provides blood to the lateral and posterior portions of the left ventricle
2. The right coronary artery (RCA) fills the groove between the atria and ventricles and gives rise to the acute marginal artery, ending as the posterior descending artery
   a. The RCA sends blood to the sinus and atrioventricular nodes and to the right atrium
   b. The posterior descending artery supplies the posterior and inferior wall of the left ventricle and the posterior portion of the right ventricle
3. Coronary arteries receive blood primarily during ventricular relaxation (diastole)

C. Circulation
1. From the inferior and superior venae cavae to the right atrium
2. Through the tricuspid valve to the right ventricle
3. Through the pulmonary valve to the pulmonary artery, to the lungs, through the pulmonary veins to the left atrium
4. Through the mitral valve to the left ventricle
5. Through the aortic valve to the aorta and the systemic circulation
6. The goal of nursing management in cardiovascular disorders is to increase blood supply and thus oxygenation to the tissues

D. Electrical conduction
   1. The heart contains specialized muscle fibers that spontaneously generate and conduct their own electrical impulses
   2. The sinoatrial (SA) mode, internodal tracts, atrioventricular (AV) node, bundle of His, right and left bundle branches, and Purkinje fibers make up the system that initiates the heartbeat and coordinates chamber contraction
   3. Impulses follow a right-to-left, top-to-bottom path.
   4. A normal electrical impulse is initiated at the SA node, the heart's intrinsic pacemaker
   5. Once generated, the normal impulse must move forward through the conduction system to the ventricles
   6. Numerous events occur almost simutaneously after initiation of the impulse at the SA node
      a. Atrial depolarization
      b. Atrial contraction
      c. Impulse transmission to the node
      d. Impulse transmission to the Bundle of His, bundle branches and Purkinje fibers
      e. Ventricular depolarization
      f. Ventricular contraction
      g. Ventricular repolarization

E. Cardiac function
   1. Cardiac output (CO) is the total amount of blood ejected per minute
   2. Stroke volume (SV) is the amount of blood ejected with each beat
   3. Cardiac output equals stroke volume times heart rate (CO = SV × HR)
   4. Alterations in CO affect every body system

F. Blood vessels
   1. Arteries are three-layered vessels (intima, media, adventitia) that carry oxygenated blood from the heart to the tissues
   2. Arterioles are small-resistance vessels that feed into capillaries
   3. Capillaries join arterioles to venules (larger, lower-pressured vessels than arterioles), where nutrients and wastes are exchanged
   4. Venules join capillaries to veins
   5. Veins are large-capacity, low-pressure vessels that return unoxygenated blood to the heart

II. Physical assessment findings

A. Subjective data associated with cardiovascular disorders
   1. Dyspnea
   2. PAROXYSMAL NOCTURNAL DYSPNEA (PND)
   3. ORTHOPNEA
   4. Chest and leg pain
   5. Fatigue and weakness

    6. Cough
    7. Syncope
    8. Palpitations

B. Objective data associated with cardiovascular disorders
    1. Blood pressure
    2. Pulse rates
    3. Skin color and temperature
    4. Heart sounds
    5. Edema
    6. Arrhythmias
    7. JUGULAR VENOUS DISTENTION (JVD)
    8. Respiratory distress
    9. Vascular BRUITS
    10. POINT OF MAXIMUM IMPULSE (PMI)
    11. Jaundice
    12. Pruritus

III. Diagnostic tests and procedures

A. Electrocardiography (ECG)
    1. Definition and purpose
        a. Noninvasive test of the heart
        b. Graphical representation of the heart's electrical activity
    2. Nursing interventions and responsibilities
        a. Determine the patient's ability to lie still
        b. Reassure the patient that electrical shock will not occur

B. Ambulatory electrocardiography (Holter monitoring)
    1. Definition and purpose
        a. Noninvasive test of the heart
        b. Recording of the heart's electrical activity for 24 hours
    2. Nursing interventions and responsibilities
        a. Instruct the patient to keep an activity diary
        b. Advise the patient not to bathe or shower, operate machinery, or use a microwave oven or an electric shaver while wearing the monitor

C. Cardiac catheterization
    1. Definition and purpose
        a. Fluoroscopic procedure using a radiopaque dye
        b. Examination of the intracardiac structures, pressures, oxygenation, and cardiac output after the dye is injected
    2. Nursing interventions and responsibilities before the procedure
        a. Withhold the patient's food and fluids after midnight
        b. Take baseline vital signs (VS) and peripheral pulses
        c. Obtain written, informed consent
        d. Inform the patient about possible nausea, chest pain, flushing of the face, or throat irritation from the injection

   e. Note the patient's allergies to seafood, iodine, or radiopaque dyes
  3. Nursing interventions and responsibilities after the procedure
   a. Monitor VS, peripheral pulses, and the injection site for bleeding
   b. Maintain a pressure dressing and bed rest
   c. Force fluids unless contraindicated
   d. Allay the patient's anxiety

D. Echocardiography
  1. Definition and purpose
   a. Noninvasive examination of the heart
   b. Test that uses echoes from sound waves to visualize intracardiac structures and direction of blood flow
  2. Nursing interventions and responsibilities
   a. Determine the patient's ability to lie still
   b. Explain the procedure

E. Exercise testing (stress)
  1. Definition and purpose
   a. Noninvasive test of the heart
   b. Study of the heart's electrical activity during prescribed levels of exercise
  2. Nursing interventions and responsibilities
   a. Withhold food and fluids for 1 hour before the test
   b. Instruct the patient to wear loose-fitting clothing and supportive shoes
   c. Explain the procedure

F. Nuclear cardiology
  1. Definition and purpose
   a. Visual examination of the heart using radioisotopes
   b. Imaging of myocardial perfusion and contractility after I.V. injection of isotopes
  2. Nursing interventions and responsibilities
   a. Explain the procedure
   b. Allay the patient's anxiety
   c. Determine the patient's ability to lie still during the procedure

G. Coronary arteriography
  1. Definition and purpose
   a. Fluoroscopic procedure using a radiopaque dye
   b. Examination of the coronary arteries
  2. Nursing interventions and responsibilities before the procedure
   a. Note the patient's allergies to iodine, seafood, or radiopaque dyes
   b. Monitor the patient's VS
   c. Allay the patient's anxiety
   d. Inform the patient about possible flushing of the face or throat irritation from the injection

3. Nursing interventions and responsibilities after the procedure
  a. Check the insertion site for bleeding
  b. Assess peripheral pulses
  c. Maintain a pressure dressing and bed rest

H. Digital subtraction angiography
  1. Definition and purpose
    a. Invasive procedure using a computer system and fluoroscopy with an image intensifier
    b. Complete visualization of the arterial blood supply to a specific area
  2. Nursing interventions and responsibilities before the procedure
    a. Obtain written, informed consent
    b. Monitor the patient's VS
  3. Nursing interventions and responsibilities after the procedure
    a. Check the insertion site for bleeding
    b. Instruct the patient to drink at least 1 liter of fluid

I. Hemodynamic monitoring
  1. Definition and purpose
    a. Procedure using a balloon-tipped, flow-directed catheter (Swan-Ganz)
    b. Examination of intracardiac pressures and cardiac output
  2. Nursing interventions and responsibilities before the procedure
    a. Obtain written, informed consent
    b. Explain the procedure and its purpose to the patient
  3. Nursing interventions and responsibilities after the procedure
    a. Check the insertion site for signs of infection
    b. Monitor the pressure tracings and record readings

J. Chest X-ray
  1. Definition and purpose
    a. Noninvasive examination of the heart and lungs
    b. Radiographic picture of the heart and lungs
  2. Nursing interventions and responsibilities
    a. Determine the patient's ability to hold the breath
    b. Ensure that the patient removes jewelry

K. Blood chemistries
  1. Definition and purpose
    a. Laboratory test of a blood sample
    b. Analysis for sodium, potassium, magnesium, calcium, glucose, phosphorus, cholesterol, triglycerides, uric acid, bicarbonate, creatinine, blood urea nitrogen (BUN), bilirubin, creatinine phosphokinase (CPK), CPK isoenzymes, lactic dehydrogenase (LDH), LDH isoenzymes, serum aspartate aminotransferase (AST, formerly serum glutamic oxaloacetic transaminase [SGOT]), and serum alanine aminotransferase (ALT, formerly serum glutamic pyruvic transaminase [SGPT])

2. Nursing interventions and responsibilities
   a. Note any drugs that may alter test results
   b. Restrict the patient's exercise before the blood sample is drawn
   c. Withhold intramuscular injections or note the time of the injection on the laboratory slip
   d. Withhold food and fluids, as ordered
   e. Assess the venipuncture site for bleeding

L. Hematologic studies
   1. Definition and purpose
      a. Laboratory test of a blood sample
      b. Analysis for red blood cells (RBCs), white blood cells (WBCs), erythrocyte sedimentation rate (ESR), prothrombin time (PT), partial thromboplastin time (PTT), platelets, hemoglobin (Hgb), and hematocrit (Hct)
   2. Nursing interventions and responsibilities
      a. Note any drugs that might alter test results before the procedure
      b. Assess the venipuncture site for bleeding after the procedure

M. Arterial blood gas (ABG) analysis
   1. Definition and purpose
      a. Test of arterial blood
      b. Assessment of tissue oxygenation, ventilation, and acid-base status
   2. Nursing interventions and responsibilities before the procedure
      a. Document the patient's temperature
      b. Note whether the patient needs supplemental oxygen or mechanical ventilation
   3. Nursing interventions and responsibilities after the procedure
      a. Check the site for bleeding
      b. Maintain a pressure dressing

N. Doppler ultrasound
   1. Definition and purpose
      a. Noninvasive procedure that transforms echoes from sound waves into audible sounds
      b. Examination of blood flow in peripheral circulation
   2. Nursing interventions and responsibilities
      a. Determine the patient's ability to lie still
      b. Explain the procedure

O. Venogram
   1. Definition and purpose
      a. Visualization of the veins after I.V. injection of a dye
      b. Diagnosis of deep vein thrombosis or incompetent valves
   2. Nursing interventions and responsibilities before the procedure
      a. Withhold food and fluids after midnight
      b. Record the patient's baseline VS and peripheral pulses
      c. Obtain written, informed consent

d. Note the patient's allergies to seafood, iodine, or radiopaque dyes
e. Inform the patient about possible flushing of the face or throat irritation from the injection
3. Nursing interventions and responsibilities after the procedure
   a. Check the injection site for bleeding and hematoma
   b. Force fluids unless contraindicated

IV. Psychosocial impact of cardiovascular disorders

A. Developmental impact
   1. Fear of rejection
   2. Lowered self-esteem
   3. Fear of dying
   4. Role conflict

B. Economic impact
   1. Disruption or loss of employment
   2. Cost of hospitalization, medications, and special diets

C. Occupational and recreational impact
   1. Restrictions in work activity
   2. Changes in leisure activity
   3. Restrictions in physical activity (walking, climbing stairs)
   4. Restrictions in activity related to environmental temperature; for example, hot or cold weather may interfere with the patient's ability to take walks or go outside

D. Social impact
   1. Changes in dietary habits, such as dining out
   2. Changes in sexual function
   3. Changes in role performance, including work and family roles
   4. Social isolation

V. Risk factors for developing cardiovascular disorders

A. Modifiable risk factors (impact of cardiovascular disorders can be reduced by altering these)
   1. Smoking
   2. Hypertension
   3. Hypercholesterolemia
   4. Obesity
   5. Physical inactivity
   6. Emotional stress

B. Nonmodifiable risk factors
   1. Sex
   2. Family history of cardiovascular illness
   3. Childhood history of cardiovascular illness
   4. Ethnicity

5. Race _____
6. Aging

VI. Nursing diagnostic categories for a patient with a cardiovascular disorder

A. Probable nursing diagnostic categories
   1. Decreased cardiac output
   2. Pain
   3. Altered cardiopulmonary tissue perfusion
   4. Altered peripheral tissue perfusion
   5. Altered cerebral tissue perfusion

B. Possible nursing diagnostic categories
   1. Fluid volume excess
   2. Activity intolerance
   3. Fear
   4. Anxiety
   5. Ineffective individual coping
   6. Compromised family coping
   7. Self-esteem disturbance
   8. Altered role performance
   9. Body image disturbance
   10. Sexual dysfunction
   11. Noncompliance
   12. Chronic low self-esteem
   13. Situational low self-esteem
   14. Fatigue

VII. Cardiac surgery

A. Definitions
   1. Coronary artery bypass graft (CABG) — surgical revascularization of the coronary arteries using the saphenous veins or the internal mammary artery to bypass an obstruction caused by atherosclerosis
   2. Valve replacement — surgical replacement of stenotic or incompetent valves with a mechanical or bioprosthetic valve, such as Starr-Edwards "ball-in-cage" valves, porcine valves, or Bjork-Shiley "tilting disk" valves
   3. Valvular annuloplasty — surgical repair or reconstruction of the leaflets and annulus of the valve
   4. Mitral valve commissurotomy — surgical opening of the fused portion of the mitral valve leaflets, using a dilator
   5. Valvuloplasty — surgical repair or reconstruction of the valve
   6. Percutaneous transluminal valvuloplasty — dilation of calcified and stenotic valvular leaflets, using a balloon catheter

B. Preoperative nursing interventions and responsibilities
   1. Complete patient and family preoperative teaching
      a. Determine the patient's understanding of the procedure
      b. Describe the operating room (OR), postanesthesia care unit (PACU), and preoperative and postoperative routines
      c. Demonstrate postoperative turning, coughing, and deep-breathing (TCDB), splinting, leg exercises, and range-of-motion (ROM) exercises
      d. Explain the postoperative need for drainage tubes, surgical dressings, oxygen therapy, I.V. therapy, and pain control
   2. Allay the patient's and family's anxiety about surgery
   3. Document the patient's history and physical assessment data base
   4. Obtain baseline hemodynamic variables, ECG readings, and ABG studies
   5. Complete a preoperative checklist
   6. Administer preoperative medications

C. Postoperative nursing interventions and responsibilities
   1. Assess cardiac, respiratory, and neurologic status
   2. Assess fluid balance
   3. Assess pain and administer analgesics, as prescribed
   4. Administer oxygen and maintain an endotracheal tube to the ventilator
   5. Monitor VS, urine output (UO), intake/output (I/O), laboratory studies, ECG, hemodynamic variables, daily weight, and pulse oximetry
   6. Monitor and maintain the waterseal chest drainage system for mediastinal and pleural chest tubes
   7. Monitor and maintain the position and patency of drainage tubes and catheters, such as a nasogastric (NG) tube, indwelling urinary (Foley) catheter, and wound drainage and chest tubes
   8. Administer I.V. fluids and transfusion therapy, as prescribed
   9. Inspect and change the surgical dressing, as directed
   10. Keep the patient in semi-Fowler's position
   11. Provide incentive spirometry after extubation or endotracheal suction
   12. Reinforce TCDB and splinting of the incision
   13. Administer antiarrhythmics, anticoagulants, vasopressors, beta adrenergics, diuretics, or cardiac glycosides, as prescribed
   14. Monitor the patient for arrhythmias
   15. Check peripheral circulation: color, temperature, pulses, and complaints of abnormal sensations, such as numbness or tingling
   16. Have a temporary pacemaker near the bed
   17. Administer antibiotics, as prescribed
   18. Assess for return of peristalsis
   19. Provide the prescribed diet, as tolerated
   20. Assist the patient with active and passive ROM and isometric exercises, as tolerated

21. Allay the patient's anxiety
22. Encourage the patient to express feelings about changes in body image or a fear of dying
23. Provide information about support groups, such as Mended Hearts

D. Possible surgical complications
1. Bleeding from the mediastinal tube
2. Myocardial infarction (MI)
3. Decreased cardiac output
4. Arrhythmias
5. Cardiac tamponade
6. Heart block
7. Embolism
8. Valve malfunction

E. Postoperative teaching goals (instructions to the patient and family)
1. Keep follow-up appointments
2. Exercise regularly
3. Stop smoking
4. Maintain a normal weight
5. Know the action, side effects, and scheduling of medications
6. Recognize the signs and symptoms of infection and bleeding
7. Avoid driving and heavy lifting for 6 weeks
8. Complete incision care daily
9. Elevate the leg with the saphenous graft when seated
10. Wear antiembolism stockings
11. Follow a low-sodium diet

VIII. Abdominal aneurysm resection

A. Definition—surgical removal of a portion of weakened arterial wall with an end-to-end anastomosis to a prosthetic graft

B. Preoperative nursing interventions and responsibilities
1. Complete patient and family preoperative teaching
   a. Determine the patient's understanding of the procedure
   b. Describe the OR, PACU, and preoperative and postoperative routines
   c. Demonstrate postoperative TCDB, splinting, and leg and ROM exercises
   d. Explain the postoperative need for drainage tubes, surgical dressings, oxygen therapy, I.V. therapy, and pain control
2. Complete a preoperative checklist
3. Administer preoperative medications, as prescribed
4. Allay the patient's and family's anxiety about surgery
5. Document the patient's history and physical assessment data base

C. Postoperative nursing interventions and responsibilities
1. Assess cardiac, respiratory, and neurologic status

  2. Assess fluid balance
  3. Assess pain and administer analgesics, as prescribed
  4. Administer I.V. fluids and transfusion therapy, as prescribed
  5. Administer oxygen and maintain an endotracheal tube to the ventilator
  6. Provide incentive spirometry after extubation or endotracheal suction
  7. Reinforce TCDB and splinting of the incision
  8. Monitor VS, UO, I/O, central venous pressure (CVP), laboratory studies, ECG, hemodynamic variables, and pulse oximetry
  9. Monitor and maintain the position and patency of NG tubes and Foley catheters
 10. Administer antibiotics, as prescribed
 11. Assess for scrotal and retroperitoneal bleeding
 12. Check peripheral circulation: color, temperature, complaints of abnormal sensation, and pulses in extremities
 13. Inspect and change the surgical dressing, as directed
 14. Keep the patient flat; set up a turning schedule, turning from side to side regularly
 15. Assist the patient with active and passive ROM and isometric exercises, as tolerated
 16. Assess for return of peristalsis
 17. Provide the prescribed diet, as tolerated
 18. Measure and record the patient's abdominal girth
 19. Allay the patient's anxiety

D. Possible surgical complications
  1. Renal failure
  2. Atelectasis
  3. Graft hemorrhage

E. Postoperative teaching goals (instructions to the patient and family)
  1. Keep follow-up appointments
  2. Exercise regularly
  3. Stop smoking
  4. Maintain a normal weight
  5. Know the action, side effects, and scheduling of medications
  6. Recognize the signs and symptoms of infection
  7. Avoid lifting, bending, and driving for 6 weeks or as allowed by the physician
  8. Complete incision care daily
  9. Monitor blood pressure daily
 10. Identify ways to reduce stress
 11. Follow a low-sodium, low-cholesterol diet

IX. Vascular grafting

A. Definition — surgical revascularization of an artery
   1. Uses a synthetic or autogenous graft
   2. Bypasses or resects the diseased segment

B. Types of revascularization
   1. Femoropopliteal
   2. Aortofemoral
   3. Aortoiliac
   4. Femorofemoral
   5. Axillofemoral

C. Preoperative nursing interventions and responsibilities
   1. Complete patient and family preoperative teaching
      a. Determine the patient's understanding of the procedure
      b. Describe the OR, PACU, and preoperative and postoperative routines
      c. Demonstrate postoperative TCDB, splinting, and leg and ROM exercises
      d. Explain the postoperative need for drainage tubes, surgical dressings, oxygen therapy, I.V. therapy, and pain control
   2. Complete a preoperative checklist
   3. Administer preoperative medications, as prescribed
   4. Allay the patient's and family's anxiety about surgery
   5. Document the patient's history and physical assessment data base
   6. Obtain a baseline assessment of peripheral circulation
   7. Administer antibiotics, as prescribed

D. Postoperative nursing interventions and responsibilities
   1. Assess cardiac and neurovascular status
   2. Assess pain and administer analgesics, as prescribed
   3. Administer I.V. fluids and transfusion therapy, as prescribed
   4. Monitor VS, UO, I/O, laboratory studies, neurovascular checks, and pulse oximetry
   5. Monitor and maintain the position and patency of NG tubes and Foley catheters
   6. Administer anticoagulants, as prescribed
   7. Inspect and change the surgical dressing, as directed
   8. Keep the patient in semi-Fowler's position; avoid positioning on or flexion at the graft site
   9. Provide a bed cradle
   10. Check peripheral circulation: temperature, color, pulses, and complaints of abnormal sensations in extremities distal to the graft site
   11. Measure and record the patient's ankle, calf, and thigh circumferences
   12. Provide incentive spirometry
   13. Reinforce TCDB and splinting of the incision
   14. Assess for return of peristalsis

15. Provide the prescribed diet, as tolerated
16. Measure and record the patient's abdominal girth
17. Assist the patient with active and passive ROM and isometric exercises, as tolerated
18. Allay the patient's anxiety
19. Encourage the patient to express feelings about changes in body image
20. Increase ambulation, as tolerated

E. Possible surgical complications
   1. Thrombosis
   2. Embolism
   3. Graft rejection
   4. Hemorrhage

F. Postoperative teaching goals (instructions to the patient and family)
   1. Keep follow-up appointments
   2. Exercise regularly
   3. Stop smoking
   4. Maintain a normal weight, and follow any dietary restrictions
   5. Know the action, side effects, and scheduling of medications
   6. Recognize the signs and symptoms of infection
   7. Avoid pressure on or flexion at the graft site
   8. Avoid wearing constrictive clothing
   9. Complete incision care daily
   10. Protect the graft site from injury
   11. Check pulses distal to the graft site daily
   12. Adhere to long-term anticoagulant therapy
   13. Wear properly fitting shoes
   14. Provide proper foot care daily

X. Hypertension

A. Definition — constant elevation of systolic or diastolic blood pressure (greater than 140/90 mm Hg)

B. Possible etiology
   1. Unknown etiology for primary hypertension
   2. Renal disease
   3. Pheochromocytoma
   4. Cushing's disease

C. Pathophysiology
   1. Narrowing of the arterioles, which increases peripheral resistance
   2. Increased force needed to circulate blood, which elevates blood pressure

D. Possible clinical manifestations
   1. Asymptomatic
   2. Elevated blood pressure

   3. Headache
   4. Visual disturbances
   5. Left ventricular hypertrophy
   6. Renal failure
   7. Dizziness
   8. Papilledema
   9. Congestive heart failure (CHF)
  10. Cerebral ischemia

E. Possible diagnostic test findings
   1. Blood pressure: sustained readings greater than 140/90 mm Hg
   2. ECG: Left ventricular hypertrophy
   3. Chest X-ray: Cardiomegaly
   4. Ophthalmoscopic examination: retinal changes, such as severe vasoconstriction and retinopathy
   5. Blood chemistry: elevated sodium and cholesterol levels

F. Medical management
   1. Diet: low-sodium, low-calorie, low-cholesterol, and low-fat; restrict alcohol and caffeine
   2. I.V. therapy: heparin lock
   3. Activity: as tolerated
   4. Monitoring: VS, ECG, UO, and I/O
   5. Laboratory studies: sodium, potassium, and cholesterol
   6. Diuretics: furosemide (Lasix), spironolactone (Aldactone), hydrochlorothiazide (HydroDIURIL)
   7. Antihypertensives: methyldopa (Aldomet), hydralazine (Apresoline), prazosin (Minipress), doxazosin mesylate (Cardura)
   8. Vasodilators: sodium nitroprusside (Nipride)
   9. Calcium blockers: nifedipine (Procardia), verapamil (Calan), diltiazem (Cardizem), nicardipine (Cardene)
  10. Beta-adrenergic blockers: propranolol (Inderal), metoprolol (Lopressor), carteolol hydrochloride (Cartrol), penbutolol sulfate (Levatol)
  11. ACE inhibitors: captopril (Capoten), enalapril (Vasotec), lisinopril (Prinivil)

G. Nursing interventions and responsibilities
   1. Maintain the patient's prescribed diet
   2. Assess cardiovascular status
   3. Monitor and record VS, UO, I/O, laboratory studies, and daily weight
   4. Administer medications, as prescribed
   5. Encourage the patient to express feelings about daily stress
   6. Maintain a quiet environment
   7. Provide information about the American Heart Association

H. Teaching goals (instructions to the patient and family)
   1. Keep follow-up appointments
   2. Exercise regularly

    3. Stop smoking
    4. Maintain a normal weight
    5. Know the action, side effects, and scheduling of medications
    6. Identify ways to reduce stress
    7. Follow dietary restrictions and recommendations
    8. Maintain a quiet environment

I. Possible medical complications
    1. Cerebrovascular accident (CVA)
    2. Visual changes
    3. Renal failure
    4. CHF
    5. Hypertensive crisis

J. Possible surgical interventions: none

XI. Coronary artery disease: arteriosclerosis and atherosclerosis

A. Definitions
    1. Arteriosclerosis — loss of elasticity of the arteries' intimal layer (sometimes called hardening of the arteries)
    2. Atherosclerosis — accumulation in the arteries of fatty plaque made of lipids

B. Possible etiology
    1. Aging
    2. Stress
    3. Genetics
    4. Depletion of estrogen

C. Pathophysiology
    1. Narrowing or obstruction of the coronary arteries by an embolus, vasospasm, or accumulated plaque
    2. Decreased perfusion and inadequate myocardial oxygen supply

D. Possible clinical manifestations
    1. Hypertension
    2. Angina
    3. MI
    4. CHF
    5. Death

E. Possible diagnostic test findings
    1. ECG or Holter monitoring: ST depression, T wave inversion
    2. Stress test: abnormal ECG, chest pain
    3. Coronary arteriography: plaque formation
    4. Blood chemistry: increased cholesterol

F. Medical management
   1. Diet: low-calorie, low-sodium, low-cholesterol, and low-fat; increased dietary fiber
   2. I.V. therapy: heparin lock
   3. Oxygen therapy
   4. Monitoring: VS, UO, CVP, ECG, hemodynamic variables, I/O, and neurovascular checks
   5. Laboratory studies: sodium, potassium, cholesterol, CPK, LDH, AST, CPK isoenzymes, LDH isoenzymes, and ABGs
   6. Weight reduction
   7. Arterial line for blood pressure monitoring
   8. Intraaortic balloon pump (IABP)
   9. Thrombolytic therapy: streptokinase (Streptase)
   10. Percutaneous transluminal coronary angioplasty (PTCA)
   11. Foley catheter
   12. Antihyperlipidemic agents: clofibrate (Atromid-S), lovastatin (Mevacor), nicotinic acid (Niacin), gemifibrozil (Lopid)
   13. Nitrates: nitroglycerin (Nitro Bid), isosorbide dinitrate (Isordil)
   14. Beta-adrenergic blockers: propranolol (Inderal), nadolol (Corgard)
   15. Calcium blockers: nifedipine (Procardia), verapamil (Calan), diltiazem (Cardizem)
   16. Analgesic: morphine (MS Contin)
   17. Antianxiety agent: diazepam (Valium)
   18. Hypocholesterolemics: cholestyramine (Questran), colestipol hydrochoride (Colestid)
   19. Laser angioplasty
   20. Atherectomy

G. Nursing interventions and responsibilities
   1. Maintain the patient's prescribed diet
   2. Administer oxygen and medications, as prescribed
   3. Assess cardiovascular status
   4. Monitor and record VS, UO, hemodynamic variables, I/O, ECG, and laboratory studies
   5. Encourage the patient to express anxiety, fears, or concerns
   6. Provide information about the American Heart Association

H. Teaching goals (instructions to the patient and family)
   1. Keep follow-up appointments
   2. Exercise regularly
   3. Stop smoking
   4. Maintain a normal weight
   5. Know the action, side effects, and scheduling of medications
   6. Identify ways to reduce stress
   7. Know the difference between angina and MI
   8. Adhere to activity limitations
   9. Limit daily alcohol intake to 2 ounces

10. Monitor blood pressure daily
11. Follow dietary restrictions and recommendations

I. Possible medical complications
   1. Angina
   2. MI
   3. CHF

J. Possible surgical interventions: CABG (see page 9)

XII. Angina

A. Definition
   1. Angina is chest pain caused by inadequate myocardial oxygen supply
   2. Complaints of chest pain have increased significance in a patient with a peripheral vascular problem

B. Possible etiology
   1. Atherosclerosis
   2. Vasospasm
   3. Aortic stenosis
   4. Activity or disease that increases metabolic demands

C. Pathophysiology
   1. Narrowing of the coronary arteries, which results from plaque accumulation in the intimal lining
   2. Obstruction of blood flow, which diminishes myocardial oxygen supply

D. Possible clinical manifestations
   1. Substernal, crushing, compressing pain
      a. May radiate to the arms
      b. Usually lasts 3 to 5 minutes
      c. Usually occurs after exertion, emotional excitement, or exposure to cold but also can develop when the patient is at rest
   2. Dyspnea
   3. Palpitations
   4. Epigastric distress
   5. Tachycardia
   6. Diaphoresis
   7. Anxiety

E. Possible diagnostic test findings
   1. ECG: ST depression, T wave inversion during acute pain
   2. Stress test: abnormal ECG, chest pain
   3. Coronary arteriography: plaque accumulation
   4. Blood chemistry: increased cholesterol
   5. Cardiac enzymes: within normal limits
   6. Holter monitoring: ST depression, T wave inversion

F. Medical management
   1. Diet: low-calorie, low-sodium, and low-cholesterol
   2. I.V. therapy: heparin lock
   3. Oxygen therapy
   4. Position: semi-Fowler's
   5. Monitoring: VS, UO, ECG, hemodynamic variables, I/O, and neurovascular checks
   6. Laboratory studies: ABGs, sodium, potassium, CPK with isoenzymes, LDH with isoenzymes, and AST
   7. PTCA
   8. Thrombolytic therapy: streptokinase (Streptase)
   9. Arterial line for blood pressure monitoring
   10. Nitrates: nitroglycerin (Nitro-Bid), isosorbide dinitrate (Isordil)
   11. Beta-adrenergic blockers: propranolol (Inderal), nadolol (Corgard), atenolol (Tenormin), metoprolol (Lopressor)
   12. Calcium blockers: verapamil (Calan), diltiazem (Cardizem), nifedipine (Procardia), nicardipine (Cardene)

G. Nursing interventions and responsibilities
   1. Maintain the patient's prescribed diet
   2. Administer oxygen and medications, as prescribed
   3. Assess cardiovascular status
   4. Monitor and record VS, UO, hemodynamic variables, I/O, and laboratory studies
   5. Assess for chest pain
   6. Encourage the patient to express anxiety, fears, or concerns
   7. Advise the patient to rest if pain begins
   8. Obtain an ECG reading during an acute attack
   9. Keep the patient in semi-Fowler's position
   10. Provide information about the American Heart Association

H. Teaching goals (instructions to the patient and family)
   1. Keep follow-up appointments
   2. Exercise regularly
   3. Stop smoking
   4. Maintain a normal weight
   5. Know the action, side effects, and scheduling of medications
   6. Identify ways to reduce stress
   7. Know the difference between angina and MI
   8. Avoid activities or situations that cause angina, such as exertion, heavy meals, emotional upsets, and exposure to cold
   9. Alternate rest periods with activity
   10. Follow dietary restrictions and recommendations
   11. Seek medical attention if pain lasts more than 20 minutes
   12. Monitor blood pressure daily

I. Possible medical complications
  1. Arrhythmias
  2. CHF
  3. MI

J. Possible surgical interventions: CABG (see page 9)

XIII. Myocardial infarction

A. Definition — death of a portion of the myocardial muscle cells caused by a lack of oxygen from inadequate perfusion

B. Possible etiology
  1. Atherosclerosis
  2. Decreased perfusion
  3. Embolism or thrombus
  4. Coronary artery spasm

C. Pathophysiology
  1. Narrowing and eventual obstruction of the coronary arteries from plaque accumulation
  2. Death of the myocardial cells from inadequate perfusion and oxygenation

D. Possible clinical manifestations
  1. Crushing substernal pain
    a. May radiate to the jaw, back, and arms
    b. Lasts longer than anginal pain
    c. Is unrelieved by rest or nitroglycerin
    d. May not be present (asymptomatic, or "silent," MI)
  2. Dyspnea
  3. Nausea and vomiting
  4. Anxiety
  5. Diaphoresis
  6. Pallor
  7. Arrhythmias
  8. Elevated temperature

E. Possible diagnostic test findings
  1. ECG: enlarged Q wave, elevated ST segment, T wave inversion
  2. Blood chemistry: increased CPK, LDH, AST, lipids; positive CPK-MB fraction; flipped LDH-1 (LDH-1 levels exceed LDH-2 levels, the reversal of their normal patterns)
  3. Hematology: increased WBC count

F. Medical management
  1. Diet: low-calorie, low-cholesterol, low-fat
  2. Antiarrhythmics: quinidine gluconate (Quinaglute), lidocaine (Xylocaine), procainamide (Pronestyl)

3. Anticoagulant: aspirin
4. Antihypertensives: hydralazine (Apresoline), methyldopa (Aldomet)
5. IABP
6. Left ventricular assist device (LVAD)
7. Thrombolytic therapy: anistreplase (Eminase), anisoylated plasminogen streptokinase activator complex (APSAC), streptokinase (Streptase)
8. Monitoring: VS, UO, ECG, and hemodynamic variables
9. Oxygen therapy
10. Laboratory studies: ABGs, CPK, CPK isoenzymes, LDH, LDH isoenzymes, AST, WBC, sodium, potassium, and glucose
11. Position: semi-Fowler's
12. I.V. therapy: heparin lock
13. PTCA
14. Arterial line for blood pressure monitoring
15. Laserangioplasty
16. Vascular stents
17. Atherectomy

G. Nursing interventions and responsibilities
1. Maintain the patient's prescribed diet
2. Assess cardiovascular and respiratory status
3. Monitor and record VS, UO, I/O, hemodynamic variables, laboratory studies, and ECG results
4. Maintain bed rest
5. Administer oxygen and medications, as prescribed
6. Obtain an ECG reading during acute pain
7. Allay the patient's anxiety
8. Keep the patient in semi-Fowler's position
9. Provide information about the American Heart Association

H. Teaching goals (instructions to the patient and family)
1. Keep follow-up appointments
2. Know the action, side effects, and scheduling of medications
3. Identify ways to reduce stress
4. Exercise regularly
5. Stop smoking
6. Follow dietary restrictions and recommendations
7. Participate in a cardiac rehabilitation program
8. Maintain a normal weight
9. Know the difference between angina and MI
10. Alternate rest periods with activity

I. Possible medical complications
1. Arrhythmias
2. Cardiogenic shock
3. CHF
4. Papillary muscle rupture

5. Pericarditis

J. Possible surgical interventions: CABG (see page 9)

XIV. Congestive heart failure: left-sided

A. Definition—failure of the left side of the heart to pump enough blood to meet metabolic demands

B. Possible etiology
   1. Atherosclerosis
   2. Fluid overload
   3. MI
   4. Valvular stenosis
   5. Valvular insufficiency
   6. Hypertension
   7. Cardiac conduction defects

C. Pathophysiology
   1. Decreased myocardial contractility or increased myocardial workload, either of which increases left ventricular pressure and left atrial pressure and reduces cardiac output
   2. Impaired oxygenation and respiratory manifestations of fluid overload

D. Possible clinical manifestations
   1. Dyspnea
   2. PND
   3. Crackles
   4. Cough
   5. Gallop rhythm: S_3, S_4
   6. Arrhythmias
   7. Fatigue
   8. Anxiety
   9. Orthopnea
   10. Tachycardia
   11. Tachypnea

E. Possible diagnostic test findings
   1. Chest X-ray: increased pulmonary congestion, left ventricular hypertrophy
   2. Echocardiography: increased size of cardiac chambers and decreased wall motion
   3. Hemodynamic monitoring: increased pulmonary capillary wedge pressure (PCWP), CVP, and pulmonary artery pressure (PAP); decreased cardiac output
   4. ABGs: hypoxemia, hypercapnea
   5. ECG: left ventricular hypertrophy
   6. Blood chemistry: decreased potassium, sodium; increased BUN, creatinine

F. Medical management
   1. Diet: low-sodium; limit fluids
   2. I.V. therapy: electrolyte replacement; heparin lock
   3. Oxygen therapy
   4. Position: semi-Fowler's
   5. Activity: bed rest; active ROM and isometric exercises
   6. Monitoring: VS, UO, I/O, ECG, and hemodynamic variables
   7. Laboratory studies: ABGs, sodium, potassium, BUN, and creatinine
   8. Foley catheter
   9. IABP
   10. LVAD
   11. Analgesic: morphine sulfate (Roxanol)
   12. Diuretics: furosemide (Lasix), ethacrynic acid (Edecrin)
   13. Vasodilator: sodium nitroprusside (Nipride)
   14. Cardiac inotropes: dopamine hydrochloride (Intropin), dobutamine (Dobutrex)
   15. Cardiac glycoside: digoxin (Lanoxin)
   16. Nitrates: isosorbide dinitrate (Isordil), nitroglycerin (Nitro-Bid)
   17. ACE inhibitors: captopril (Capoten), enalapril (Vasotec), lisinopril (Prinivil)
   18. Phosphodiesterase inhibitor: amrinone lactate (Inocor)
   19. Specialized bed: active or static, low air loss (Kin Air, Flexicair)

G. Nursing interventions and responsibilities
   1. Maintain the patient's prescribed diet
   2. Restrict oral fluids
   3. Administer I.V. fluids, oxygen, and medications, as prescribed
   4. Provide suctioning and TCDB
   5. Assess cardiovascular and respiratory status
   6. Weigh the patient daily
   7. Keep the patient in semi-Fowler's position
   8. Monitor and record VS, UO, CVP, hemodynamic variables, I/O, and laboratory studies
   9. Assess peripheral edema
   10. Encourage the patient to express feelings, such as a fear of dying
   11. Provide information about the American Heart Association

H. Teaching goals (instructions to the patient and family)
   1. Keep follow-up appointments
   2. Stop smoking
   3. Maintain a normal weight
   4. Know the action, side effects, and scheduling of medications
   5. Supplement the diet with foods high in potassium and low in sodium
   6. Recognize the signs and symptoms of fluid overload
   7. Adhere to activity limitations
   8. Alternate rest periods with activity
   9. Follow dietary restrictions and recommendations

   I. Possible medical complications
      1. Digoxin toxicity
      2. Fluid overload
      3. Cardiogenic shock
      4. Pulmonary edema
      5. Hypokalemia

   J. Possible surgical interventions: none

XV. Congestive heart failure: right-sided

   A. Definition — failure of the right side of the heart to pump enough blood to meet metabolic demands

   B. Possible etiology
      1. Atherosclerosis
      2. Left-sided CHF
      3. Chronic obstructive pulmonary disease (COPD)
      4. Valvular stenosis
      5. Valvular insufficiency

   C. Pathophysiology
      1. Increased pressure from left-sided CHF
      2. Increased venous congestion in the systemic circulation with fluid overload

   D. Possible clinical manifestations
      1. JVD
      2. Anorexia
      3. Nausea
      4. Ascites
      5. Hepatomegaly
      6. Dependent edema
      7. Weight gain
      8. Signs of left-sided CHF
      9. Gallop rhythm: S_3, S_4
    10. Tachycardia
    11. Fatigue

   E. Possible diagnostic test findings
      1. Chest X-ray: pulmonary congestion, cardiomegaly, pleural effusions
      2. Echocardiogram: increased size of chambers, decrease in wall motion
      3. Hemodynamic monitoring: increased PCWP, PAP, CVP; decreased cardiac output
      4. ABGs: hypoxemia
      5. ECG: left and right ventricular hypertrophy
      6. Blood chemistry: decreased sodium, potassium; increased BUN, creatinine

F. Medical management
1. Diet: low-sodium; limit fluids
2. I.V. therapy: electrolyte replacement, heparin lock
3. Oxygen therapy
4. Position: semi-Fowler's
5. Activity: bed rest, active ROM and isometric exercises
6. Monitoring: VS, UO, I/O, ECG, and hemodynamic variables
7. Laboratory studies: ABGs, sodium, potassium, BUN, and creatinine
8. Foley catheter
9. IABP
10. Thoracentesis
11. Paracentesis
12. Analgesic: morphine sulfate (Roxanol)
13. Diuretics: furosemide (Lasix), ethacrynic acid (Edecrin)
14. Vasodilator: sodium nitroprusside (Nipride)
15. Cardiac inotropes: dopamine hydrochloride (Intropin), dobutamine (Dobutrex)
16. Cardiac glycoside: digoxin (Lanoxin)
17. Nitrates: isosorbide dinitrate (Isordil), nitroglycerin (Nitro-Bid)

G. Nursing interventions and responsibilities
1. Maintain the patient's prescribed diet
2. Restrict oral fluids
3. Administer I.V. fluids, oxygen, and medications, as prescribed
4. Provide suctioning and TCDB
5. Assess cardiovascular and respiratory status
6. Assess peripheral edema
7. Keep the patient in semi-Fowler's position
8. Monitor and record VS, UO, I/O, hemodynamic variables, and laboratory studies
9. Weigh the patient daily
10. Encourage the patient to express feelings, such as a fear of dying
11. Measure and record the patient's abdominal girth

H. Teaching goals (instructions to the patient and family)
1. Keep follow-up appointments
2. Stop smoking
3. Maintain a normal weight
4. Know the action, side effects, and scheduling of medications
5. Supplement the diet with foods high in potassium and low in sodium
6. Recognize the signs and symptoms of fluid overload
7. Adhere to activity limitations
8. Alternate rest periods with activity
9. Follow dietary restrictions and recommendations

I. Possible medical complications
1. Digoxin toxicity

2. Fluid overload
3. Cardiogenic shock
4. Pulmonary edema
5. Hypokalemia
6. Hypernatremia

J. Possible surgical interventions: none

XVI. Acute pulmonary edema

A. Definition — most extreme form of left-sided heart failure; results in increased pressure in the capillaries of the lungs and acute transudation of fluid

B. Possible etiology
1. Atherosclerosis
2. MI
3. Myocarditis
4. Valvular disease
5. Smoke inhalation
6. Drug overdose: heroin, barbiturates, morphine sulfate
7. Overload of I.V. fluids

C. Pathophysiology
1. Alveolar and interstitial edema from the heart's failure to pump adequately
2. Impaired oxygenation and hypoxia

D. Possible clinical manifestations
1. Dyspnea
2. Paroxysmal cough
3. Blood-tinged, frothy sputum
4. Orthopnea
5. Tachypnea
6. Agitation
7. Restlessness
8. Intense fear
9. Chest pain
10. Syncope
11. Tachycardia
12. Cold, clammy skin
13. Gallop rhythm: S_3, S_4
14. JVD

E. Possible diagnostic test findings
1. Chest X-ray: interstitial edema
2. ABGs: respiratory alkalosis or acidosis
3. ECG: tachycardia, ventricular enlargement

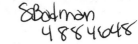

4. Hemodynamic monitoring: increased PCWP, CVP, PAP; decreased cardiac output

F. Medical management
   1. Diet: low-sodium; limit fluids
   2. I.V. therapy: electrolyte replacement, heparin lock
   3. Oxygen therapy
   4. Intubation and mechanical ventilation
   5. Tourniquets: rotating
   6. Position: high-Fowler's
   7. Activity: bed rest; active ROM and isometric exercises
   8. Monitoring: VS, UO, I/O, ECG, and hemodynamic variables
   9. Laboratory studies: sodium, potassium, ABGs, BUN, and creatinine
   10. Foley catheter, endotracheal tube suctioning
   11. Analgesic: morphine sulfate (Roxanol)
   12. Diuretics: furosemide (Lasix), ethacrynic acid (Edecrin)
   13. Vasodilator: sodium nitroprusside (Nipride)
   14. Cardiac inotropes: dopamine hydrochloride (Intropin), dobutamine (Dobutrex)
   15. Cardiac glycoside: digoxin (Lanoxin)
   16. Nitrates: isosorbide dinitrate (Isordil), nitroglycerin (Nitro-Bid)
   17. Bronchodilators: aminophylline (Somophyllin)
   18. Pulse oximetry

G. Nursing interventions and responsibilities
   1. Withhold food and fluids, as directed
   2. Administer I.V. fluids, oxygen, and medications, as prescribed
   3. Provide suctioning and TCDB
   4. Assess cardiovascular and respiratory status
   5. Keep the patient in high-Fowler's position
   6. Monitor and record VS, UO, I/O, hemodynamic variables, laboratory studies, and daily weight
   7. Allay the patient's anxiety
   8. Encourage the patient to express feelings, such as a fear of suffocation
   9. Note the color, amount, and consistency of sputum
   10. Apply rotating tourniquets

H. Teaching goals (instructions to the patient and family)
   1. Stop smoking
   2. Maintain a normal weight
   3. Know the action, side effects, and scheduling of medications
   4. Recognize the signs and symptoms of respiratory distress
   5. Note signs of fluid overload
   6. Adhere to activity limitations
   7. Alternate rest periods with activity
   8. Follow dietary restrictions and recommendations
   9. Sleep with the head of the bed elevated

10. Supplement the diet with foods high in potassium and low in sodium
11. Identify ways to reduce stress

I. Possible medical complications
  1. Digoxin toxicity
  2. Fluid overload
  3. Pulmonary embolism
  4. Hypokalemia
  5. Hypernatremia

J. Possible surgical interventions: none

XVII. Cardiogenic shock

A. Definition — failure of the heart to pump adequately, thereby reducing cardiac output and compromising tissue perfusion

B. Possible etiology
  1. MI
  2. Myocarditis
  3. Advanced heart block
  4. CHF

C. Pathophysiology
  1. Decreased stroke volume and cardiac output; increased left ventricular volume
  2. Compensatory increases in heart rate and contractility, which raise the demand for myocardial oxygen
  3. Imbalance between oxygen supply and demand, which increases myocardial ischemia and further compromises the heart's pumping action

D. Possible clinical manifestations
  1. Hypotension (systolic pressure of less than 90 mm Hg)
  2. Oliguria (urine output of less than 30 ml/hour)
  3. Cold, clammy skin
  4. Tachycardia
  5. Restlessness
  6. Hypoxia
  7. Tachypnea
  8. Anxiety
  9. Arrhythmias
  10. Disorientation and confusion

E. Possible diagnostic test findings
  1. ABGs: metabolic acidosis, hypoxemia
  2. ECG: MI (enlarged Q wave, ST elevation)
  3. Blood chemistry: increased BUN, creatinine

4. Hemodynamic monitoring: decreased stroke volume and cardiac output; increased PCWP, CVP, PAP

F. Medical management
1. Diet: withhold food and fluids
2. I.V. therapy: electrolyte replacement, heparin lock
3. Oxygen therapy
4. Intubation and mechanical ventilation
5. Position: semi-Fowler's
6. Activity: bed rest; passive ROM and isometric exercises
7. Monitoring: VS, UO, I/O, ECG, hemodynamic variables, and level of consciousness
8. Laboratory studies: potassium, sodium, BUN, creatinine, and ABGs
9. Foley catheter, endotracheal tube suction
10. IABP
11. Diuretics: furosemide (Lasix), ethacrynic acid (Edecrin)
12. Vasodilator: sodium nitroprusside (Nipride)
13. Cardiac inotropes: dopamine hydrochloride (Intropin), dobutamine (Dobutrex), amrinone lactate (Inocor)
14. Cardiac glycoside: digoxin (Lanoxin)
15. Vasopressor: norepinephrine (Levophed)
16. Adrenergic agent: epinephrine hydrochloride (Adrenalin)
17. Hemopump
18. Pulse oximetry

G. Nursing interventions and responsibilities
1. Withhold food and fluids, as directed
2. Administer I.V. fluids, oxygen, and medications, as prescribed
3. Provide suctioning and TCDB
4. Assess cardiovascular and respiratory status and fluid balance
5. Keep the patient in semi-Fowler's position
6. Monitor and record VS, UO, I/O, hemodynamic variables, level of consciousness, and laboratory studies
7. Encourage the patient to express feelings, such as a fear of dying
8. Allay the patient's anxiety

H. Teaching goals (instructions to the patient and family)
1. Keep follow-up appointments
2. Exercise regularly
3. Stop smoking
4. Maintain a normal weight
5. Know the action, side effects, and scheduling of medications
6. Identify ways to reduce stress
7. Recognize the signs and symptoms of fluid overload
8. Adhere to activity limitations
9. Alternate rest periods with activity
10. Follow dietary restrictions and recommendations

I. Possible medical complications
   1. Arrhythmias
   2. Cardiac arrest
   3. Infection

J. Possible surgical interventions: CABG (see page 9)

XVIII. Mitral stenosis

A. Definition — narrowing of the mitral valve opening

B. Possible etiology: rheumatic endocarditis

C. Pathophysiology
   1. Thickening and calcification of valvular tissue, thereby narrowing the mitral valve opening and limiting blood flow from the left atrium to the left ventricle
   2. Increased pressure in the left atrium, leading to pulmonary hypertension and left atrial hypertrophy
   3. Right ventricular failure, producing pulmonary congestion

D. Possible clinical manifestations
   1. Fatigue
   2. Low cardiac output
   3. Dyspnea on exertion
   4. Right-sided heart failure
   5. Cough
   6. Peripheral edema
   7. Atrial fibrillation
   8. Orthopnea
   9. JVD
   10. Tachycardia
   11. PND
   12. Hemoptysis

E. Possible diagnostic test findings
   1. Chest X-ray: enlargement of the left atrium and right ventricle; pulmonary congestion
   2. Echocardiogram: thickening of the mitral valve and left atrial enlargement
   3. Cardiac catheterization: increased left atrial pressure, PCWP; decreased cardiac output
   4. Angiography: mitral stenosis

F. Medical management
   1. Diet: low-sodium; limit fluids
   2. I.V. therapy: heparin lock
   3. Oxygen therapy
   4. Position: semi-Fowler's

5. Activity: bed rest; active ROM and isometric exercises
6. Monitoring: VS, UO, I/O, ECG, and hemodynamic variables
7. Laboratory studies: sodium, potassium, PT, PTT, and ABGs
8. Foley catheter
9. Cardiac glycoside: digoxin (Lanoxin)
10. Nitrates: isosorbide dinitrate (Isordil), nitroglycerin (Nitro-Bid)
11. Diuretics: furosemide (Lasix), ethacrynic acid (Edecrin)
12. Antiarrhythmics: quinidine (Cardioquin), procainamide (Pronestyl)
13. Anticoagulants: warfarin sodium (Coumadin)
14. Antibiotics: pencillin G potassium (Pentids)
15. Percutaneous transluminal valvuloplasty

G. Nursing interventions and responsibilities
1. Maintain the patient's prescribed diet; restrict oral fluids
2. Administer I.V. fluids, oxygen, and medications, as prescribed
3. Assess cardiovascular and respiratory status
4. Keep the patient in semi-Fowler's position
5. Monitor and record VS, UO, I/O, hemodynamic variables, laboratory studies, and ECG readings
6. Encourage the patient to express feelings, such as a fear of dying
7. Assess pain
8. Allay the patient's anxiety
9. Assess peripheral edema

H. Teaching goals (instructions to the patient and family)
1. Keep follow-up appointments
2. Stop smoking
3. Maintain a normal weight
4. Know the action, side effects, and scheduling of medications
5. Identify ways to reduce stress
6. Recognize the signs and symptoms of CHF
7. Adhere to activity limitations; alternate rest periods with activity
8. Monitor for infection, avoid exposure to people with infections, and seek treatment if infection develops
9. Follow dietary restrictions and recommendations
10. Test stools for occult blood

I. Possible medical complications
1. Thrombosis
2. Embolism
3. CHF
4. Atrial fibrillation

J. Possible surgical interventions
1. Valve replacement (see page 9)
2. Open mitral commissurotomy (see page 9)

XIX. Mitral regurgitation (mitral insufficiency)

A. Definition — incomplete closure of the mitral valve

B. Possible etiology
1. Congenital defect
2. Rheumatic fever
3. Trauma
4. Papillary muscle dysfunction
5. Bacterial endocarditis

C. Pathophysiology
1. Valvular incompetence
2. Backflow of blood to the left atrium
3. Increased left atrial pressure, pulmonary hypertension, and left atrial hypertrophy

D. Possible clinical manifestations
1. Shortness of breath
2. Cough
3. Fatigue
4. Dyspnea on exertion
5. Peripheral edema
6. Atrial fibrillation
7. Angina pectoris
8. Orthopnea
9. Hemoptysis

E. Possible diagnostic test findings
1. Chest X-ray: enlargement of the left atrium and the left ventricle
2. ECG: atrial fibrillation, left atrial hypertension, and left ventricular hypertrophy
3. Echocardiogram: enlargement of the left atrium, abnormal movement of the mitral valve
4. Cardiac catheterization: increased left atrial and left ventricular pressure
5. Angiography: regurgitation

F. Medical management
1. Diet: low-sodium; limit fluids
2. I.V. therapy: heparin lock
3. Oxygen therapy
4. Position: semi-Fowler's
5. Monitoring: VS, UO, I/O, ECG, and hemodynamic variables
6. Laboratory studies: sodium, potassium, BUN, creatinine, and ABGs
7. Foley catheter
8. Cardiac glycoside: digoxin (Lanoxin)
9. Nitrates: isosorbide dinitrate (Isordil), nitroglycerin (Nitro-Bid)
10. Diuretics: furosemide (Lasix), ethacrynic acid (Edecrin)

11. Antiarrhythmics: quinidine (Cardioquin), procainamide (Pronestyl)
12. Anticoagulants: warfarin sodium (Coumadin)

G. Nursing interventions and responsibilities
   1. Maintain the patient's prescribed diet; limit oral fluids
   2. Administer I.V. fluids, oxygen, and medications, as prescribed
   3. Assess cardiovascular and respiratory status
   4. Keep the patient in semi-Fowler's position
   5. Monitor and record VS, UO, I/O, hemodynamic variables, laboratory studies, and ECG readings
   6. Encourage the patient to express feelings, such as a fear of dying
   7. Assess pain
   8. Assess peripheral edema
   9. Allay the patient's anxiety
  10. Provide information about the American Heart Association

H. Teaching goals (instructions to the patient and family)
   1. Keep follow-up appointments
   2. Stop smoking
   3. Maintain a normal weight
   4. Know the action, side effects, and scheduling of medications
   5. Identify ways to reduce stress
   6. Test stools for occult blood
   7. Adhere to activity limitations; alternate rest periods with activity
   8. Monitor for infection, avoid exposure to people with infections, and seek treatment if infection develops
   9. Follow dietary restrictions and recommendations
  10. Know the difference between angina and MI

I. Possible medical complications
   1. Embolism
   2. Thrombosis
   3. CHF
   4. Ruptured papillary muscle

J. Possible surgical interventions
   1. Mitral valve replacement (see page 9)
   2. Valvuloplasty (see page 9)

XX. Aortic stenosis

A. Definition—narrowing of the aortic valve

B. Possible etiology
   1. Syphilis
   2. Rheumatic fever
   3. Atherosclerosis
   4. Congenital malformations

C. Pathophysiology
   1. Fibrosis and calcification of valvular tissue, which narrows the valve opening and limits blood flow
   2. Increased left ventricular pressure, which causes hypertrophy of the left ventricle and lowers cardiac output
   3. Increased congestion in the lungs, resulting in right ventricular failure

D. Possible clinical manifestations
   1. Angina pectoris
   2. Syncope
   3. Pulmonary hypertension
   4. Left-sided heart failure
   5. Fatigue
   6. Orthopnea
   7. PND

E. Possible diagnostic test findings
   1. Chest X-ray: aortic valve calcification, left ventricular enlargement
   2. ECG: left bundle branch block, first-degree heart block, left ventricular hypertrophy
   3. Echocardiogram: thickened left ventricular wall, thickened aortic valve that moves abnormally
   4. Cardiac catheterization: increased left ventricular pressure

F. Medical management
   1. Diet: low-sodium; limit fluids
   2. I.V. therapy: heparin lock
   3. Monitoring: VS, UO, I/O, ECG, and hemodynamic variables
   4. Laboratory studies: sodium, potassium, BUN, creatinine, and ABGs
   5. Cardiac glycoside: digoxin (Lanoxin)
   6. Nitrates: isosorbide dinitrate (Isordil), nitroglycerin (Nitro-Bid)
   7. Diuretics: furosemide (Lasix), ethacrynic acid (Edecrin)
   8. Percutaneous transluminal valvuloplasty

G. Nursing interventions and responsibilities
   1. Maintain the patient's prescribed diet; limit fluids
   2. Assess cardiovascular and respiratory status
   3. Monitor and record VS, UO, I/O, hemodynamic variables, laboratory studies, and ECG readings
   4. Administer I.V. therapy and medications, as prescribed
   5. Encourage the patient to express feelings, such as a fear of dying
   6. Assess pain
   7. Allay the patient's anxiety
   8. Provide information about the American Heart Association

H. Teaching goals (instructions to the patient and family)
   1. Keep follow-up appointments
   2. Stop smoking

3. Maintain a normal weight
4. Know the action, side effects, and scheduling of medications
5. Identify ways to reduce stress
6. Recognize the signs and symptoms of CHF
7. Adhere to activity limitations; alternate rest periods with activity
8. Follow dietary restrictions and recommendations

I. Possible medical complications
   1. CHF
   2. Pulmonary edema

J. Possible surgical interventions
   1. Aortic valve replacement (see page 9)
   2. Commissurotomy (see page 9)

XXI. Aortic regurgitation (aortic insufficiency)

A. Definition—incomplete closure of the aortic valve

B. Possible etiology
   1. Rheumatic fever
   2. Infective endocarditis
   3. Syphilis
   4. Atherosclerosis
   5. Congenital defect

C. Pathophysiology
   1. Retrograde flow of blood from the aorta to the left ventricle
   2. Left ventricular hypertrophy

D. Possible clinical manifestations
   1. Signs of left-sided heart failure
   2. Dyspnea on exertion
   3. Dizziness
   4. Neck pain
   5. Orthopnea
   6. Angina pectoris
   7. Tachycardia
   8. PND

E. Possible diagnostic test findings
   1. Chest X-ray: enlarged left ventricle, aortic valve calcification
   2. ECG: left ventricular hypertrophy, sinus tachycardia
   3. Echocardiogram: left ventricular enlargement, abnormal valve movement
   4. Cardiac catheterization: increased left atrial and left ventricular pressures
   5. Cardiac angiography: regurgitation

F. Medical management
   1. Diet: low-sodium; limit fluids
   2. I.V. therapy: heparin lock
   3. Monitoring: VS, UO, I/O, ECG, and hemodynamic variables
   4. Laboratory studies: ABGs, sodium, potassium, BUN, and creatinine
   5. Foley catheter
   6. Antibiotic: penicillin G potassium (Pentids)
   7. Cardiac glycoside: digoxin (Lanoxin)
   8. Nitrates: isosorbide dinitrate (Isordil), nitroglycerin (Nitro-Bid)
   9. Diuretics: furosemide (Lasix), ethacrynic acid (Edecrin)
   10. Vasodilators: hydralazine (Apresoline), nifedipine (Procardia)
   11. ACE inhibitors: captopril (Capoten), enalapril (Vasotec), lisinopril (Prinivil)

G. Nursing interventions and responsibilities
   1. Maintain the patient's prescribed diet; restrict oral fluids
   2. Administer I.V. fluids and medications, as prescribed
   3. Assess cardiovascular and respiratory status
   4. Monitor and record VS, UO, I/O, hemodynamic variables, and laboratory studies
   5. Assess pain
   6. Encourage the patient to express feelings, such as a fear of dying
   7. Allay the patient's anxiety
   8. Provide information about the American Heart Association

H. Teaching goals (instructions to the patient and family)
   1. Keep follow-up appointments
   2. Stop smoking
   3. Maintain a normal weight
   4. Know the action, side effects, and scheduling of medications
   5. Identify ways to reduce stress
   6. Recognize the signs and symptoms of CHF
   7. Adhere to activity limitations; alternate rest periods with activity
   8. Monitor for infection
   9. Follow dietary restrictions and recommendations
   10. Know the difference between angina and MI

I. Possible medical complications
   1. CHF
   2. Thrombosis
   3. Embolism
   4. Infection

J. Possible surgical interventions
   1. Valvuloplasty (see page 9)
   2. Valve replacement (see page 9)

XXII. Peripheral vascular disease

A. Definition — chronic inadequate blood flow in the lower extremities

B. Types
   1. Arteriosclerosis obliterans
   2. Raynaud's phenomena
   3. Buerger's disease

C. Possible etiology
   1. Atherosclerosis
   2. Vasospasm
   3. Inflammation

D. Pathophysiology
   1. Arterial thickening and loss of elasticity, narrowing the diameter of the artery
   2. Decreased perfusion and blood clot formation, causing arterial blockage and ischemia (common sites are the femoral, popliteal, and iliac arteries and the aorta)

E. Possible clinical manifestations
   1. INTERMITTENT CLAUDICATION
   2. Pain in extremities at rest
   3. Trophic changes: thickened nails; absence of hair; taut, shiny skin
   4. Diminished or absent pulses in extremities (a unilateral finding has greater significance than bilateral findings)
   5. Temperature changes in extremities
   6. Color changes in extremities: rubor, cyanosis, pallor
   7. Ulcerations in extremities

F. Possible diagnostic test findings
   1. Arteriography: location of obstructing plaque
   2. Doppler studies: decreased blood flow and arterial pressure
   3. Blood chemistry: increased lipids

G. Medical management
   1. Diet: low-fat, low-calorie
   2. Activity: active ROM and isometric exercises, as tolerated
   3. Monitoring: VS, I/O, and neurovascular checks
   4. Laboratory studies: serum lipids, PTT, and PT
   5. Bed cradle
   6. Analgesic: aspirin
   7. Vasodilators: papaverine (Pavabid), isoxsuprine (Vasodilan)
   8. Anticoagulant: warfarin sodium (Coumadin)
   9. Lipid reducers: cholestryamine (Questran), clofibrate (Atromid-S)
   10. Percutaneous transluminal angioplasty
   11. Laser angioplasty
   12. Vascular stents

13. Thrombolytic therapy: urokinase (Abbokinase)

H. Nursing interventions and responsibilities
1. Maintain the patient's prescribed diet
2. Assess cardiovascular status
3. Monitor and record VS, UO, I/O, and laboratory studies
4. Administer medications, as prescribed
5. Encourage the patient to express feelings about changes in body image
6. Check peripheral circulation: pulses, color, temperature, and complaints of abnormal sensations, such as numbness or tingling
7. Encourage walking and other leg exercises
8. Provide daily foot care

I. Teaching goals (instructions to the patient and family)
1. Keep follow-up appointments
2. Exercise regularly
3. Stop smoking
4. Maintain a normal weight
5. Know the action, side effects, and scheduling of medications
6. Recognize the signs and symptoms of decreased peripheral circulation
7. Identify ways to reduce stress
8. Alternate rest periods with activity
9. Monitor for skin breakdown
10. Follow dietary restrictions and recommendations
11. Care for the feet daily
12. Avoid activities or situations that will exacerbate the condition, such as temperature extremes, prolonged standing, constrictive clothing, or crossing the legs at the knee when seated

J. Possible medical complications
1. Gangrene
2. Septicemia
3. Pressure sores
4. Acute vascular occlusion

K. Possible surgical interventions
1. Bypass grafting (see page 12)
2. Endarterectomy (see page 97)
3. SYMPATHECTOMY
4. Amputation (see page 55)
5. Embolectomy (see page 271)

XXIII. Thrombophlebitis

A. Definition – inflammation of the venous wall, resulting in clot formation

B. Possible etiology
1. Venous stasis (from varicose veins, pregnancy, CHF, prolonged bed rest)

   2. Hypercoagulability (from cancer, blood dyscrasias, oral contraceptives)
   3. Injury to the venous wall (from I.V. injections, fractures, antibiotics)

C. Pathophysiology
   1. Massing of red blood cells in a fibrin network
   2. Obstruction by enlarged thrombus, leading to venous insufficiency (common sites are deep veins and superficial veins)

D. Possible clinical manifestations
   1. Superficial veins: red, warm skin that is tender to touch
   2. Deep veins: edema, positive Homans' sign, tender to touch, cramping pain

E. Possible diagnostic test findings
   1. Venography: venous-filling defects
   2. Ultrasound: decreased blood flow
   3. Phlebography: venous-filling defects
   4. Hematology: increased WBC count

F. Medical management
   1. Position: elevation of the affected extremity
   2. Activity: bed rest; active and passive ROM and isometric exercises
   3. Monitoring: VS and neurovascular checks
   4. Laboratory studies: WBC, PT, and PTT
   5. Antiembolism stockings; warm, moist compresses
   6. Anticoagulants: warfarin sodium (Coumadin), heparin sodium (Lipo-Hepin)
   7. Fibrinolytic agents: streptokinase (Streptase)
   8. Vasodilators: papaverine (Pavabid), isoxsuprine (Vasodilan)
   9. Anti-inflammatory agent: aspirin

G. Nursing interventions and responsibilities
   1. Assess cardiovascular status
   2. Keep the patient in bed, and elevate the affected extremity
   3. Monitor and record VS, neurovascular checks, and laboratory studies
   4. Administer medications, as prescribed
   5. Assess for Homans' sign
   6. Assess for bleeding
   7. Apply warm, moist compresses
   8. Measure and record the circumference of thighs and calves

H. Teaching goals (instructions to the patient and family)
   1. Keep follow-up appointments
   2. Exercise, as directed
   3. Stop smoking
   4. Maintain a normal weight
   5. Know the action, side effects, and scheduling of medications
   6. Identify ways to reduce stress
   7. Recognize the signs and symptoms of bleeding

8. Avoid prolonged sitting or standing, constrictive clothing, or crossing the legs when seated
9. Do not take oral contraceptives

I. Possible medical complications
   1. Pulmonary embolism
   2. CVA

J. Possible surgical interventions
   1. Vena cava filter (plication of inferior vena cava; see page 272)
   2. Vein ligation and stripping
   3. Thrombectomy

XXIV. Bacterial endocarditis

A. Definition—inflammation and infection of the endocardial lining

B. Possible etiology
   1. Bacterial infection: Beta-hemolytic streptococcus, *Staphylococcus aureus*
   2. Rheumatic heart disease
   3. Dental extractions
   4. Invasive monitoring

C. Pathophysiology
   1. Formation of bacterial colonies on the endocardial lining, destroying heart valve leaflets
   2. Disrupted blood flow, resulting in murmurs
   3. Vegetations that seed the bloodstream with bacteria

D. Possible clinical manifestations
   1. Elevated temperature
   2. Heart murmur
   3. Diaphoresis
   4. Malaise
   5. Dyspnea
   6. Tachycardia
   7. Clubbing of fingers and toes
   8. Petechiae
   9. Night sweats
   10. Splinter hemorrhages in nailbeds

E. Possible diagnostic test findings
   1. Blood cultures: positive for specific organism
   2. Hematology: increased WBCs, ESR; decreased Hct
   3. Echocardiography: valvular damage, vegetations

F. Medical management
   1. I.V. therapy: hydration, heparin lock

    2. Oxygen therapy

    3. Activity: bed rest

    4. Monitoring: VS, UO, I/O, and neurovascular checks

    5. Laboratory studies: blood cultures, WBC, and Hct

    6. Antibiotics: penicillin G potassium (Pentids), vancomycin hydrochloride (Vancocin)

    7. Fluids: increased intake

    8. Antipyretic: aspirin

    9. Anticoagulant: warfarin sodium (Coumadin)

G. Nursing interventions and responsibilities

    1. Force fluids

    2. Administer I.V. fluids, oxygen, and medications, as prescribed

    3. Assess cardiovascular status

    4. Monitor and record VS, UO, I/O, and laboratory studies

    5. Encourage the patient to express feelings, such as a fear of dying

    6. Allay the patient's anxiety

H. Teaching goals (instructions to the patient and family)

    1. Keep follow-up appointments

    2. Stop smoking

    3. Maintain a normal weight

    4. Know the action, side effects, and scheduling of medications

    5. Identify ways to reduce stress

    6. Recognize the signs and symptoms of endocarditis

    7. Follow activity limitations; alternate rest periods with activity, and adhere to the prescribed exercise regimen

    8. Avoid exposure to people with infections; monitor self for infection, particularly after a dental or gynecologic exam, and seek treatment if infection develops

    9. Wear a medical identification bracelet

I. Possible medical complications

    1. Embolism

    2. CHF

    3. Mycotic aneurysm

J. Possible surgical intervention: valve replacement (see page 9)

XXV. Abdominal aortic aneurysm

A. Definition—dilation of or localized weakness in the medial layer of an artery

B. Possible etiology

    1. Atherosclerosis

    2. Congenital defect

    3. Trauma

    4. Syphilis

    5. Hypertension
    6. Infection

C. Pathophysiology
    1. Degenerative changes from atherosclerosis, weakening the medial layer
    2. Continued weakening from the force of blood flow, resulting in outpouching of the artery
    3. Four types: saccular, fusiform, dissecting, false

D. Possible clinical manifestations
    1. Asymptomatic
    2. Lower abdominal pain, low back pain
    3. Abdominal mass to the left of the midline
    4. Abdominal pulsations
    5. Bruits
    6. Diminished femoral pulses
    7. Systolic blood pressure in the legs lower than that in the arms

E. Possible diagnostic test findings
    1. Chest X-ray: aneurysm
    2. ECG: differentiation of aneurysm from MI
    3. Echocardiography: aneurysm
    4. Aortography: aneurysm

F. Medical management
    1. Activity: bed rest
    2. Monitoring: VS, UO, I/O, and neurovascular checks
    3. Analgesic: oxycodone (Tylox)
    4. Beta-adrenergic blocker: propranolol (Inderal)
    5. Antihypertensives: methyldopa (Aldomet), hydralazine (Apresoline), prazosin (Minipress)

G. Nursing interventions and responsibilities
    1. Assess cardiovascular status
    2. Monitor and record VS, UO, I/O, neurovascular checks, and laboratory studies
    3. Administer medications, as prescribed
    4. Encourage the patient to express feelings, such as a fear of dying
    5. Assess pain
    6. Check peripheral circulation: pulses, temperature, color, and complaints of abnormal sensations
    7. Allay the patient's anxiety
    8. Observe the patient for signs of shock, such as anxiety; restlessness; decreased pulse pressure; increased thready pulse; and pale, cool, moist, clammy skin
    9. Palpate the abdomen for distention

H. Teaching goals (instructions to the patient and family)
    1. Keep follow-up appointments

2. Stop smoking
3. Know the action, side effects, and scheduling of medications
4. Identify ways to reduce stress
5. Recognize the signs and symptoms of decreased peripheral circulation, such as change in skin color or temperature, complaints of numbness or tingling, and absent pulses
6. Adhere to activity limitations; alternate rest periods with activity, and adhere to prescribed exercise regimen
7. Maintain a quiet environment

I. Possible medical complication: rupture of aneurysm

J. Possible surgical intervention: resection of aneurysm (see page 11)

Points to remember

The focus of nursing management in cardiovascular disorders is to increase blood supply—and thus oxygenation—to tissues.

Alterations in cardiac output affect every system in the body.

The impact of cardiovascular disease can be reduced by altering modifiable risk factors.

Complaints of chest pain have increased significance in a patient with a peripheral vascular problem.

A unilateral finding in the assessment of peripheral circulation has greater significance than bilateral findings.

Glossary

The following terms are defined in Appendix A, page 354.

bruit

intermittent claudication

jugular venous distention

orthopnea

paroxysmal nocturnal dyspnea

point of maximum impulse

Study questions

To evaluate your understanding of this chapter, answer the following questions in the space provided; then compare your responses with the correct answers in Appendix B, pages 357 and 358.

1. How is cardiac output measured? _____

_____

2. Which nursing interventions are appropriate after cardiac catheterization?

_____

_____

3. Which risk factors for cardiovascular disorders can be modified? _____

_____

_____

4. Which medications might be administered to a patient after cardiac surgery?

_____

_____

5. What are key postoperative assessments of circulation for a patient who had

   vascular graft surgery? _____

_____

6. What are the dietary recommendations for hypertension? _____

_____

_____

7. Which ECG changes would appear in a patient with coronary artery dis-

   ease? _____

_____

8. How might a patient with angina describe the pain? _____

_____

_____

Study questions *(continued)*

9. What are the possible blood chemistry findings in a patient experiencing an acute MI? _____

10. Which myocardial changes lead to left-sided heart failure? _____

11. What are the clinical manifestations of acute pulmonary edema? _____

12. Which acid-base imbalance would a patient in cardiogenic shock experience?

13. What would a chest X-ray reveal about a patient with mitral stenosis?

14. What is the difference between aortic stenosis and aortic regurgitation?

15. What are three possible clinical manifestations of PVD? _____

CHAPTER 2

Musculoskeletal System

Learning objectives

Check off the following items once you've mastered them:

☐ Describe the psychosocial impact of musculoskeletal disorders.

☐ Differentiate between modifiable and nonmodifiable risk factors in the development of a musculoskeletal disorder.

☐ List three probable and three possible nursing diagnoses for a patient with a musculoskeletal disorder.

☐ Identify the nursing interventions and responsibilities for a patient with a musculoskeletal disorder.

☐ Write three goals for teaching a patient with a musculoskeletal disorder.

I. Anatomy and physiology

A. Skeleton
1. Consists of 206 bones (long, short, flat, or irregular)
2. Stores calcium, magnesium, and phosphorus; marrow produces red blood cells (RBCs)
3. Works with muscles to provide support, locomotion, and protection of internal organs

B. Skeletal muscles
1. Provide body movement and posture by tightening and shortening
2. Attach to bones by tendons
3. Begin contracting with the stimulus of a muscle fiber by a motor neuron
4. Derive energy for muscle contraction from hydrolysis of adenosine triphosphate (ATP) to adenosine diphosphate (ADP) and phosphate
5. Retain some contraction to maintain muscle tone
6. Relax with the breakdown of acetylcholine by cholinesterase

C. Ligaments
1. Are tough bands of collagen fibers that connect bones
2. Encircle a joint to add strength and stability

D. Tendons
1. Are nonelastic collagen cords
2. Connect muscles to bones

E. Joints
1. Are the articulation of two bone surfaces
2. Provide stabilization and permit locomotion; degree of joint movement is called range of motion (ROM)

F. Synovium
1. Is the membrane that lines a joint's inner surfaces
2. Secretes synovial fluid and antibodies
3. Reduces friction in joints (in conjunction with cartilage)

G. Cartilage
1. Serves as a smooth surface for articulating bones
2. Absorbs shock to joints
3. Atrophies with limited ROM or in the absence of weight bearing

H. Bursa
1. Is a fluid-filled sac
2. Serves as padding to reduce friction
3. Facilitates the motion of body structures that rub against each other

II. Physical assessment findings

A. Subjective data associated with musculoskeletal disorders
  1. Pain
  2. Numbness
  3. Joint stiffness
  4. Swelling
  5. Fatigue
  6. Fever
  7. Difficulty with movement

B. Objective data associated with musculoskeletal disorders
  1. Abnormal vital signs (VS)
  2. Inflammation
  3. Edema
  4. Skin breakdown
  5. Skeletal deformity
  6. Limited ROM
  7. Poor posture
  8. Muscle weakness and rigidity
  9. Abnormal skin color and temperature
  10. Paresthesia
  11. Nodules
  12. Erythema
  13. TOPHI
  14. Abnormal peripheral pulses
  15. Muscle spasms

III. Diagnostic tests and procedures

A. Electromyography (EMG)
  1. Definition and purpose
    a. Noninvasive test of muscle activity
    b. Graphical recording of the muscle at rest and during contraction
  2. Nursing interventions and responsibilities
    a. Explain that the patient will be asked to flex and relax muscles during the procedure
    b. Instruct the patient that the procedure may cause some minor discomfort but is not painful
    c. Administer analgesics, as prescribed, after the procedure

B. Arthroscopy
  1. Definition and purpose – direct visualization of a joint after injection of local anesthesia
  2. Nursing interventions and responsibilities before the procedure
    a. Administer prophylactic antibiotics, as prescribed
    b. Explain the procedure, skin preparation, and use of local anesthetics

3. Nursing interventions and responsibilities after the procedure
   a. Apply a pressure dressing to the injection site
   b. Monitor neurovascular status
   c. Apply ice to the affected joint
   d. Limit weight bearing or joint use until allowed by the physician
   e. Administer analgesics, as prescribed

C. Arthrocentesis
   1. Definition and purpose — needle aspiration of synovial fluid from a joint under local anesthesia to examine a specimen or remove the fluid
   2. Nursing interventions and responsibilities before the procedure
      a. Administer prophylactic antibiotics, as prescribed
      b. Explain the procedure to the patient
   3. Nursing interventions and responsibilities after the procedure
      a. Maintain a pressure dressing on the aspiration site
      b. Monitor neurovascular status
      c. Apply ice to the affected area
      d. Limit weight bearing or joint use until allowed by the physician
      e. Administer analgesics, as prescribed

D. Bone scan
   1. Definition and purpose
      a. Procedure using I.V. injection of a radioisotope
      b. Visual imaging of bone metabolism
   2. Nursing interventions and responsibilities before the procedure
      a. Determine the patient's ability to lie still during the scan
      b. Advise the patient that radioisotope will be injected intravenously
      c. Explain that the patient will be required to drink several glasses of fluid during the waiting period to enhance excretion of isotope not absorbed by bone tissue

E. Myelogram
   1. Definition and purpose
      a. Procedure using an injection of radiopaque dye by lumbar puncture
      b. Fluoroscopic visualization of the subarachnoid space, spinal cord, and vertebral bodies
   2. Nursing interventions and responsibilities before the procedure
      a. Note the patient's allergies to iodine, seafood, and radiopaque dyes
      b. Inform the patient about possible throat irritation and flushing of the face from the injection
   3. Nursing interventions and responsibilities after the procedure
      a. Maintain bed rest, with the patient lying flat
      b. Inspect the insertion site for bleeding
      c. Monitor neurovital signs
      d. Force fluids

F. X-ray examination
   1. Definition and purpose – noninvasive radiographic examination of bones and joints
   2. Nursing interventions and responsibilities
      a. Use caution when moving a patient with a suspected fracture
      b. Explain the procedure to the patient
      c. Make sure that the patient is not pregnant

G. Blood chemistry
   1. Definition and purpose
      a. Laboratory test of a blood sample
      b. Analysis for potassium, sodium, calcium, phosphorus, glucose, bicarbonate, blood urea nitrogen (BUN), creatinine, protein, albumin, osmolality, creatine phosphokinase (CPK), serum aspartate aminotransferase (AST, formerly SGOT), aldolase, rheumatoid factor, complement fixation, lupus erythematosus cell preparation (LE prep), antinuclear antibody (ANA), anti-DNA, and C-reactive protein
   2. Nursing interventions and responsibilities
      a. Withhold food and fluid before the procedure
      b. Monitor the venipuncture site for bleeding after the procedure

H. Hematologic studies
   1. Definition and purpose
      a. Laboratory test of a blood sample
      b. Analysis for white blood cells (WBCs), RBCs, platelets, prothrombin time (PT), partial thromboplastin time (PTT), erythrocyte sedimentation rate (ESR), hemoglobin (Hgb), and hematocrit (Hct)
   2. Nursing interventions and responsibilities
      a. Note current drug therapy to anticipate possible interference with test results
      b. Assess the venipuncture site for bleeding after the procedure

IV. Psychosocial impact of musculoskeletal disorders

A Developmental impact
   1. Decreased self-esteem
   2. Fear of rejection
   3. Changes in body image
   4. Embarrassment from changes in body structure and function
   5. Dependence

B. Economic impact
   1. Disruption or loss of employment
   2. Cost of vocational retraining
   3. Cost of hospitalizations
   4. Cost of home health care
   5. Cost of special equipment

C. Occupational and recreational impact
1. Restrictions in work activity
2. Changes in leisure activity
3. Restrictions in physical activity

D. Social impact
1. Social isolation
2. Changes in role performance

V. Risk factors for developing musculoskeletal disorders

A. Modifiable risk factors
1. Occupations that require heavy lifting or use of machinery
2. Occupational or recreational activities that include repetitive motion of joints
3. Vegetarian diets
4. Immobility
5. Medication history
6. Stress
7. Contact sports
8. Obesity

B. Nonmodifiable risk factors
1. Aging
2. Menopause
3. Family history of musculoskeletal illness
4. History of musculoskeletal injury
5. History of immune disorders

VI. Nursing diagnostic categories for a patient with a musculoskeletal disorder

A. Probable nursing diagnostic categories
1. Impaired physical mobility
2. Altered peripheral tissue perfusion
3. Impaired skin integrity
4. Pain
5. Toileting self-care deficit
6. Feeding self-care deficit
7. Bathing self-care deficit

B. Possible nursing diagnostic categories
1. Sexual dysfunction
2. Powerlessness
3. Constipation
4. Body image disturbance
5. Social isolation
6. Disuse syndrome

VII. Joint surgery

A. Definition
   1. Arthrodesis — surgical removal of cartilage from joint surfaces to fuse a joint into a functional position
   2. Synovectomy — removal of the synovial membrane from a joint, using an arthroscope, to reduce pain
   3. Arthroplasty (total joint replacement) — surgical replacement of a joint with a metal, plastic, or porous prosthesis

B. Preoperative nursing interventions and responsibilities
   1. Complete patient and family preoperative teaching
      a. Determine the patient's understanding of the procedure
      b. Describe the operating room (OR), postanesthesia care unit (PACU), and preoperative and postoperative routines
      c. Demonstrate postoperative turning, coughing, and deep breathing (TCDB), splinting, and leg and ROM exercises
      d. Explain the postoperative need for drainage tubes, surgical dressings, oxygen therapy, I.V. therapy, and pain control
   2. Complete a preoperative checklist
   3. Administer preoperative medications, as prescribed
   4. Allay the patient's and family's anxiety about surgery
   5. Document the patient's history and physical assessment data base
   6. Administer antibiotics, as prescribed

C. Postoperative nursing interventions and responsibilities
   1. Assess cardiac and respiratory status
   2. Assess pain and administer postoperative analgesic, as prescribed
   3. Administer I.V. fluids and transfusion therapy, as prescribed
   4. Allay the patient's anxiety
   5. Inspect the surgical dressing and change, as directed
   6. Reinforce TCDB
   7. Keep the patient in semi-Fowler's position
   8. Provide incentive spirometry
   9. Maintain activity: active and passive ROM for unaffected limbs and isometric exercises, as tolerated
   10. Monitor VS, urine output (UO), intake and output (I/O), laboratory studies, neurovascular checks, and pulse oximetry
   11. Monitor and maintain the position and patency of wound drainage tubes
   12. Encourage the patient to express feelings about limited mobility
   13. Assess movement limitations
   14. Elevate the affected extremity
   15. Administer antibiotics, as prescribed
   16. Assess for return of peristalsis
   17. Give solid foods and liquids, as tolerated
   18. Administer stool softeners, as prescribed

19. Provide routine cast care (arthrodesis)
20. Provide specific care for total knee replacement
    a. Maintain continuous passive motion (CPM)
    b. Apply a knee immobilizer before getting the patient out of bed
21. Provide specific care for total hip replacement
    a. Maintain hips in abduction
    b. Limit hip flexion to 90° when sitting
    c. Turn to the affected or unaffected side, as ordered

D. Possible surgical complications
   1. Infection
   2. Hemorrhage

E. Postoperative teaching goals (instructions to the patient and family)
   1. Keep follow-up appointments
   2. Exercise regularly
   3. Maintain a normal weight
   4. Know the action, side effects, and scheduling of medications
   5. Recognize the signs and symptoms of infection
   6. Avoid jogging, jumping, and lifting
   7. Complete incision care daily
   8. Continue cast care (arthrodesis)
   9. Use crutches, a walker, or a cane
   10. Follow recommendations for total hip replacement
       a. Avoid sitting in low or soft chairs
       b. Do not cross the legs
       c. Use an elevated toilet seat

VIII. External fixation

A. Definition—fracture immobilization in which transfixing pins are inserted through the bone above and below the fracture and then attached to a rigid external metal frame

B. Preoperative nursing interventions and responsibilities
   1. Complete patient and family preoperative teaching
      a. Determine the patient's understanding of the procedure
      b. Describe the OR, PACU, and preoperative and postoperative routines
      c. Demonstrate postoperative TCDB, splinting, and leg and ROM exercises
      d. Explain the postoperative need for drainage tubes, surgical dressings, oxygen therapy, I.V. therapy, and pain control
   2. Complete a preoperative checklist
   3. Administer preoperative medications, as prescribed
   4. Allay the patient's and family's anxiety about surgery
   5. Document the patient's history and physical assessment data base
   6. Monitor for fracture complications

7. Maintain the position of the affected extremity with sandbags and pillows
8. Maintain traction or splint

C. Postoperative nursing interventions and responsibilities
1. Assess pain and administer postoperative analgesics, as prescribed
2. Assess for return of peristalsis; give solid foods and liquids, as tolerated
3. Administer I.V. fluids
4. Allay the patient's anxiety
5. Reinforce TCDB
6. Keep the patient in semi-Fowler's position
7. Provide incentive spirometry
8. Maintain activity: active and passive ROM for unaffected limbs, isometric exercises, and quadriceps setting, as tolerated
9. Monitor VS, UO, I/O, laboratory studies, and neurovascular checks
10. Encourage the patient to express feelings about changes in body image
11. Check wound and pin sites for infection
12. Provide pin care
13. Maintain balanced suspension traction
14. Do not adjust clamps

D. Possible surgical complications
1. Infection of wound and pin sites
2. Osteomyelitis
3. Hemorrhage
4. Chronic pain

E. Postoperative teaching goals (instructions to the patient and family)
1. Keep follow-up appointments
2. Exercise regularly
3. Attend physical therapy sessions
4. Maintain fixator as set
5. Maintain a normal weight
6. Know the action, side effects, and scheduling of medications
7. Recognize the signs and symptoms of soft tissue and bone infection
8. Adhere to activity limitations
9. Complete wound and pin care daily
10. Use crutches, a walker, or a cane

IX. Amputation

A. Definition
1. Surgical removal of all or part of a limb
2. Two types of amputation
   a. Closed (flap)
   b. Open (guillotine)

B. Preoperative nursing interventions and responsibilities
1. Complete patient and family preoperative teaching
   a. Determine the patient's understanding of the procedure
   b. Describe the OR, PACU, and preoperative and postoperative routines
   c. Demonstrate postoperative TCDB, splinting, and leg and ROM exercises
   d. Explain the postoperative need for drainage tubes, surgical dressings, oxygen therapy, I.V. therapy, and pain control
2. Complete a preoperative checklist
3. Administer preoperative medications, as prescribed
4. Allay the patient's and family's anxiety about surgery
5. Document the patient's history and physical assessment data base
6. Administer antibiotics, as prescribed
7. Prepare the patient for the possibility of phantom limb sensation or phantom pain

C. Postoperative nursing interventions and responsibilities
1. Assess cardiac and respiratory status
2. Assess pain and administer postoperative analgesics, as prescribed
3. Administer I.V. fluids and transfusion therapy, as prescribed
4. Allay the patient's anxiety
5. Inspect the surgical dressing and change, as directed
6. Reinforce TCDB
7. Keep the patient in semi-Fowler's position
8. Assess for return of peristalsis; give solid foods and liquids, as tolerated
9. Provide incentive spirometry
10. Maintain activity: active and passive ROM for unaffected limbs and isometric exercises, as tolerated
11. Monitor VS, UO, I/O, laboratory studies, neurovascular checks, and pulse oximetry
12. Monitor and maintain the position and patency of wound drainage tubes
13. Encourage the patient to express feelings about changes in body image and phantom limb sensation and pain
14. Administer antibiotics, as prescribed
15. Elevate the affected extremity for 24 hours only
16. Rewrap the stump before getting the patient out of bed
17. Prevent hip flexion
18. Inspect the stump for bleeding, infection, and edema
19. Maintain a rigid dressing for the stump prosthesis
20. Irrigate the wound and change the stump dressing, as directed
21. Reinforce physical therapy attendance

D. Possible surgical complications
1. Hemorrhage
2. Infection

3. Contractures
4. Skin breakdown

E. Postoperative teaching goals (instructions to the patient and family)
1. Keep follow-up appointments
2. Exercise regularly
3. Maintain a normal weight
4. Know the action, side effects, and scheduling of medications
5. Recognize the signs and symptoms of infection and skin breakdown
6. Complete stump care daily
7. Use a prosthesis
8. Maintain a stump conditioning program
9. Avoid using powder or lotion on the stump
10. Demonstrate proper wrapping of the stump
11. Use crutches, a walker, or a cane
12. Protect the stump from injury

X. Release of transverse carpal ligament

A. Definition – surgical ligation of the transverse carpal ligament to relieve compression of the median nerve in the carpal canal of the wrist

B. Postoperative nursing interventions and responsibilities
1. Complete patient and family preoperative teaching
   a. Determine the patient's understanding of the procedure
   b. Describe the OR, PACU, and preoperative and postoperative routines
   c. Demonstrate postoperative TCDB, splinting, and leg and ROM exercises
   d. Explain the postoperative need for drainage tubes, surgical dressings, oxygen therapy, I.V. therapy, and pain control
2. Complete a preoperative checklist
3. Administer preoperative medications, as prescribed
4. Allay the patient's and family's anxiety about surgery
5. Document the patient's history and physical assessment data base
6. Use a splint to increase the patient's comfort

C. Postoperative nursing interventions and responsibilities
1. Assess pain and administer postoperative analgesics, as prescribed
2. Assess for return of peristalsis; give solid foods and liquids, as tolerated
3. Administer I.V. fluids
4. Allay the patient's anxiety
5. Inspect the surgical dressing and change, as directed
6. Reinforce TCDB
7. Keep the patient in a semi-Fowler's position
8. Provide incentive spirometry
9. Maintain activity: active and passive ROM and isometric exercises to affected and unaffected extremities, as tolerated

10. Monitor VS, UO, I/O, laboratory studies, and neurovascular checks
11. Elevate the hand and apply ice
12. Administer steroids, as prescribed
13. Administer antibiotics, as prescribed
14. Assist with activities of daily living (ADLs)
15. Prevent injury to the affected hand
16. Apply splint
17. Reinforce immobilization of the affected hand

D. Possible surgical complications
1. Infection
2. Paralysis

E. Postoperative teaching goals (instructions to the patient and family)
1. Keep follow-up appointments
2. Exercise regularly
3. Continue active ROM exercises of the affected hand
4. Maintain a normal weight
5. Know the action, side effects, and scheduling of medications
6. Recognize the signs and symptoms of infection
7. Avoid heavy lifting
8. Complete incision care daily
9. Use a splint
10. Monitor the affected hand for return of sensation and motor function

XI. Open reduction internal fixation (ORIF)

A. Definition — surgical reduction and stabilization of a fracture, using orthopedic devices or hardware (such as Austin-Moore prosthesis, Smith-Petersen nail, Jewett nail, intramedullary nails, and compression screws)

B. Postoperative nursing interventions and responsibilities
1. Complete patient and family preoperative teaching
   a. Determine the patient's understanding of the procedure
   b. Describe the OR, PACU, and preoperative and postoperative routines
   c. Demonstrate postoperative TCDB, splinting, and leg and ROM exercises
   d. Explain the postoperative need for drainage tubes, surgical dressings, oxygen therapy, I.V. therapy, and pain control
2. Complete a preoperative checklist
3. Administer preoperative medications, as prescribed
4. Allay the patient's and family's anxiety about surgery
5. Document the patient's history and physical assessment data base
6. Monitor the patient for fracture complications
7. Keep the affected extremity in position with sandbags and pillows
8. Maintain traction or splint

C. Postoperative nursing interventions and responsibilities
   1. Assess cardiac and respiratory status
   2. Assess pain and administer postoperative analgesics, as prescribed
   3. Assess for return of peristalsis; give solid foods and liquids, as tolerated
   4. Administer I.V. fluids and transfusion therapy, as prescribed
   5. Allay the patient's anxiety
   6. Inspect the surgical dressing and change, as directed
   7. Reinforce TCDB
   8. Keep the patient in semi-Fowler's position: no higher than 30°
   9. Provide incentive spirometry
   10. Maintain activity: bed rest, active and passive ROM for unaffected limbs, isometric exercises, and progressive ambulation
   11. Monitor VS, UO, I/O, laboratory studies, neurovascular checks, and pulse oximetry
   12. Monitor and maintain the position and patency of drainage tubes
   13. Use abductor pillow and trochanter rolls
   14. Turn the patient to the affected or unaffected side, as ordered
   15. Maintain a high-fiber, low-calcium diet with increased fluid intake
   16. Apply antiembolism or pneumatic stockings
   17. Administer anticoagulants, as prescribed
   18. Administer antibiotics, as prescribed
   19. Administer stool softeners, as prescribed
   20. Use a fracture bedpan
   21. Provide heel and elbow protectors

D. Possible surgical complications
   1. Osteomyelitis
   2. Hemorrhage
   3. Thrombophlebitis
   4. Pneumonia
   5. Avascular necrosis
   6. Pulmonary embolism

E. Postoperative teaching goals (instructions to the patient and family)
   1. Keep follow-up appointments
   2. Exercise regularly
   3. Maintain a normal weight
   4. Know the action, side effects, and scheduling of medications
   5. Recognize the signs and symptoms of infection
   6. Avoid jogging, jumping, lifting, crossing the legs, and sitting in soft, low chairs
   7. Complete incision care daily
   8. Use crutches, a walker, or a cane after fixation with Austin-Moore prosthesis
   9. Apply antiembolism stockings
   10. Use an elevated toilet seat

XII. Laminectomy

A. Definition — surgical excision of vertebral posterior arch

B. Preoperative nursing interventions and responsibilities
   1. Complete patient and family preoperative teaching
      a. Determine the patient's understanding of the procedure
      b. Describe the OR, PACU, and preoperative and postoperative routines
      c. Demonstrate postoperative TCDB, splinting, and leg and ROM exercises
      d. Explain the postoperative need for drainage tubes, surgical dressings, oxygen therapy, I.V. therapy, and pain control
   2. Complete a preoperative checklist
   3. Administer preoperative medications, as prescribed
   4. Allay the patient's and family's anxiety about surgery
   5. Document the patient's history and physical assessment data base
   6. Teach the patient the logrolling technique
   7. Administer antibiotics, as prescribed

C. Postoperative nursing interventions and responsibilities
   1. Assess neurological and neurovascular status
   2. Assess pain and administer postoperative analgesics, as prescribed
   3. Assess for return of peristalsis; give solid foods and liquids, as tolerated
   4. Administer I.V. fluids
   5. Allay the patient's anxiety
   6. Inspect surgical dressings for drainage of cerebrospinal fluid (CSF) and blood
   7. Reinforce TCDB
   8. Keep the patient in a flat position
   9. Provide incentive spirometry
   10. Maintain activity: active and passive ROM and isometric exercises
   11. Monitor VS, UO, I/O, laboratory studies, and neurovascular checks
   12. Turn the patient by logrolling
   13. Prevent flexion of the neck after cervical laminectomy
   14. Administer muscle relaxants, as prescribed
   15. Administer corticosteroids, as prescribed
   16. Administer stool softeners, as prescribed

D. Possible surgical complications
   1. Urine retention
   2. Motor and sensory deficits
   3. Infection
   4. Muscle spasm
   5. Paralytic ileus

E. Postoperative teaching goals (instructions to the patient and family)
   1. Keep follow-up appointments

2. Exercise regularly
3. Maintain a normal weight
4. Know the action, side effects, and scheduling of medications
5. Recognize the signs and symptoms of infection
6. Recognize the signs and symptoms of a motor or sensory deficit
7. Avoid lifting, driving, stooping, tub bathing, and repetitive bending until allowed by the physician
8. Complete incision care daily
9. Alternate rest periods with activity
10. Wear a supportive brace
11. Complete exercises for the lower back daily
12. Sleep on the side, with hips and knees flexed
13. Sleep on a firm mattress

XIII. Spinal fusion

A. Definition—stabilization of spinous processes with bone chips from iliac crest or Harrington rod metallic implant

B. Preoperative nursing interventions and responsibilities
   1. Complete patient and family preoperative teaching
      a. Determine the patient's understanding of the procedure
      b. Describe the OR, PACU, and preoperative and postoperative routines
      c. Demonstrate postoperative TCDB, splinting, and leg and ROM exercises
      d. Explain the postoperative need for drainage tubes, surgical dressings, oxygen therapy, I.V. therapy, and pain control
   2. Complete a preoperative checklist
   3. Administer preoperative medications, as prescribed
   4. Allay the patient's and family's anxiety about surgery
   5. Document the patient's history and physical assessment data base
   6. Administer antibiotics, as prescribed
   7. Teach the patient the logrolling technique

C. Postoperative nursing interventions and responsibilities
   1. Assess cardiac, respiratory, and neurologic status
   2. Assess pain and administer postoperative analgesics, as prescribed
   3. Assess for return of peristalsis; give solid foods and liquids, as tolerated
   4. Administer I.V. fluids
   5. Allay the patient's anxiety
   6. Inspect the surgical dressing and change, as directed
   7. Reinforce TCDB
   8. Maintain the patient in the supine position
   9. Provide incentive spirometry
   10. Maintain activity: active and passive ROM and isometric exercises
   11. Monitor VS, UO, I/O, and laboratory studies

12. Check neurovascular status: color, temperature, pulses, movement, and sensation in extremities
13. Administer antipyretics, as prescribed
14. Administer antibiotics, as prescribed
15. Administer corticosteroids, as prescribed
16. Turn the patient every 2 hours using the logrolling technique
17. Administer muscle relaxants, as prescribed
18. Administer stool softeners, as prescribed

D. Possible surgical complications
   1. Urine retention
   2. Infection
   3. Muscle spasm
   4. Motor and sensory deficits
   5. Paralytic ileus

E. Postoperative teaching goals (instructions to the patient and family)
   1. Keep follow-up appointments
   2. Exercise regularly
   3. Maintain a normal weight
   4. Know the action, side effects, and scheduling of medications
   5. Recognize the signs and symptoms of infection
   6. Recognize the signs and symptoms of motor and sensory deficits
   7. Avoid lifting, driving, stooping, tub bathing, repetitive bending, and prolonged sitting until allowed by the physician
   8. Complete incision care daily
   9. Walk regularly
   10. Note spinal flexion limitations
   11. Complete exercises for lower back daily
   12. Sleep on the side with hips and knees flexed
   13. Sleep on a firm mattress

XIV. Rheumatoid arthritis

A. Definition—systemic inflammatory disease that affects the synovial lining of the joints

B. Possible etiology
   1. Unknown
   2. Autoimmune disease
   3. Genetic transmission

C. Pathophysiology
   1. Inflammation of the synovial membranes is followed by formation of PANNUS and destruction of cartilage, bone, and ligaments
   2. Pannus is replaced by fibrotic tissue and calcification, which causes SUBLUXATION of the joint

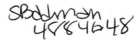

D. Possible clinical manifestations
   1. Fatigue
   2. Anorexia
   3. Malaise
   4. Elevated body temperature
   5. Painful, swollen joints
   6. Limited ROM
   7. Subcutaneous nodules
   8. Symmetrical joint swelling (mirror image of affected joints)
   9. Morning stiffness
   10. Paresthesia of the hands and the feet
   11. Crepitus
   12. Pericarditis
   13. Splenomegaly
   14. Leukopenia
   15. Enlarged lymph nodes

E. Possible diagnostic test findings
   1. X-rays: joint space narrowing, bone erosions
   2. Hematology: increased ESR, WBC, platelets
   3. Gamma globulin: increased IgM, IgG
   4. Synovial fluid analysis: increased WBC, decreased viscosity, opaque
   5. Latex fixation test: positive rheumatoid factor

F. Medical management
   1. Activity: as tolerated
   2. Monitoring: VS, UO, and I/O
   3. Analgesic: aspirin
   4. Nonsteroidal anti-inflammatory drugs (NSAID): indomethacin (Indocin), ibuprofen (Motrin), sulindac (Clinoril), piroxicam (Feldene), flurbiprofen (Ansaid), diclofenac sodium (Voltaren)
   5. Glucocorticoids: prednisone (Deltasone), hydrocortisone (Cortef)
   6. Antacids: magnesium and aluminum hydroxide (Maalox), aluminum hydroxide gel (Gelusil)
   7. Gold therapy: gold sodium thiomalate (Myochrysine)
   8. Physical therapy
   9. Heat therapy
   10. Cold therapy
   11. Plasmapheresis
   12. Laboratory studies: ESR, WBC
   13. Antirheumatic: hydroxychloroquine (HCQ, Plaquenil)
   14. Antimetabolite: methotrexate (Rheumatrex)

G. Nursing interventions and responsibilities
   1. Assess neuromuscular status
   2. Keep joints extended
   3. Monitor and record VS, UO, I/O, and laboratory studies

    4. Administer medications, as prescribed
    5. Encourage the patient to express feelings about changes in body image and self-esteem
    6. Provide skin care
    7. Minimize environmental stress
    8. Check joints for swelling, pain, and redness
    9. Provide passive ROM exercises
    10. Provide warm compresses and paraffin dips (heat therapy), as prescribed
    11. Provide information about the Arthritis Foundation

H. Teaching goals (instructions to the patient and family)
    1. Keep follow-up appointments
    2. Exercise regularly
    3. Maintain a normal weight
    4. Know the action, side effects, and scheduling of medications
    5. Identify ways to reduce stress
    6. Recognize the signs and symptoms of skin breakdown
    7. Adhere to activity limitations
    8. Alternate rest periods with activity
    9. Promote a safe environment
    10. Seek help from community agencies and resources
    11. Alter ADLs to compensate for limited ROM
    12. Complete skin and foot care daily
    13. Avoid cold, stress, and infection
    14. Use devices to assist with ADLs
    15. Use proper body mechanics
    16. Avoid unproven remedies

I. Possible medical complications: carpal tunnel syndrome

J. Possible surgical interventions
    1. Joint replacement (see page 53)
    2. Synovectomy (see page 53)

XV. Osteoarthritis (degenerative joint disease)

A. Definition—degeneration of articular cartilage, usually affecting the weight-bearing joints: spine, knees, hips

B. Possible etiology
    1. Aging
    2. Obesity
    3. Joint trauma
    4. Congenital abnormalities

C. Pathophysiology
    1. Cartilage softens with age, narrowing the joint space
    2. Normal use thins and erodes cartilage

3. Cartilage flakes enter the synovial lining, which fibroses, thus limiting joint movement

D. Possible clinical manifestations
  1. Pain relieved by resting joints
  2. Joint stiffness
  3. Heberden's nodules
  4. Limited ROM
  5. CREPITATION
  6. Increased pain in damp, cold weather
  7. Enlarged, edematous joints
  8. Smooth, taut, shiny skin

E. Possible diagnostic test findings
  1. X-rays: joint deformity, narrowing of joint space, bone spurs
  2. Arthroscopy: bone spurs, narrowing of joint space
  3. Hematology: increased ESR

F. Medical management
  1. Diet: low-calorie
  2. Activity: as tolerated
  3. Monitoring: VS, UO, and I/O
  4. Heat therapy
  5. Cold therapy
  6. Isometric exercises
  7. Weight reduction
  8. Canes, walkers
  9. Analgesic: aspirin
  10. NSAID: indomethacin (Indocin), ibuprofen (Motrin), sulindac (Clinoril), piroxicam (Feldene), flurbiprofen (Ansaid), diclofenac (Voltaren)

G. Nursing interventions and responsibilities
  1. Maintain the patient's diet
  2. Assess musculoskeletal status
  3. Keep joints extended
  4. Monitor and record VS, UO, and I/O
  5. Administer medications, as prescribed
  6. Encourage the patient to express feelings about changes in body image
  7. Provide skin care
  8. Provide rest periods
  9. Determine degree of joint mobility
  10. Maintain calorie count
  11. Assess pain
  12. Provide moist compresses and paraffin baths (heat therapy), as prescribed
  13. Teach proper body mechanics
  14. Provide passive ROM exercises
  15. Provide information about the Arthritis Foundation

H. Teaching goals (instructions to the patient and family)
1. Keep follow-up appointments
2. Exercise regularly
3. Maintain a normal weight
4. Know the action, side effects, and scheduling of medications
5. Identify ways to reduce stress
6. Recognize the signs and symptoms of skin breakdown
7. Adhere to activity limitations
8. Alternate rest periods with activity
9. Follow dietary recommendations and restrictions
10. Promote a safe environment
11. Seek help from community agencies and resources
12. Alter ADLs to compensate for limited ROM
13. Complete skin and foot care daily
14. Use proper body mechanics

I. Possible medical complications: contractures

J. Possible surgical interventions
1. Synovectomy (see page 53)
2. Arthrodesis (see page 53)
3. Joint replacement (see page 53)

XVI. Gouty arthritis

A. Definition – inflammatory joint disease caused by the deposit of uric acid crystals

B. Possible etiology
1. Genetics
2. Decreased uric acid excretion
3. Chronic renal failure
4. Myxedema
5. Polycythemia vera
6. Hyperparathyroidism

C. Pathophysiology
1. End product of purine metabolism is uric acid
2. Abnormal purine metabolism results in decreased secretion of urates and increased blood levels of uric acid
3. Uric acid forms a precipitate in areas where blood flow is slowest
4. Genetic defect in purine metabolism can cause overproduction of uric acid

D. Possible clinical manifestations
1. Joint pain
2. Redness and swelling in joints
3. Tophi in great toe, ankle, and outer ear
4. Malaise

5. Tachycardia
6. Elevated skin temperature

E. Possible diagnostic test findings
   1. Hematology: increased ESR
   2. Blood chemistry: increased uric acid
   3. Synovial fluid analysis: sodium urate crystals

F. Medical management
   1. Diet: low-purine, alkaline-ash
   2. Dietary recommendations: increase fluid intake to 3,000 ml/day
   3. Dietary restrictions: no shellfish, liver, sardines, anchovies, and kidneys; limited alcohol
   4. Activity: as tolerated
   5. Monitoring: VS, UO, and I/O
   6. Laboratory studies: uric acid, ESR
   7. Exercise program, including passive and active ROM exercises, and ambulation, as tolerated
   8. Uricosuric agents: probenecid (Benemid), sulfinpyrazone (Anturane)
   9. Xanthine-oxidase inhibitor: allopurinal (Zyloprim)
   10. Antigout: colchicine (Colsalide)
   11. Analgesic: aspirin
   12. NSAID: indomethacin (Indocin), ibuprofen (Motrin), sulindac (Clinoril), piroxicam (Feldene)

G. Nursing interventions and responsibilities
   1. Maintain the patient's diet
   2. Force fluids to 3,000 ml/day
   3. Assess integumentary status
   4. Monitor and record VS, UO, I/O, and laboratory studies
   5. Administer medications, as prescribed
   6. Allay the patient's anxiety
   7. Provide skin care
   8. Check joints for pain, edema, and ROM
   9. Provide a bed cradle
   10. Reinforce exercise of joints; show the patient how to perform the exercises
   11. Provide information about the Arthritis Foundation

H. Teaching goals (instructions to the patient and family)
   1. Keep follow-up appointments
   2. Exercise regularly
   3. Maintain a normal weight
   4. Know the action, side effects, and scheduling of medications
   5. Identify ways to reduce stress
   6. Recognize the signs and symptoms of gout
   7. Alternate rest periods with activity
   8. Follow dietary recommendations and restrictions

9. Avoid fasting
10. Limit alcohol intake
11. Complete skin and foot care daily

I. Possible medical complications
   1. Renal calculi
   2. Cartilage damage

J. Possible surgical interventions: none

XVII. Osteomyelitis

A. Definition — bacterial infection of bone and soft tissue

B. Possible etiology
   1. *Staphylococcus aureus*
   2. Hemolytic streptococcus
   3. Open trauma
   4. Infection

C. Pathophysiology
   1. Organism reaches bone through an open wound or via the bloodstream
   2. Infection causes bone destruction
   3. Bone fragments necrose (sequestra)
   4. New bone cells form over the sequestrum during healing, resulting in nonunion

D. Possible clinical manifestations
   1. Malaise
   2. Elevated body temperature
   3. Bone pain
   4. Tachycardia
   5. Localized edema and redness
   6. Muscle spasms
   7. Increased pain with movement

E. Possible diagnostic test findings
   1. Blood cultures: positive identification of organism
   2. Hematology: increased WBCs, ESR
   3. Wound culture: positive identification of organism
   4. Bone biopsy: positive
   5. Bone scan: positive

F. Medical management
   1. Diet: high-calorie, high-vitamin C and D, high-protein, and high-calcium
   2. I.V. therapy: heparin lock
   3. Activity: bed rest
   4. Monitoring: VS, UO, I/O, and neurovascular checks

5. Laboratory studies: WBC, ESR
6. Nutritional support: total parenteral nutrition (TPN)
7. Special care: wound and skin
8. Antibiotic: ciprofloxacin (Cipro)
9. Analgesic: oxycodone (Tylox)
10. Continuous wound irrigation
11. Heat therapy
12. Cast or splint for the affected body part
13. Antipyretic: aspirin

G. Nursing interventions and responsibilities
1. Maintain the patient's diet
2. Force fluids to 3,000 ml/day
3. Administer I.V. fluids
4. Assess integumentary status
5. Maintain the patency of wound irrigation
6. Monitor and record VS, UO, I/O, and laboratory studies
7. Administer TPN
8. Administer medications, as prescribed
9. Encourage the patient to express feelings about changes in body image
10. Provide skin care
11. Turn the patient every 2 hours
12. Immobilize the affected body part
13. Maintain proper body alignment
14. Maintain bedrest
15. Provide cast and splint care
16. Assess pain

H. Teaching goals (instructions to the patient and family)
1. Keep follow-up appointments
2. Exercise regularly
3. Maintain a normal weight
4. Know the action, side effects, and scheduling of medications
5. Recognize the signs and symptoms of fractures
6. Adhere to activity limitations
7. Avoid exposure to people with infections
8. Alternate rest periods with activity
9. Monitor self for infection
10. Follow dietary recommendations and restrictions
11. Promote a safe, quiet environment
12. Seek help from community agencies and resources for supportive services, such as equipment and finances
13. Alter ADLs to compensate for immobilization
14. Practice health routines that prevent infection
15. Avoid bearing weight on the affected part

I. Possible medical complications
   1. Bone necrosis
   2. Pathological fractures
   3. Sepsis

J. Possible surgical interventions
   1. Incision and drainage of bone abscess
   2. Sequestrectomy
   3. Bone graft
   4. Bone segment transfer

XVIII. Osteoporosis

A. Definition
   1. Osteoporosis is a metabolic bone dysfunction that results in reduced bone mass and increased porosity
   2. Metabolic illnesses or medications that cause osteoporosis increase the risk of skeletal fracture

B. Possible etiology
   1. Lowered estrogen levels
   2. Immobility
   3. Liver disease
   4. Calcium deficiency
   5. Vitamin D deficiency
   6. Protein deficiency
   7. Bone marrow disorders
   8. Lack of exercise
   9. Increased phosphorus
   10. Cushing's syndrome
   11. Hyperthyroidism

C. Pathophysiology
   1. Rate of bone resorption exceeds the rate of bone formation
   2. Increased phosphate stimulates parathyroid activity, which increases bone resorption
   3. Estrogens decrease bone resorption

D. Possible clinical manifestations
   1. Dowager's hump (kyphosis)
   2. Back pain: thoracic and lumbar
   3. Loss of height
   4. Unsteady gait
   5. Joint pain
   6. Weakness

E. Possible diagnostic test findings
   1. X-ray: thin, porous bone; increased vertebral curvature
   2. Photon absorptiometry: decreased bone mineral content

F. Medical management
   1. Diet: high in calcium, protein, vitamins, minerals, and boron
   2. Dietary restrictions: limit caffeine and alcohol
   3. Activity: as tolerated
   4. Monitoring: VS, UO, and I/O
   5. Laboratory studies: calcium, phosphorus
   6. Estrogen: estradiol (Estrace)
   7. Calcium supplements: calcium carbonate (Os-Cal)
   8. Vitamin and mineral supplements
   9. Exercise program
   10. Thiazide diuretics: hydrochlorothiazide (Aldactazide, Dyazide)
   11. NSAID: flurbiprofen (Ansaid)

G. Nursing interventions and responsibilities
   1. Maintain the patient's diet
   2. Assess musculoskeletal status
   3. Monitor and record VS, UO, I/O, and laboratory studies
   4. Administer medications, as prescribed
   5. Encourage the patient to express feelings about changes in body image
   6. Reinforce the importance of following an exercise program
   7. Teach proper body mechanics and posture
   8. Assess pain
   9. Provide information about the Osteoporosis Foundation

H. Teaching goals (instructions to the patient and family)
   1. Keep follow-up appointments
   2. Exercise regularly
   3. Maintain a normal weight
   4. Know the action, side effects, and scheduling of medications
   5. Alternate rest periods with activity
   6. Follow dietary recommendations and restrictions
   7. Promote a safe environment
   8. Use proper body mechanics

I. Possible medical complication: fracture

J. Possible surgical interventions: none

XIX. Osteogenic sarcoma (osteosarcoma)

A. Definition—malignant bone tumor that invades the ends of long bones

B. Possible etiology
   1. Osteoblastic activity
   2. Osteolytic activity

C. Pathophysiology
   1. Unregulated cell growth and uncontrolled cell division result in the development of a neoplasm

   2. Tumor arises from osteoblasts and dissolves the bone and soft tissue
   3. Tumor may spread to the lung

D. Possible clinical manifestations
   1. Pain
   2. Limited movement
   3. Pathologic fractures
   4. Soft tissue mass over the tumor site
   5. Warm tissue over the tumor site
   6. Elevated body temperature

E. Possible diagnostic test findings
   1. Bone scan: mass
   2. Biopsy: cytology positive for cancer cells
   3. Computerized tomography (CT) scan: mass
   4. Blood chemistry: increased alkaline phosphatase
   5. Bone marrow aspiration: cancer cells

F. Medical management
   1. Diet: high-protein
   2. I.V. therapy: heparin lock
   3. Activity: as tolerated
   4. Monitoring: VS, UO, and I/O
   5. Laboratory studies: calcium, phosphorus
   6. Antiemetics: prochlorperazine (Compazine)
   7. Nutritional support: TPN
   8. Radiation therapy
   9. Analgesic: oxycodone (Tylox)
  10. Antineoplastics: cyclophosphamide (Cytoxan), vincristine sulfate (Oncovin)
  11. Chemotherapy
  12. Antiemetic: nabilone (Cesamet)

G. Nursing interventions and responsibilities
   1. Maintain the patient's diet
   2. Assess integumentary and musculoskeletal status
   3. Monitor and record VS, UO, I/O, and laboratory studies
   4. Administer TPN
   5. Administer medications, as prescribed
   6. Encourage the patient to express feelings about changes in body image and a fear of dying
   7. Provide skin and mouth care
   8. Provide postchemotherapeutic and postradiation nursing care
      a. Provide skin, mouth, and perineal care
      b. Encourage food and fluid intake
      c. Administer antiemetics and antidiarrheals, as prescribed
      d. Monitor for bleeding, infection, and electrolyte imbalance
      e. Provide rest periods

9. Assess pain
10. Provide information about the American Cancer Society

H. Teaching goals (instructions to the patient and family)
1. Keep follow-up appointments
2. Exercise regularly
3. Maintain a normal weight
4. Know the action, side effects, and scheduling of medications
5. Recognize the signs and symptoms of a fracture
6. Avoid exposure to people with infections
7. Alternate rest periods with activity
8. Monitor self for infection
9. Promote a safe environment
10. Seek help from community agencies and resources
11. Alter ADLs to compensate for musculoskeletal deficits
12. Complete skin care daily
13. Use crutches, a cane, or a walker

I. Possible medical complications
1. Metastasis
2. Pathologic fractures

J. Possible surgical interventions: amputation (see page 55)

XX. Carpal tunnel syndrome

A. Definition — chronic compression neuropathy of the median nerve at the wrist

B. Possible etiology
1. Strenuous and repetitive use of the hands
2. Fractures and dislocations of the wrist
3. Bruising of the wrist
4. Menopause
5. Genetics
6. Pregnancy
7. Tenosynovitis
8. Rheumatoid arthritis
9. Acromegaly
10. Hyperparathyroidism
11. Obesity
12. Gout
13. Amyloidosis

C. Pathophysiology
1. Median nerve supplies sensory innervation to the palmar surface of the thumb and the first three fingers
2. Median nerve also supplies motor innervation to the wrist and finger flexion

3. Compression of the median nerve in the space between the inelastic transverse carpal ligament and the bones of the wrist (carpal tunnel) leads to pain and numbness in the thumb, index, middle, and half of the ring finger

D. Possible clinical manifestations
1. Nocturnal pain and paresthesia in the thumb and first three fingers, relieved by shaking the hand
2. Burning and tingling of the hand
3. Impaired sensation in the hand
4. Pain radiating to forearm, shoulder, neck, and chest
5. THENAR atrophy
6. Loss of fine motor movement of the hand

E. Possible diagnostic test findings
1. Tinel's sign: positive
2. Phalen's sign: positive
3. Motor nerve velocity studies: segmental, distal, median, and motor conduction delay, and conduction block at wrist

F. Medical management
1. Diet: low-sodium
2. Dietary restrictions: limit fluids
3. Position: avoid flexion of the wrist, elevate the hand
4. Activity: avoid using the hand
5. Monitoring: VS, UO, I/O, and neurovascular checks
6. Hand splint
7. Analgesic: acetaminophen (Tylenol)
8. Diuretic: furosemide (Lasix)
9. Glucocorticoid: cortisone (Cortone)
10. NSAID: ibuprofen (Motrin, Advil)
11. Vitamin: pyridoxine hydrochloride (Vitamin B_6)

G. Nursing interventions and responsibilities
1. Maintain the patient's diet
2. Assess neurovascular status
3. Elevate the patient's hand
4. Monitor and record VS
5. Administer medications, as prescribed
6. Encourage the patient to express feelings about inability to use the hand and to perform job requirements
7. Provide skin care
8. Provide ROM exercises to the splinted hand
9. Protect the hand from cold, burns, abrasions, local trauma, and chemical irritations
10. Avoid manual activity that includes dorsiflexion and volar flexion of the wrist

H. Teaching goals (instructions to the patient and family)
 1. Keep follow-up appointments
 2. Maintain ROM exercises for the hand
 3. Maintain a normal weight
 4. Know the action, side effects, and scheduling of medications
 5. Avoid activities that increase pain
 6. Recognize the signs and symptoms of skin breakdown and contracture
 7. Adhere to activity limitations
 8. Alternate rest periods with activities involving the hand
 9. Follow dietary recommendations and restrictions
 10. Alter ADLs to compensate for neuromuscular deficits
 11. Complete skin care daily
 12. Protect the hand from trauma
 13. Splint the hand
 14. Consider vocational retraining, if appropriate

I. Possible medical complications
 1. Contracture
 2. Loss of thumb abduction and opposition ("ape hand")
 3. Trophic changes of tips of thumbs and index and middle fingers

J. Possible surgical interventions: carpal tunnel release (see page 57)

XXI. Herniated nucleus pulposa (HNP, "slipped disk")

A. Definition
 1. Rupture of intervertebral disk
 2. Two types of ruptured disk
    a. Lumbrosacral (L4, L5)
    b. Cervical (C5, C6, C7)

B. Possible etiology
 1. Accidents
 2. Back or neck strain
 3. Congenital bone deformity
 4. Degeneration of disk
 5. Weakness of ligaments
 6. Heavy lifting
 7. Trauma

C. Pathophysiology
 1. Protrusion of the nucleus pulposus into the spinal canal compresses the spinal cord or nerve roots
 2. Compression of the spinal cord or nerve roots causes pain, numbness, and loss of motor function

D. Possible clinical manifestations
   1. Lumbrosacral
      a. Acute pain in the lower back radiating across the buttock and down the leg
      b. Weakness, numbness, and tingling of the foot and leg
      c. Pain on ambulation
   2. Cervical
      a. Neck stiffness
      b. Weakness, numbness, and tingling of the hand
      c. Neck pain that radiates down the arm to the hand
      d. Weakness of affected upper extremities
      e. Atrophy of biceps and triceps
      f. Straightening of normal lumbar curve with scoliosis away from the affected side

E. Possible diagnostic test findings
   1. Lasègue's sign: positive
   2. CSF analysis: increased protein
   3. Myelogram: compression of spinal cord
   4. EMG: spinal nerve involvement
   5. X-ray: narrowing of disk space
   6. Deep tendon reflexes: depressed or absent upper extremity reflexes or Achilles reflex

F. Medical management
   1. Diet: calories according to metabolic needs; increase fiber; force fluids
   2. Position: semi-Fowler's
   3. Activity: bed rest; active and passive ROM and isometric exercises
   4. Monitoring: VS, UO, I/O, neurovascular checks, and laboratory studies
   5. Heating pad; moist, hot compresses
   6. Orthopedic devices: back brace, cervical collar
   7. Analgesic: oxycodone hydrochloride (Tylox)
   8. Antacid: magnesium and aluminum hydroxide (Maalox), aluminum hydroxide gel (Gelusil)
   9. Sedative: phenobarbital (Luminal)
   10. Stool softener: docusate sodium (Colace)
   11. Pelvic traction
   12. Cervical traction
   13. Muscle relaxants: diazepam (Valium), cyclobenzaprine hydrochloride (Flexeril)
   14. Chemonucleolysis using chymopapain (Discase)
   15. NSAID: indomethacin (Indocin), ibuprofen (Motrin), sulindac (Clinoril), piroxicam (Feldene)
   16. Corticosteroid: cortisone (Cortone)
   17. Transcutaneous electrical nerve stimulation (TENS)

G. Nursing interventions and responsibilities
1. Maintain the patient's diet; increase fluid intake
2. Assess neurovascular status
3. Keep the patient in semi-Fowler's position with moderate hip and knee flexion
4. Monitor and record VS, UO, I/O, and laboratory studies
5. Administer medications, as prescribed
6. Encourage the patient to express feelings about changes in body image and about fears of disability
7. Provide skin and back care
8. Turn the patient every 2 hours, using the logrolling technique
9. Maintain bed rest and body alignment
10. Maintain traction, braces, and cervical collar
11. Promote independence in ADLs
12. Apply bedboards

H. Teaching goals (instructions to the patient and family)
1. Keep follow-up appointments
2. Exercise regularly, with special attention to exercises that strengthen and stretch the muscles
3. Maintain a normal weight
4. Know the action, side effects, and scheduling of medications
5. Recognize the signs and symptoms of neuromuscular deficits
6. Avoid lifting, sleeping prone, climbing stairs, and riding in a car until allowed by the physician
7. Alternate rest periods with activity
8. Follow dietary recommendations and restrictions
9. Alter ADLs to compensate for neuromuscular deficits
10. Use proper body mechanics and posture
11. Avoid flexion, extension, or rotation of the neck
12. Use one pillow
13. Use a back brace or cervical collar

I. Possible medical complications
1. Upper respiratory infection
2. Urinary tract infection
3. Thrombophlebitis
4. Chronic pain
5. Muscle atrophy
6. Progressive paralysis

J. Possible surgical interventions
1. Laminectomy (see page 60)
2. Spinal fusion (see page 61)
3. Microdiskectomy
4. Percutaneous lateral diskectomy

XXII. Fractures

A. Definition
  1. Break in the continuity of bone
  2. Thirteen types of fractures
     a. Complete
     b. Incomplete
     c. Comminuted
     d. Greenstick
     e. Simple
     f. Compound
     g. Transverse
     h. Spiral
     i. Oblique
     j. Depressed
     k. Compression
     l. Avulsion
     m. Pathologic
  3. Three types of fractured hip
     a. Intracapsular
     b. Extracapsular
     c. Intertrochanteric

B. Possible etiology
  1. Trauma
  2. Osteoporosis
  3. Multiple myeloma
  4. Bone tumors
  5. Immobility
  6. Malnutrition
  7. Cushing's syndrome
  8. Osteomyelitis
  9. Steroid therapy
  10. Aging

C. Pathophysiology
  1. Fracture occurs when stress placed on the bone is more than the bone can withstand
  2. Localized tissue injury results in muscle spasm, edema, hemorrhage, compressed nerves, and ecchymosis

D. Possible clinical manifestations
  1. Pain aggravated by motion
  2. Tenderness over the fracture site
  3. Loss of function or motion
  4. Edema
  5. Crepitus
  6. Ecchymosis

7. Deformity
8. False motion
9. Paresthesia
10. Affected leg that appears shorter (fractured hip)

E. Possible diagnostic test findings
  1. X-ray: break in continuity of bone
  2. Hematology: decreased Hgb and Hct

F. Medical management
  1. Diet: high-protein, high-vitamin, and low-calcium; increase fluid intake
  2. Position: elevate a fractured leg; keep the patient flat with the leg abducted for a fractured hip
  3. Activity: as tolerated for extremity fractures; active and passive ROM exercises for unaffected limbs for fractured hip; isometric exercises
  4. Monitoring: VS, UO, I/O, and neurovascular checks
  5. Laboratory studies: Hgb, Hct, phosphorus, and calcium
  6. Cast care, pin care, ice packs, incentive spirometry, abductor pillow (fractured hip)
  7. Analgesic: oxycodone hydrochloride (Tylox)
  8. Skin traction: Buck's, Bryant's, or Russell's
  9. Skeletal traction: Thomas splint with Pearson attachment, Steinmann pin, Kirschner wire, or Crutchfield tongs
  10. Closed reduction with hip spica cast (fractured hip)
  11. Cast or closed reduction (fracture)

G. Nursing interventions and responsibilities
  1. Maintain the patient's diet; increased fluid intake
  2. Assess neurovascular and respiratory status
  3. Keep the patient in a flat position with the foot of the bed elevated 25° (fractured hip)
  4. Keep the legs abducted (fractured hip)
  5. Elevate a fractured extremity
  6. Monitor and record VS, UO, I/O, and laboratory studies
  7. Administer medications, as prescribed
  8. Allay the patient's anxiety
  9. Provide skin, pin, and cast care
  10. Turn the patient to the affected or unaffected side every 2 hours as ordered (fractured hip)
  11. Keep the hip extended (fractured hip)
  12. Maintain activity, as tolerated (fractures)
  13. Promote independence in ADLs
  14. Provide active and passive ROM and isometric exercises for unaffected limbs
  15. Provide a trapeze
  16. Maintain traction

    17. Keep side rails up
    18. Provide appropriate sensory stimulation with frequent reorientation
    19. Provide TCDB and incentive spirometry
    20. Prevent constipation, as prescribed
    21. Maintain proper body alignment
    22. Inspect pin sites for infection
    23. Provide diversional activities
    24. Provide heel and elbow protectors and sheepskin
    25. Apply antiembolism stockings
    26. Use the logrolling technique to turn the patient

H. Teaching goals (instructions to the patient and family)
    1. Keep follow-up appointments
    2. Know the action, side effects, and scheduling of medications
    3. Recognize the signs and symptoms of decreased circulation and infection
    4. Adhere to activity limitations
    5. Alternate rest periods with activity
    6. Follow dietary recommendations and restrictions
    7. Promote a safe environment
    8. Alter ADLs to compensate for altered mobility and neuromuscular function
    9. Complete skin and foot care daily
    10. Use ambulation aids and devices in ADLs
    11. Complete cast care (fracture)
    12. Exercise regularly with ROM and iosmetric exercises
    13. Maintain a normal weight

I. Possible medical complications
    1. Deep vein thrombosis
    2. Anemia
    3. Fat embolism
    4. Pulmonary embolism
    5. Renal lithiasis
    6. Pneumonia
    7. Urinary tract infections
    8. Compartmental syndrome (fracture)
    9. Hypovolemic shock
    10. Nonunion
    11. Osteomyelitis (fracture)
    12. Avascular necrosis of the femoral head (fractured hip)
    13. Pressure sores

J. Possible surgical interventions
    1. ORIF (see page 58)
    2. External fixation for fractures (see page 54)

XXIII. Systemic lupus erythematosus (SLE)

A. Definition—chronic connective tissue disease involving multiple organ systems

B. Possible etiology
  1. Unknown
  2. Genetic
  3. Autoimmune disease
  4. Viral
  5. Drug-induced: procainamide (Pronestyl) and hydralazine (Apresoline)

C. Pathophysiology
  1. Defect in the body's immunologic mechanism produces serum autoantibodies directed against components of the patient's cell nuclei
  2. Deposits of antigen or antibody complexes affect connective cells throughout the body, including blood vessels, mucous membranes, joints, skin, kidneys, muscles, brain, and heart

D. Possible clinical manifestations
  1. Oral and nasopharyngeal ulcerations
  2. Alopecia
  3. Photosensitivity
  4. Early morning joint stiffness
  5. Low-grade fever
  6. Butterfly erythema on face
  7. Erythema on palms
  8. Muscle pain
  9. Abdominal pain
  10. Malaise and weakness
  11. Weight loss
  12. Lymphadenopathy
  13. Anorexia

E. Possible diagnostic test findings
  1. Hematology: decreased Hgb, Hct, WBC, platelets; increased ESR
  2. Rheumatoid factor: positive
  3. LE prep: positive
  4. Urine chemistry: proteinuria, hematuria
  5. Blood chemistry: decreased complement fixation
  6. ANA test: positive

F. Medical management
  1. Diet: high in iron, protein, and vitamins (especially vitamin C)
  2. I.V. therapy: heparin lock
  3. Activity: as tolerated
  4. Monitoring: VS, UO, and I/O
  5. Laboratory studies: Hgb, Hct, WBC, platelets, ESR, BUN, and creatinine

6. Plasmapheresis
7. Special care: seizure precautions
8. Analgesics: acetaminophen (Tylenol)
9. Antacids: magnesium and aluminum hydroxide (Maalox), aluminum hydroxide gel (Gelusil)
10. Corticosteroids: prednisone (Deltasone)
11. Antimalarials: hydroxychloroquine (Plaquenil)
12. Antipyretic: aspirin
13. NSAID: indomethacin (Indocin), ibuprofen (Motrin)
14. Antianemics: ferrous sulfate (Feosol), ferrous gluconate (Fergon)
15. Immunosuppressive agents: azathioprine (Imuran), cyclophosphamide (Cytoxan)
16. Vitamins and minerals

G. Nursing interventions and responsibilities
1. Maintain the patient's diet
2. Assess musculoskeletal and renal status
3. Monitor and record VS, UO, I/O, laboratory studies, and daily weight
4. Administer medications, as prescribed
5. Encourage the patient to express feelings about changes in body image and the chronicity of the disease
6. Provide skin and mouth care
7. Avoid exposing the patient to sunlight
8. Minimize environmental stress
9. Maintain seizure precautions
10. Provide rest periods
11. Prevent infection
12. Maintain a quiet environment
13. Do not use dusting powder on the patient
14. Promote independence in ADLs
15. Provide postchemotherapeutic and postradiation nursing care
   a. Provide skin, mouth, and perineal care
   b. Encourage dietary intake
   c. Administer antiemetics and antidiarrheals, as prescribed
   d. Monitor for bleeding, infection, and electrolyte imbalance
16. Provide information about the Lupus Foundation

H. Teaching goals (instructions to the patient and family)
1. Keep follow-up appointments
2. Exercise regularly
3. Stop smoking
4. Maintain a normal weight
5. Know the action, side effects, and scheduling of medications
6. Identify ways to reduce stress
7. Recognize the signs and symptoms of renal failure
8. Avoid exposure to people with infections
9. Alternate rest periods with activity

    10. Monitor self for infection
    11. Follow dietary recommendations and restrictions
    12. Maintain a quiet environment
    13. Seek help from community agencies and resources
    14. Alter ADLs to compensate for fatigue and joint pain
    15. Complete skin and mouth care daily
    16. Avoid over-the-counter medications
    17. Avoid exposure to sunlight
    18. Do not use hair spray or hair coloring
    19. Do not take oral contraceptives
    20. Use liquid cosmetics to cover rashes
    21. Reinforce independence in ADLs

I. Possible medical complications
    1. Necrosis of glomerular capillaries
    2. Inflammation of cerebral and ocular blood vessels
    3. Necrosis of lymph nodes
    4. Vasculitis of gastrointestinal tract and pleura
    5. Degeneration of the skin's basal layer
    6. Congestive heart failure (CHF)
    7. Seizures
    8. Depression
    9. Infection
    10. Peripheral neuropathy

J. Possible surgical interventions: none

Points to remember

Metabolic illnesses or medications that cause osteoporosis increase the risk of skeletal fracture.

Alterations in mobility that result from a musculoskeletal disorder may affect a patient's developmental, economic, occupational, recreational, and social activities.

Pain control is a primary focus for the nursing management of a patient with a musculoskeletal disorder.

Glossary

The following terms are defined in Appendix A, page 354.

crepitation

pannus

subluxation

thenar

tophi

Study questions

To evaluate your understanding of this chapter, answer the following questions in the space provided; then compare your responses with the correct answers in Appendix B, pages 358 and 359.

1. What is the purpose of an EMG? _____

_____

2. How should the patient be positioned after a total hip replacement?

_____

_____

3. What is a key postoperative teaching goal for a patient with an external fixation? _____

_____

4. When should the nurse rewrap the stump after an amputation? _____

_____

_____

5. How should the nurse turn the patient who has had a laminectomy?

_____

_____

6. In what position should the patient who has had a spinal fusion sleep?

_____

_____

7. How does the pain of rheumatoid arthritis differ from that of osteoarthritis?

_____

_____

8. Which pharmacologic agents are used to treat gouty arthritis? _____

_____

_____

Study questions *(continued)*

9. What is the pathophysiologic basis for osteomyelitis? _____

_____

_____

10. What is a possible complication of osteoporosis? _____

_____

_____

11. What is osteosarcoma? _____

_____

12. A patient with carpal tunnel syndrome should avoid which activities?

_____

_____

13. What are the clinical manifestations of HNP? _____

_____

_____

14. What are the 3 types of hip fractures? _____

_____

15. What is a key clinical manifestation of SLE? _____

_____

_____

CHAPTER 3

Nervous System

Learning objectives

Check off the following items once you've mastered them:

☐ Describe the psychosocial impact of nervous system disorders.

☐ Differentiate between modifiable and nonmodifiable risk factors in the development of a nervous system disorder.

☐ List three probable and three possible nursing diagnoses for a patient with a nervous system disorder.

☐ Identify the nursing interventions and responsibilities for a patient with a nervous system disorder.

☐ Write three goals for teaching a patient with a nervous system disorder.

I. Anatomy and physiology

A. Neuron

1. The nerve cell, or neuron, is the basic functional unit of the nervous system
2. The neuron is composed of a cell body, dendrites, and an axon, surrounded by a myelin sheath
3. The neuron conducts impulses across a synapse to muscles, glands, and organs
4. Neurotransmitters (acetylcholine and norepinephrine) help conduct impulses across the synapse

B. Central nervous system (CNS)

1. The CNS includes the brain and the spinal cord
   a. Brain
      (1) The *cerebrum* is divided into two hemispheres that contain four lobes each
         (a) The frontal lobe is the site of personality, intellectual functioning, and motor speech
         (b) The parietal lobe is the site of sensation, integration of sensory information, and spatial relationships
         (c) The temporal lobe is the site of hearing, taste, smell, and speech
         (d) The occipital lobe is the site of vision
      (2) The *diencephalon* is composed of the thalamus and the hypothalamus
         (a) The thalamus relays sensory impulses of pain, temperature, and touch to the cortex
         (b) The hypothalamus controls temperature, respiration, blood pressure, and emotional states
      (3) The *brain stem* is composed of the midbrain, pons, and medulla oblongata
         (a) The medulla oblongata contains the vomiting, vasomotor, respiratory, and cardiac centers
         (b) Pyramidal tracts decussate at the medulla oblongata
      (4) The *cerebellum* coordinates muscle tone and movement, equilibrium, and posture
      (5) Blood is supplied to the brain via the internal carotid arteries, vertebral arteries, and circle of Willis
   b. Spinal cord
      (1) The spinal cord is composed of grey matter and white matter
         (a) *Grey matter* forms an H-shaped core in the spinal cord
         (b) *White matter* includes the spinal cord's ascending (sensory) and descending (motor) tracts
      (2) The spinal cord's reflex arc is an involuntary response to a stimulus

2. The CNS is covered and protected by the meninges, which are composed of three membranous layers
   a. Dura mater
   b. Pia mater
   c. Arachnoid membrane
3. Four ventricles produce and circulate cerebrospinal fluid (CSF)
   a. CSF surrounds and protects the brain and spinal cord
   b. CSF exchanges nutrients and wastes at the cellular level

C. Peripheral nervous system (PNS)
   1. The PNS and the CNS together constitute the nervous system
   2. The PNS comprises 12 pairs of cranial nerves, 31 pairs of spinal nerves, and the autonomic nervous system
      a. The cranial nerves consist of the olfactory, optic, oculomotor, trochlear, trigeminal, abducent, facial, acoustic, glossopharyngeal, vagus, accessory, and hypoglossal nerves
      b. Spinal nerves carry mixed impulses (motor and sensory) to and from the spinal cord
      c. The autonomic nervous system regulates smooth muscle, cardiac muscle, and glands; it is composed of the sympathetic and parasympathetic nervous systems
         (1) Sympathetic activity results in adrenergic responses
         (2) Parasympathetic activity results in cholinergic responses

II. Physical assessment findings

A. Subjective data associated with nervous system disorders
   1. Memory impairment
   2. Numbness and tingling
   3. Muscle weakness
   4. Twitching and spasm
   5. Ringing in the ears
   6. Difficulty chewing, swallowing, talking, and walking
   7. Headache
   8. Dizziness
   9. Fainting
   10. Loss of balance and coordination
   11. Nausea and vomiting
   12. Pain
   13. Mental confusion or excitement
   14. Blurred or double vision
   15. Change in bowel and bladder patterns
   16. Sexual dysfunction
   17. Tremors
   18. Stiff neck
   19. Drooping eyelids

B. Objective data associated with nervous system disorders
1. Paresthesia
2. Change in level of consciousness
3. Ataxic gait
4. Dyskinesia
5. Tinnitus
6. Dysphagia
7. Aphasia
8. Seizures
9. Diplopia
10. PAPILLEDEMA
11. Change in visual fields
12. Loss of vision
13. Abnormal temperature
14. Pulse changes
15. Abnormal respirations
16. Hypertension
17. Change in muscle reflexes
18. Abnormal pupil size and reaction
19. Positive Babinski's reflex
20. Loss of cough, gag, corneal, oculocephalic, and oculovestibular reflexes
21. PTOSIS

III. Diagnostic tests and procedures

A. Electroencephalography (EEG)
1. Definition and purpose
a. Noninvasive test of the brain
b. Graphical representation of the brain's electrical activity
2. Nursing interventions and responsibilities before the procedure
a. Determine the patient's ability to lie still
b. Reassure the patient that electrical shock will not occur
c. Explain that the patient will be subjected to stimuli, such as lights and sounds
d. Withhold medications and caffeine 8 hours before the procedure

B. Computerized tomography (CT)
1. Definition and purpose
a. Noninvasive scan after injection of a contrast dye
b. Visualization of the brain and its structures
2. Nursing interventions and responsibilities before the procedure
a. Note the patient's allergies to iodine, seafood, and radiopaque dyes
b. Allay the patient's anxiety
c. Inform the patient about possible throat irritation and flushing of the face

C. Magnetic resonance imaging (MRI)
   1. Definition and purpose
      a. Noninvasive scan using magnetic and radio waves
      b. Visualization of the brain and its structures
   2. Nursing interventions and responsibilities before the procedure
      a. Be aware that patients with pacemakers, surgical and orthopedic clips, or shrapnel should not be scanned
      b. Remove jewelry and metal objects from the patient
      c. Determine the patient's ability to lie still
      d. Administer sedation, as prescribed

D. Cerebral angiogram
   1. Definition and purpose
      a. Fluoroscopic procedure using a radiopaque dye
      b. Examination of the cerebral arteries
   2. Nursing interventions and responsibilities before the procedure
      a. Note the patient's allergies to iodine, seafood, or radiopaque dyes
      b. Inform the patient about possible throat irritation and flushing of the face
   3. Nursing interventions and responsibilities after the procedure
      a. Monitor vital signs (VS)
      b. Allay the patient's anxiety
      c. Check the insertion site for bleeding
      d. Monitor NEUROVITAL signs

E. Lumbar puncture (LP)
   1. Definition and purpose
      a. Invasive procedure
      b. Collection of CSF from the lumbar subarachnoid space and measurement of CSF pressure and injection of radiopaque dye for myelogram
   2. Nursing interventions and responsibilities before the procedure
      a. Determine the patient's ability to lie still in a flexed, lateral, recumbent position
      b. Explain the procedure to the patient
   3. Nursing interventions and responsibilities after the procedure
      a. Keep the patient flat in bed for 24 hours
      b. Administer analgesics, as prescribed
      c. Check the puncture site for bleeding
      d. Monitor neurovital signs
      e. Force fluids

F. CSF analysis
   1. Definition and purpose
      a. Laboratory test of CSF obtained via LP

b. Microscopic examination of CSF for blood, white blood cells (WBCs), immunoglobulins, bacteria, protein, glucose, and electrolytes
2. Nursing interventions and responsibilities
    a. Label specimens properly and send to the laboratory immediately
    b. Adhere to nursing responsibilities after an LP

G. Electromyography (EMG)
  1. Definition and purpose
    a. Noninvasive test of muscles
    b. Graphical recording of the electrical activity of a muscle at rest and during contraction
  2. Nursing interventions and responsibilities
    a. Explain that the patient must flex and relax the muscles during the procedure
    b. Explain that the patient will feel some discomfort but not pain
    c. Administer analgesics, as prescribed, after the procedure

H. Myelogram
  1. Definition and purpose
    a. Injection of radiopaque dye by LP
    b. Visualization of the subarachnoid space, spinal cord, and vertebrae under fluoroscopy
  2. Nursing interventions and responsibilities before the procedure
    a. Note the patient's allergies to iodine, seafood, and radiopaque dyes
    b. Inform the patient about possible throat irritation and flushing of the face
  3. Nursing interventions and responsibilities after the procedure
    a. Keep the patient flat in bed, as directed
    b. Check the puncture site for bleeding
    c. Monitor neurovital signs
    d. Force fluids

I. Brain scan
  1. Definition and purpose
    a. Procedure that involves injection of a radiopaque dye
    b. Visual imaging of blood flow and distribution and brain structures
  2. Nursing interventions and responsibilities before the procedure
    a. Note the patient's allergies to iodine, seafood, and radiopaque dyes
    b. Inform the patient about possible throat irritation and flushing of the face
    c. Determine the patient's ability to lie still during the procedure

J. Skull X-rays
  1. Definition and purpose
    a. Noninvasive examination
    b. Radiographic picture of head and neck bones
  2. Nursing interventions and responsibilities before the procedure

    a. Determine the patient's ability to lie still during the procedure
    b. Explain the events that will occur during the procedure

K. Positron emission tomography (PET)
  1. Definition and purpose
    a. Imaging that involves injection of a radioisotope
    b. Visualization of oxygen uptake, blood flow, and glucose metabolism
  2. Nursing interventions and responsibilities
    a. Determine the patient's ability to lie still during the procedure
    b. Withhold alcohol, tobacco, and caffeine for 24 hours before the procedure
    c. Withhold medications, as directed, before the procedure
    d. Check the injection site for bleeding after the procedure

L. Blood chemistry
  1. Definition and purpose
    a. Laboratory test of a blood sample
    b. Analysis for potassium, sodium, calcium, phosphorus, protein, albumin, osmolality, glucose, bicarbonate, blood urea nitrogen (BUN), and creatinine
  2. Nursing interventions and responsibilities
    a. Withhold food and fluids before the procedure
    b. Monitor the site for bleeding after the procedure

M. Hematologic studies
  1. Definition and purpose
    a. Laboratory test of a blood sample
    b. Analysis for WBCs, red blood cells (RBCs), erythrocyte sedimentation rate (ESR), prothrombin time (PT), partial thromboplastin time (PTT), platelets, hemoglobin (Hgb), and hematocrit (Hct)
  2. Nursing interventions and responsibilities
    a. Note current drug therapy before the procedure
    b. Check the venipuncture site for bleeding after the procedure

IV. Psychosocial impact of nervous system disorders

A. Developmental impact
  1. Changes in body image
  2. Loss of control over body functions
  3. Fear of rejection
  4. Embarrassment from changes in body structure and function
  5. Decreased self-esteem
  6. Fear of dying
  7. Dependence

B. Economic impact
  1. Disruption or loss of employment

    2. Cost of hospitalizations
    3. Cost of home health care
    4. Cost of special equipment

C. Occupational and recreational impact
    1. Restrictions in work activity
    2. Changes in leisure activity
    3. Restrictions in physical activity
    4. Need for vocational retraining

D. Social impact
    1. Changes in eating modes
    2. Changes in elimination patterns and modes
    3. Social isolation
    4. Changes in sexual function
    5. Changes in role performance

V. Risk factors for developing nervous system disorders

A. Modifiable risk factors
    1. Exposure to chemical or environmental pollutants
    2. Substance abuse
    3. Participation in contact sports
    4. Hypertension

B. Nonmodifiable risk factors
    1. Aging
    2. Family history of neurologic disease
    3. History of cardiac disease
    4. History of head injury
    5. Exposure to viral or bacterial infection

VI. Nursing diagnostic categories for a patient with a nervous system disorder

A. Probable nursing diagnostic categories
    1. Impaired physical mobility
    2. Feeding self-care deficit
    3. Bathing/hygiene self-care deficit
    4. Dressing/grooming self-care deficit
    5. Toileting self-care deficit
    6. Sensory-perceptual alteration: visual
    7. Sensory-perceptual alteration: tactile
    8. Altered thought processes
    9. Social isolation
    10. Impaired home maintenance management
    11. Unilateral neglect
    12. Body image disturbance

13. Self-esteem disturbance

B. Possible nursing diagnostic categories
1. Sexual dysfunction
2. Altered urinary elimination
3. Impaired verbal communication
4. Bowel incontinence
5. Altered nutrition: less than body requirements
6. Ineffective airway clearance
7. Ineffective individual coping
8. Potential for injury
9. Altered cerebral tissue perfusion
10. Powerlessness
11. Potential for violence

VII. Craniotomy

A. Definition
1. Surgical opening in the skull to excise a tumor, evacuate a blood clot, relieve intracranial pressure, or repair an aneurysm
2. Classified as supratentorial or infratentorial

B. Preoperative nursing interventions and responsibilities
1. Complete patient and family preoperative teaching
   a. Determine the patient's understanding of the procedure
   b. Describe the operating room (OR), postanesthesia care unit (PACU), and preoperative and postoperative routines; demonstrate postoperative turning, coughing, and deep breathing (TCDB), splinting, leg exercises, and range-of-motion (ROM) exercises
   c. Explain the postoperative need for drainage tubes, surgical dressings, oxygen therapy, I.V. therapy, and pain control
2. Complete a preoperative checklist
3. Administer preoperative medications, as prescribed
4. Allay the patient's and family's anxiety about surgery
5. Document the patient's history and physical assessment data base
6. Administer antibiotics, as prescribed
7. Prepare the patient for preoperative shaving of the head

C. Postoperative nursing interventions and responsibilities
1. Assess cardiac, respiratory, and neurologic status, including level of consciousness
2. Assess pain and administer postoperative analgesics, as prescribed
3. Assess for return of peristalsis; give solid foods and liquids, as tolerated
4. Administer I.V. fluids and total parenteral nutrition (TPN)
5. Allay the patient's anxiety
6. Inspect the surgical dressing and change, as directed
7. Reinforce TCDB

8. Keep the patient in semi-Fowler's position
9. Provide incentive spirometry
10. Maintain activity: as tolerated or passive ROM exercises
11. Administer oxygen and maintain endotracheal tube (ET) to ventilator
12. Monitor VS, urine output (UO), intake and output (I/O), central venous pressure (CVP), laboratory studies, ECG, neurovital signs, neurovascular checks, intracranial pressure (ICP), and pulse oximetry
13. Monitor and maintain the position and patency of drainage tubes: nasogastric (NG), indwelling urinary (Foley), wound drainage
14. Assess cough and gag reflexes
15. Encourage the patient to express feelings about changes in body image or a fear of dying
16. Check for signs of diabetes insipidus
17. Provide eye care
18. Allow a rest period between each nursing activity
19. Observe for signs of increasing ICP
20. Administer corticosteroids, as prescribed
21. Administer anticonvulsants, as prescribed
22. Administer laxatives, as prescribed
23. Administer antacids, as prescribed
24. Maintain seizure precautions

D. Possible surgical complications
   1. Increased ICP
   2. Seizures
   3. Respiratory distress
   4. Diabetes insipidus
   5. Motor and sensory deficits
   6. Infection
   7. Meningitis

E. Postoperative teaching goals (instructions to the patient and family)
   1. Keep follow-up appointments
   2. Exercise regularly
   3. Stop smoking
   4. Maintain a normal weight
   5. Know the action, side effects, and scheduling of medications
   6. Recognize the signs and symptoms of infection, seizure activity, and change in level of consciousness
   7. Adhere to activity limitations
   8. Complete incision care daily
   9. Provide a safe environment

VIII. Endarterectomy

A. Definition—surgical removal of atheromas from arteries and a patch graft repair of the vessel

B. Preoperative nursing interventions and responsibilities
1. Complete patient and family preoperative teaching
   a. Determine the patient's understanding of the procedure
   b. Describe the OR, PACU, and preoperative and postoperative routines
   c. Demonstrate postoperative TCDB, splinting, and leg and ROM exercises
   d. Explain the postoperative need for drainage tubes, surgical dressings, oxygen therapy, I.V. therapy, and pain control
2. Complete a preoperative checklist
3. Administer preoperative medications, as prescribed
4. Allay the patient's and family's anxiety about surgery
5. Document the patient's history and physical assessment data base
6. Administer antibiotics, as prescribed
7. Protect the surgical site from trauma
8. Obtain a preoperative vascular assessment

C. Postoperative nursing interventions and responsibilities
1. Assess cardiac, respiratory, and neurologic status
2. Assess pain and administer postoperative analgesics, as prescribed
3. Assess for return of peristalsis; give solid foods and liquids, as tolerated
4. Administer I.V. fluids
5. Allay the patient's anxiety
6. Inspect the surgical dressing and change, as directed
7. Reinforce TCDB
8. Keep the patient in semi-Fowler's position
9. Provide incentive spirometry
10. Maintain activity: as tolerated, active or passive ROM and isometric exercises
11. Administer oxygen
12. Monitor VS, UO, I/O, laboratory studies, neurovital signs, neurovascular checks, and pulse oximetry
13. Monitor and maintain the position and patency of drainage tubes: NG, Foley, and wound drainage
14. Check the surgical site for bleeding
15. Maintain a pressure dressing
16. Provide special care for carotid endarterectomy
    a. Check neck edema
    b. Assess ability to swallow

D. Possible surgical complications
1. Bleeding
2. Embolism

3. Thrombosis
4. Neurologic deficits
5. Infection

E. Postoperative teaching goals (instructions to the patient and family)
   1. Keep follow-up appointments
   2. Exercise regularly
   3. Stop smoking
   4. Maintain a normal weight
   5. Know the action, side effects, and scheduling of medications
   6. Recognize the signs and symptoms of infection and of motor and sensory deficits
   7. Adhere to activity limitations
   8. Complete incision care daily

IX. Parkinson's disease (paralysis agitans)

A. Definition — progressive degenerative disease of the extrapyramidal system associated with dopamine deficiency

B. Possible etiology
   1. Unknown
   2. Neuromuscular imbalance of dopamine and acetylcholine
   3. Cerebral vascular disease
   4. Drug-induced: phentolamine (Regitine), reserpine (Serpasil), methyldopa (Aldomet)
   5. Dopamine deficiency

C. Pathophysiology
   1. Nerve cells in the basal ganglia are destroyed, resulting in decreased muscular function
   2. Dopamine in the substantia nigra degenerates
   3. Lack of dopamine results in the loss of inhibitory synaptic transmitter for muscle tone and coordination

D. Possible clinical manifestations
   1. "Pill rolling" tremors
   2. Shuffling gait
   3. Stiff joints
   4. Masklike facial expression
   5. Dyskinesia
   6. Dysphagia
   7. Drooling
   8. "Cogwheel" rigidity
   9. Fatigue
   10. Stooped posture
   11. Tremors at rest
   12. Small handwriting

E. Possible diagnostic test findings
   1. EEG: minimal slowing
   2. CT scan: normal

F. Medical management
   1. Diet: high-residue, high-calorie, and high-protein; soft foods
   2. Physical therapy
   3. Activity: as tolerated
   4. Monitoring: VS, UO, I/O, and neurovital signs
   5. Anticholinergics: benztropine mesylate (Cogentin), trihexyphenidyl (Artane)
   6. Antiparkinsonian agents: levodopa (Larodopa), carbidopa-levodopa (Sinemet), benztropine mesylate (Cogentin)
   7. Antispasmodic: procyclidine (Kemadrin)
   8. Antidepressant: amitriptyline (Elavil)
   9. Antiviral: amantadine (Symmetrel)
  10. MAO-B inhibitor: selegiline hydrochloride (Eldepryl)
  11. Dopamine receptor agonists: pergolide mesylate (Permax), bromocriptine mesylate (Parlodel)

G. Nursing interventions and responsibilities
   1. Maintain the patient's diet
   2. Assess neurovascular and respiratory status
   3. Position the patient to prevent contractures
   4. Monitor and record VS, UO, and I/O
   5. Administer medications, as prescribed
   6. Encourage the patient to express feelings about changes in body image
   7. Promote daily ambulation
   8. Maintain a patent airway
   9. Provide active and passive ROM exercises
  10. Provide skin care daily
  11. Provide oral hygiene
  12. Reinforce gait training
  13. Reinforce independence in care
  14. Provide information about the American Parkinson's Disease Association, Inc.; the Parkinson Disease Foundation; and the National Parkinson's Foundation

H. Postoperative teaching goals (instructions to the patient and family)
   1. Keep follow-up appointments
   2. Exercise regularly
   3. Know the action, side effects, and scheduling of medications
   4. Recognize the signs and symptoms of respiratory distress
   5. Alternate rest periods with activity
   6. Promote a safe environment
   7. Seek help from community agencies and resources
   8. Take measures to prevent choking

    a. Cut food into small pieces
    b. Suction the mouth frequently
    c. Eat soft foods
  9. Avoid foods high in vitamin B_{15}: tuna, pork, dried beans, salmon, and beef liver
 10. Increase intake of roughage and fluids to prevent constipation

I. Possible medical complications
  1. Depression
  2. Corneal ulceration
  3. Injury
  4. Aspiration
  5. Constipation

J. Possible surgical intervention: stereotaxic thalamotomy to relieve tremor and rigidity

X. Multiple sclerosis

A. Definition — progressive disease of impaired motor nerve conduction

B. Possible etiology
  1. Unknown
  2. Autoimmune disease
  3. Viral

C. Pathophysiology
  1. Scattered demyelinization occurs in the brain and spinal cord
  2. Degeneration of myelin sheath results in patches of sclerotic tissue and impaired conduction of motor nerve impulses

D. Possible clinical manifestations
  1. Weakness
  2. Nystagmus
  3. Scanning speech
  4. ATAXIA
  5. Diplopia
  6. Paresthesia
  7. Blurred vision
  8. Impaired sensation
  9. Feelings of euphoria
 10. Paralysis
 11. Urinary incontinence
 12. Intention tremor
 13. Inability to sense or gauge body position

E. Possible diagnostic test findings
  1. CSF analysis: increased IgG, protein, WBCs
  2. CT scan: normal except in chronic illness, when atrophy is found

3. MRI: normal except in chronic illness, when atrophy is found
4. Evoked potentials: slowing of nerve conduction
5. Oligoclonal banding: positive
6. EMG: abnormal

F. Medical management
1. Diet: high-calorie, high-protein, and high-vitamin; gluten-free; low-fat
2. Activity: as tolerated
3. Monitoring: VS, UO, I/O, and neurovital signs
4. Speech therapy
5. Plasmapheresis
6. Muscle relaxant: baclofen (Lioresal)
7. Physical therapy
8. Glucocorticoids: prednisone (Deltasone), dexamethasone (Decadron), corticotropin (ACTH)
9. Antacids: magnesium and aluminum hydroxide (Maalox), aluminum hydroxide gel (ALternaGEL)
10. Fluids: increased intake
11. Antineoplastic (immunosuppressant): cyclophosphamide (Cytoxan)
12. Skeletal muscle relaxant: quinine sulfate (Quinamm)

G. Nursing interventions and responsibilities
1. Maintain the patient's diet
2. Force fluids
3. Assess neurologic status
4. Monitor and record: VS, UO, I/O, and neurovital signs
5. Administer medications, as prescribed
6. Encourage the patient to express feelings about changes in body image
7. Maintain active and passive ROM exercises
8. Establish bowel and bladder program
9. Maintain activity, as tolerated
10. Protect the patient from falls
11. Maintain a stress-free environment
12. Provide information about the National Multiple Sclerosis Society

H. Postoperative teaching goals (instructions to the patient and family)
1. Keep follow-up appointments
2. Exercise regularly
3. Know the action, side effects, and scheduling of medications
4. Identify ways to reduce stress
5. Recognize the signs and symptoms of exacerbation
6. Avoid exposure to people with infections
7. Alternate rest periods with activity
8. Monitor self for infection
9. Follow dietary recommendations and restrictions
10. Maintain a safe, quiet environment
11. Seek help from community agencies and resources

  12. Minimize environmental stress
  13. Use assistive devices in activities of daily living (ADLs), such as specialized eating utensils, and wheelchair ramps
  14. Reinforce independence
  15. Avoid temperature extremes

I. Possible medical complications
  1. Urinary tract infection
  2. Respiratory tract infection
  3. Contractures
  4. Depression
  5. Paraplegia
  6. Quadriplegia

J. Possible surgical intervention: contralateral thalamotomy

XI. Myasthenia gravis

A. Definition — neuromuscular disorder that results in weakness of voluntary muscles

B. Possible etiology
  1. Insufficient acetylcholine
  2. Autoimmune disease
  3. Excessive cholinesterase

C. Pathophysiology
  1. Disturbance occurs in transmission of nerve impulses at the myoneural junction
  2. Transmission defect results from deficiency in release of acetylcholine or deficient number of acetylcholine receptor sites
  3. Thymus gland may remain active, triggering autoimmune reaction

D. Possible clinical manifestations
  1. Muscle weakness that increases with activity and decreases with rest
  2. Dysphagia
  3. Diplopia
  4. Dysarthria
  5. Ptosis
  6. Strabismus
  7. Impaired speech
  8. Respiratory distress
  9. Masklike expression
  10. Drooling

E. Possible diagnostic test findings
  1. Neostigmine (Prostigmin) or edrophonium (Tensilon) test: relief of symptoms after medication administration
  2. EMG: decreased amplitude of evoked potentials

3. Thymus scan: hyperplasia or thymoma

F. Medical management
   1. Diet: high-calorie; soft foods
   2. Activity: as tolerated
   3. Monitoring: VS, UO, I/O, and neurovital signs
   4. Glucocorticoids: prednisone (Deltasone), dexamethasone (Decadron), corticotropin (ACTH)
   5. Antacids: magnesium and aluminum hydroxide (Maalox), aluminum hydroxide gel (ALternaGEL)
   6. Anticholinesterases: neostigmine (Prostigmin), pyridostigmine bromide (Mestinon), ambenonium chloride (Mytelase)
   7. Plasmapheresis
   8. Immunosuppressant: azathioprine (Imuran)
   9. Antineoplastic: cyclophosphamide (Cytoxan)

G. Nursing interventions and responsibilities
   1. Maintain the patient's diet; encourage small, frequent meals
   2. Assess neurologic and respiratory status
   3. Assess swallow and gag reflexes
   4. Monitor and record VS, UO, I/O, and neurovital signs
   5. Administer medications, as prescribed
   6. Encourage the patient to express feelings about changes in body image and about difficulty in communicating verbally
   7. Determine the patient's activity tolerance
   8. Provide rest periods
   9. Provide oral hygiene
   10. Protect the patient from falls
   11. Watch the patient for choking while eating
   12. Provide information about the Myasthenia Gravis Foundation

H. Postoperative teaching goals (instructions to the patient and family)
   1. Keep follow-up appointments
   2. Exercise regularly
   3. Know the action, side effects, and scheduling of medications
   4. Identify ways to reduce stress
   5. Recognize the signs and symptoms of respiratory distress and myasthenic crisis
   6. Adhere to activity limitations
   7. Avoid exposure to people with infections
   8. Alternate rest periods with activity
   9. Monitor self for infection
   10. Maintain a safe, quiet environment
   11. Seek help from community agencies and resources
   12. Minimize environmental stress
   13. Avoid hot foods and tonic preparations containing quinine

I. Possible medical complications
   1. Myasthenic crisis
      a. Increased symptoms of muscular weakness from undermedication or stress
      b. Symptoms improve with edrophonium (Tensilon)
   2. Cholinergic crisis
      a. Increased symptoms of muscular weakness and side effects of anticholinesterase medications from overmedication with cholinergic drugs
      b. Symptoms worsen with edrophonium (Tensilon)

J. Possible surgical intervention: thymectomy

XII. Guillain-Barré syndrome (polyradiculitis, acute infectious polyneuritis)

A. Definition – peripheral polyneuritis characterized by ascending paralysis

B. Possible etiology
   1. Unknown
   2. Virus
   3. Infection
   4. Autoimmune disease

C. Pathophysiology
   1. Preceding infection synthesizes lymphocytes, which attack the myelin sheath, causing demyelinization
   2. Demyelinization is followed by inflammation around nerve roots, veins, and capillaries
   3. Inflammatory process compresses nerve roots

D. Possible clinical manifestations
   1. Generalized weakness
   2. Paralysis that starts in the legs
   3. Ascending paralysis
   4. Respiratory paralysis
   5. Tachycardia
   6. Hypertension
   7. Increased temperature
   8. Ptosis
   9. Facial weakness
   10. Dysphagia
   11. Dysarthria

E. Possible diagnostic test findings
   1. CSF analysis: increased protein
   2. EMG: slowed nerve conduction

F. Medical management
   1. Diet: high-calorie, high-protein
   2. Position: semi-Fowler's
   3. Activity: bed rest, active and passive ROM and isometric exercises
   4. Monitoring: VS, UO, I/O, and neurovital signs
   5. Plasmapheresis
   6. Nutritional support: gastrostomy feedings, NG feedings
   7. Intubation and mechanical ventilation
   8. Physical therapy
   9. Foley catheter, chest physiotherapy (CPT), postural drainage, and suction
   10. Antibiotics: amoxicillin (Amoxil), ampicillin (Omnipen), gentamicin (Garamycin)
   11. Glucocorticoids: prednisone (Deltasone), dexamethasone (Decadron), corticotropin (ACTH)
   12. Antacids: magnesium and aluminum hydroxide (Maalox), aluminum hydroxide gel (ALternaGEL)
   13. IgG antibody: Immune Globulin IV (Gammagard)
   14. Pulse oximetry

G. Nursing interventions and responsibilities
   1. Maintain the patient's diet
   2. Administer oxygen
   3. Provide suction and TCDB
   4. Assess respiratory and neurologic status
   5. Maintain the position and patency of NG and endotracheal tubes
   6. Keep the patient in semi-Fowler's position
   7. Monitor and record VS, UO, I/O, neurovital signs, and pulse oximetry
   8. Administer medications, as prescribed
   9. Encourage the patient to express feelings about powerlessness, changes in body image, and difficulty in communicating verbally
   10. Assess muscle strength
   11. Assess gag and swallow reflexes
   12. Provide eye and mouth care
   13. Establish alternate means of communicating with the patient
   14. Protect the patient from falls
   15. Prevent skin breakdown
   16. Provide ROM exercises
   17. Assess for Homans' sign
   18. Establish a bowel and bladder program
   19. Apply antiembolism stockings
   20. Turn the patient every 2 hours
   21. Provide information about the Guillain-Barré Foundation

H. Teaching goals (instructions to the patient and family)
   1. Keep follow-up appointments
   2. Stop smoking

3. Know the action, side effects, and scheduling of medications
4. Identify ways to reduce stress
5. Recognize the signs and symptoms of respiratory distress
6. Avoid exposure to people with infections
7. Alternate rest periods with activity
8. Monitor self for infection
9. Follow dietary recommendations and restrictions
10. Maintain a safe, quiet environment
11. Seek help from community agencies and resources
12. Minimize environmental stress
13. Exercise hands, arms, and legs regularly

I. Possible medical complications
1. Respiratory failure
2. Contractures
3. Aspiration
4. Pneumonia

J. Possible surgical interventions: none

XIII. Seizure disorders

A. Definition
1. Involuntary muscle contractions caused by abnormal discharge of electrical impulses from nerve cells
2. Classification of seizures
   a. Simple partial (Jacksonian)
   b. Complex partial
   c. Partial evolving to secondarily generalized
   d. Generalized (tonic-clonic, tonic, clonic, absence, atonic-akinetic, myoclonic)
   e. Unclassified

B. Possible etiology
1. Idiopathic origin
2. Head injury
3. Hypoglycemia
4. Brain tumor
5. Infection
6. Anoxia

C. Pathophysiology
1. Many neurons fire in a synchronous pattern, resulting in a transient physiologic disturbance
2. Physiologic disturbances include abnormal movements, abnormal sensations, and a change in the level of consciousness

D. Possible clinical manifestations
1. Aura

2. Loss of consciousness
3. Dyspnea
4. Fixed and dilated pupils
5. Incontinence

E. Possible diagnostic test findings
   1. EEG: abnormal wave patterns, focus of seizure activity
   2. CT scan: a space-occupying lesion
   3. MRI: pathologic changes
   4. Brain-mapping: identification of seizure areas

F. Medical management
   1. Diet: ketogenic
   2. I.V. therapy: heparin lock
   3. Activity: bed rest
   4. Monitoring: VS, UO, I/O, and neurovital signs
   5. Laboratory studies: glucose, potassium, and phenytoin levels
   6. Special care: seizure precautions
   7. Anticonvulsants: phenytoin (Dilantin), ethosuximide (Zarontin), phenobarbital (Luminal), diazepam (Valium)

G. Nursing interventions and responsibilities
   1. Maintain the patient's diet
   2. Assess neurologic and respiratory status
   3. Monitor and record VS, UO, I/O, neurovital signs, and laboratory studies
   4. Administer medications, as prescribed
   5. Encourage the patient to express feelings about powerlessness
   6. Maintain seizure precautions
   7. Protect the patient during seizure activity
   8. Observe and record seizure activity
      a. Initial movement
      b. Respiratory pattern
      c. Duration of seizure
      d. Loss of consciousness
      e. Aura
      f. Incontinence
      g. Pupillary changes
   9. Assess postictal state
   10. Maintain a patent airway
   11. Protect the patient from falls
   12. Provide information about the Epilepsy Foundation of America; the National Epilepsy League, Inc.; and the National Association to Control Epilepsy

H. Teaching goals (instructions to the patient and family)
   1. Keep follow-up appointments
   2. Know the action, side effects, and scheduling of medications

3. Identify ways to reduce stress
4. Recognize the signs and symptoms of seizure activity
5. Adhere to activity limitations
6. Avoid drinking alcohol
7. Alternate rest periods with activity
8. Follow dietary recommendations and restrictions
9. Promote a safe environment
10. Seek help from community agencies and resources
11. Wear a medical identification bracelet
12. Identify and time seizure activity
13. Prevent injury during seizure activity

I. Possible medical complications
1. Musculoskeletal injury
2. Hypoxia
3. Status epilepticus

J. Possible surgical intervention: excision of epileptogenic area (rare)

XIV. Increased ICP

A. Definition—elevated ICP beyond the normal pressure exerted by blood, brain, and CSF within the skull

B. Possible etiology
1. Tumor
2. Abscess
3. Space-occupying lesion
4. Edema
5. Hemorrhage
6. Hydrocephalus
7. Head injury

C. Pathophysiology
1. Because the skull cannot expand, an increase in brain tissue, CSF, or blood results in increased ICP
2. Increased ICP results in decreased cerebral circulation and anoxia, which can lead to permanent brain damage

D. Possible clinical manifestations
1. Restlessness
2. Hypertension
3. Bradycardia
4. Pupillary changes
   a. Sluggish reaction
   b. Dilation
5. Weakness
6. Decreased level of consciousness
7. Widening pulse pressure

8. Abnormal posturing
   a. Decortication
   b. DECEREBRATION
9. Headache
10. Vomiting
11. Papilledema

E. Possible diagnostic test findings
   1. ICP measurement via ventriculostomy, epidural sensor, and subarachnoid screw: increased pressure
   2. LP: contraindicated

F. Medical management
   1. Diet: withhold food and fluids, as ordered
   2. I.V. therapy: electrolyte replacement, heparin lock
   3. Oxygen therapy
   4. Intubation and mechanical ventilation with hyperventilation
   5. Gastrointestinal decompression: NG tube
   6. Position: semi-Fowler's
   7. Activity: bedrest, passive ROM exercises
   8. Monitoring: VS, UO, I/O, ECG, ICP, neurovital signs, and arterial pressure
   9. Laboratory studies: potassium, sodium, glucose, osmolality, BUN, and creatinine
   10. Foley catheter
   11. ICP monitoring: ventriculostomy, subarachnoid screw, epidural sensor
   12. Diuretics: mannitol (Osmitrol), furosemide (Lasix)
   13. Antacids: magnesium and aluminum hydroxide (Maalox)
   14. CSF drainage via ventriculostomy
   15. Anticonvulsant: phenytoin (Dilantin)
   16. Glucocorticoid: dexamethasone (Decadron)
   17. Histamine antagonists: cimetidine (Tagamet), ranitidine (Zantac)
   18. Barbiturate-induced coma
   19. Seizure precautions
   20. Pulse oximetry
   21. Mucosal barrier fortifier: sucralfate (Carafate)

G. Nursing interventions and responsibilities
   1. Maintain fluid restrictions
   2. Administer I.V. fluids
   3. Administer oxygen
   4. Provide suction, TCDB
   5. Assess neurologic and respiratory status
   6. Maintain the position and patency of the NG tube; provide low suctioning
   7. Maintain the position and patency of the ET tube and Foley catheter
   8. Keep the patient in semi-Fowler's position

9. Monitor and record VS, UO, I/O, ICP, neurovital signs, laboratory studies, and pulse oximetry
10. Administer medications, as prescribed
11. Allay the patient's anxiety
12. Maintain neutral alignment
13. Turn the patient every 2 hours
14. Prevent jugular venous constriction
15. Allow a period of rest between each nursing activity
16. Maintain a quiet environment
17. Continue bed rest
18. Prevent Valsalva's maneuver
19. Provide mouth and skin care
20. Provide appropriate sensory input and stimuli with frequent reorientation
21. Assist with ADLs; make referrals to appropriate community agencies
22. Maintain seizure precautions

H. Teaching goals (instructions to the patient and family)
1. Keep follow-up appointments
2. Exercise regularly
3. Know the action, side effects, and scheduling of medications
4. Recognize the signs and symptoms of decreased level of consciousness and seizures
5. Alternate rest periods with activity
6. Maintain a safe, quiet environment
7. Seek help from community agencies and resources for supportive services
8. Minimize environmental stress
9. Set limits for impulsive behavior
10. Continue fluid restrictions
11. Identify ways to reduce stress
12. Adhere to activity limitations

I. Possible medical complications
1. Tentorial herniation
2. Herniation through foramen magnum
3. Coma
4. Seizure
5. Death

J. Possible surgical intervention: craniotomy for surgical decompression (see page 95)

XV. Head injury

A. Definition — classified by the type of fracture, hemorrhage, or trauma to the brain
1. Fractures

       a. Depressed
       b. Comminuted
       c. Linear
   2. Hemorrhages
       a. Epidural
       b. Subdural
       c. Intracerebral
       d. Subarachnoid
   3. Trauma
       a. Concussion
       b. Contusion

B. Possible etiology
   1. Auto accidents
   2. Falls
   3. Assaults
   4. Blunt trauma
   5. Penetrating trauma

C. Pathophysiology: brain injury or bleeding within the brain results in edema and hypoxia

D. Possible clinical manifestations
   1. Disorientation to time, place, or person
   2. Paresthesia
   3. Positive Babinski's reflex
   4. Decreased level of consciousness
   5. Otorrhea
   6. Rhinorrhea
   7. Unequal pupil size
   8. Loss of pupil reaction

E. Possible diagnostic test findings
   1. Skull X-ray: skull fracture
   2. CT scan: hemorrhage, cerebral edema, or shift of midline structures
   3. MRI: hemorrhage, cerebral edema, or shift of midline structures
   4. Cerebral angiography: intracerebral, subdural, epidural hematoma
   5. Echoencephalogram: shift of midline structures

F. Medical management
   1. Diet: restricted fluids
   2. I.V. therapy: electrolyte replacement; heparin lock
   3. Oxygen therapy
   4. Intubation and mechanical ventilation with hyperventilation
   5. Gastrointestinal decompression: NG tube
   6. Position: semi-Fowler's
   7. Activity: bed rest; active and passive ROM exercises

8. Monitoring: VS, UO, I/O, ECG, hemodynamic variables, ICP, CVP, neurovital signs, and arterial line
9. Laboratory studies: potassium, sodium, osmolality, arterial blood gases (ABGs), Hgb, and Hct
10. Foley catheter
11. Analgesic: codeine phosphate (Paveral)
12. Diuretics: mannitol (Osmitrol), furosemide (Lasix)
13. Antacids: magnesium and aluminum hydroxide (Maalox), aluminum hydroxide gel (ALternaGEL)
14. Anticonvulsant: phenytoin (Dilantin)
15. Glucocorticoid: dexamethasone (Decadron)
16. Histamine antagonists: cimetidine (Tagamet), ranitidine (Zantac)
17. Cervical collar
18. Reflex checks: oculocephalic, oculovestibular, corneal, cough, and gag
19. Mucosal barrier fortifier: sucralfate (Carafate)
20. Pulse oximetry

G. Nursing interventions and responsibilities
1. Restrict fluids
2. Administer I.V. fluids
3. Administer oxygen
4. Provide suction, TCDB
5. Assess neurologic and respiratory status
6. Maintain position, patency, and low suction of NG tube
7. Maintain position and patency of ET and Foley catheter
8. Keep the patient in semi-Fowler's position
9. Monitor and record VS, UO, I/O, hemodynamic variables, ICP, CVP, specific gravity, urine glucose and ketones, laboratory studies, and pulse oximetry
10. Maintain seizure precautions
11. Administer medications, as prescribed
12. Encourage the patient to express feelings about changes in body image
13. Assess for CSF leak: otorrhea, rhinorrhea
14. Assess pain
15. Check for signs of diabetes insipidus
16. Check cough and gag reflex
17. Provide appropriate sensory input and stimuli with frequent reorientation
18. Provide means of communication
19. Observe for signs of increasing ICP
20. Provide eye, skin, and mouth care
21. Turn the patient every 2 hours
22. Assist with ADLs
23. Provide information about the National Head Injury Foundation

H. Teaching goals (instructions to the patient and family)
1. Keep follow-up appointments

2. Exercise regularly
3. Know the action, side effects, and scheduling of medications
4. Recognize the signs and symptoms of decreased level of consciousness and seizures
5. Alternate rest periods with activity
6. Maintain a safe, quiet environment
7. Seek help from community agencies and resources
8. Minimize environmental stress
9. Set limits for impulsive behavior
10. Adhere to fluid restrictions

I. Possible medical complications
1. Shock
2. Meningitis
3. Increased ICP
4. Stress ulcer
5. Diabetes insipidus
6. Infection

J. Possible surgical intervention: craniotomy for evacuation of hematomas (see page 95)

XVI. Cerebrovascular accident (CVA)

A. Definition—disruption of cerebral circulation that results in motor and sensory deficits

B. Possible etiology
1. Cerebral arteriosclerosis
2. Syphilis
3. Trauma
4. Hypertension
5. Thrombosis
6. Embolism
7. Hemorrhage
8. Vasospasm

C. Pathophysiology
1. Disruption of cerebral blood flow causes cerebral anoxia
2. Cerebral anoxia results in cerebral infarction
3. Infarction results in edema

D. Possible clinical manifestations
1. Syncope
2. Change in level of consciousness
3. Paresthesia
4. Headache
5. Aphasia
6. Seizures

    7. Labile emotional responses
    8. Paralysis

E. Possible diagnostic test findings
    1. LP: increased pressure, bloody CSF
    2. CT scan: intracranial bleeding, infarct, or shift of midline structures
    3. EEG: focal slowing in area of lesion
    4. MRI: intracranial bleeding, infarct, or shift of midline structures
    5. Brain scan: decreased perfusion
    6. Digital subtraction angiography: occlusion or narrowing of vessels

F. Medical management
    1. Diet: low-sodium, increased potassium
    2. I.V. therapy: heparin lock
    3. Oxygen therapy
    4. Intubation and mechanical ventilation
    5. Gastrointestinal decompression: NG tube
    6. Position: semi-Fowler's
    7. Activity: bed rest, active and passive ROM and isometric exercises
    8. Monitoring: VS, UO, I/O, ECG, ICP, and neurovital signs
    9. Laboratory studies: sodium, potassium, glucose, ABGs, PT, and PTT
   10. Nutritional support: TPN
   11. Foley catheter, incentive spirometry
   12. Seizure precautions
   13. Analgesic: codeine phosphate (Paveral)
   14. Diuretics: mannitol (Osmitrol), furosemide (Lasix)
   15. Antacids: magnesium and aluminum hydroxide (Maalox), aluminum hydroxide gel (ALternaGEL)
   16. Anticonvulsant: phenytoin (Dilantin)
   17. Glucocorticoid: dexamethasone (Decadron)
   18. Histamine antagonists: cimetidine (Tagamet), ranitidine (Zantac)
   19. Antihypertensive: diazoxide (Hyperstat)
   20. Anticoagulant: warfarin sodium (Coumadin)
   21. Pulse oximetry
   22. Physical therapy

G. Nursing interventions and responsibilities
    1. Maintain the patient's diet
    2. Administer I.V. fluids
    3. Administer oxygen
    4. Provide suction, TCDB
    5. Assess neurovascular, cardiac, and respiratory status
    6. Maintain position, patency, and low suction of NG tube
    7. Keep the patient in semi-Fowler's position
    8. Monitor and record VS, UO, I/O, ICP, neurovital signs, laboratory studies, and pulse oximetry
    9. Administer TPN

10. Administer medications, as prescribed
11. Encourage the patient to express feelings about changes in body image and about difficulty in communicating verbally
12. Maintain a quiet environment
13. Assess for receptive and expressive aphasia
14. Assess for hemianopia
15. Protect the patient from falls and injury
16. Apply antiembolism stockings
17. Maintain seizure precautions
18. Provide passive ROM exercises
19. Turn and position the patient every 2 hours
20. Provide means of communication
21. Provide skin and mouth care
22. Provide information about the American Heart Association and the National Stroke Foundation

H. Teaching goals (instructions to the patient and family)
1. Keep follow-up appointments
2. Exercise regularly
3. Stop smoking
4. Maintain a normal weight
5. Know the action, side effects, and scheduling of medications
6. Identify ways to reduce stress
7. Recognize the signs and symptoms of seizures
8. Adhere to activity limitations
9. Alternate rest periods with activity
10. Follow dietary recommendations and restrictions
11. Maintain a safe, quiet environment
12. Seek help from community agencies and resources
13. Minimize environmental stress
14. Reinforce established methods of communication (aphasic patient)
15. Monitor blood pressure
16. Use assistive devices in ADLs

I. Possible medical complications
1. Cerebral edema
2. Vasospasm
3. Pneumonia
4. Increased ICP
5. Problems from immobility
   a. Thrombophlebitis
   b. Pulmonary embolism
   c. Osteoporosis
   d. Urinary stasis

J. Possible surgical interventions
1. Carotid endarterectomy (see page 97)

2. Craniotomy for evacuation of a clot (see page 95)
3. Craniotomy for superior temporal artery—middle cerebral artery anastamosis (see page 95)

XVII. Cerebral aneurysm

A. Definition
  1. Dilation or localized weakness of the middle layer of an artery
  2. Classified by aneurysm type
     a. Saccular (berry)
     b. Fusiform
     c. Mycotic

B. Possible etiology
  1. Atherosclerosis
  2. Trauma
  3. Congenital weakness
  4. Syphilis

C. Pathophysiology
  1. Enlargement of aneurysm compresses nerves
  2. Enlargement of the aneurysm finally results in dissolution of the wall and rupture of the aneurysm
  3. Rupture of the aneurysm results in subarachnoid hemorrhage
  4. Release of serotonin, prostaglandins, and catecholamines from blood precipitates vasospasm

D. Possible clinical manifestations
  1. Diplopia
  2. Ptosis
  3. Headache
  4. Hemiparesis
  5. Nuchal rigidity
  6. Decreased level of consciousness
  7. Seizure activity
  8. Blurred vision

E. Possible diagnostic test findings
  1. CT scan: shift of intracranial midline structures, blood in subarachnoid space
  2. MRI: shift of intracranial midline structures, blood in subarachnoid space
  3. Cerebral angiogram: identification of vasospasm and vasculature associated with aneurysm
  4. LP (contraindicated with increased ICP): increased pressure, protein, WBC; bloody and xanthochromic CSF

F. Medical management
  1. I.V. therapy: heparin lock

2. Oxygen therapy
3. Position: semi-Fowler's
4. Activity: bed rest; passive ROM exercises
5. Monitoring: VS, UO, I/O (fluid restrictions), ICP, neurovital signs, and arterial line
6. Precautions: aneurysm and seizure
7. Antacids: magnesium and aluminum hydroxide (Maalox), aluminum hydroxide gel (ALternaGEL)
8. Anticonvulsant: phenytoin (Dilantin)
9. Glucocorticoid: dexamethasone (Decadron)
10. Histamine antagonists: cimetidine (Tagamet), ranitidine (Zantac)
11. Stool softener: docusate sodium (Colace)
12. Antifibrolytic: aminocaproic acid (Amicar)
13. Antihypertensives: methylodopa (Aldomet), hydralazine (Apresoline)
14. Ergot alkaloid: methysergide (Sansert)
15. Calcium channel blocker: nimodipine hydrochloride (Nimotop)
16. Intubation and mechanical ventilation
17. Pulse oximetry
18. Mucosal barrier fortifier: sucralfate (Carafate)

G. Nursing interventions and responsibilities
1. Maintain fluid restriction
2. Administer oxygen
3. Assess neurologic status
4. Keep the patient in semi-Fowler's position
5. Monitor and record VS, UO, I/O, ICP, and pulse oximetry
6. Administer medication, as prescribed
7. Encourage the patient to express feelings about a fear of dying
8. Allay the patient's anxiety
9. Maintain a quiet, darkened environment
10. Assess pain
11. Allow a rest period between nursing activities
12. Maintain bed rest
13. Prevent Valsalva's maneuver
14. Assess for signs of increased ICP
15. Maintain seizure and aneurysm precautions
16. Provide passive ROM exercises
17. Limit visitors
18. Provide skin care
19. Assist with ADLs
20. Prevent constipation
21. Assess for meningeal irritation

H. Teaching goals (instructions to the patient and family)
1. Keep follow-up appointments
2. Know the action, side effects, and scheduling of medications
3. Identify ways to reduce stress

4. Recognize the signs and symptoms of decreasing level of consciousness and seizures
5. Adhere to activity limitations
6. Promote a safe environment
7. Maintain a quiet environment
8. Minimize environmental stress
9. Alter ADLs to compensate for neurologic deficits
10. Prevent constipation

I. Possible medical complications
1. Vasospasm
2. Rebleeding of the aneurysm
3. Increased ICP
4. Rupture of the aneurysm
5. Hydrocephalus
6. Brain herniation

J. Possible surgical interventions
1. Craniotomy for clipping or wrapping of an aneurysm (see page 95)
2. Craniotomy for evacuation of hematomas (see page 95)

XVIII. Brain tumor

A. Definition—malignant or benign tumor of the brain that may be primary or metastatic

B. Possible etiology
1. Genetic
2. Environmental

C. Pathophysiology
1. Unregulated cell growth and uncontrolled cell division result in the development of a neoplasm
2. Tumors are classified according to tissue of origin
a. Gliomas
b. Meningiomas
c. Metastatic
3. Tumors can be infiltrative and destroy surrounding tissue or be encapsulated and displace brain tissue
4. Presence of lesion and compression of blood vessels produces ischemia, edema, and increased ICP

D. Possible clinical manifestations
1. Tumor in any brain area
a. Headache
b. Vomiting
c. Papilledema
2. Tumor in the frontal lobe
a. Personality changes

      b. Aphasia

      c. Memory loss

  3. Tumor in the temporal lobe

      a. Seizures

      b. Aphasia

  4. Tumor in the parietal lobe

      a. Motor seizures

      b. Sensory impairment

  5. Tumor in the occipital lobe

      a. Visual impairment

      b. Homonymous hemianopia

      c. Visual hallucinations

  6. Tumor in the cerebellum

      a. Impaired equilibrium

      b. Impaired coordination

E. Possible diagnostic test findings
   1. EEG: seizure activity
   2. CT scan: location and size of tumor
   3. Skull X-ray: location and size of tumor
   4. Angiography: location and size of tumor
   5. LP (contraindicated with increased ICP): increased protein

F. Medical management
   1. Diet: high-protein, high-calorie
   2. I.V. therapy: heparin lock
   3. Oxygen therapy
   4. Position: semi-Fowler's
   5. Activity: bed rest
   6. Monitoring: VS, UO, I/O, ICP, and neurovital signs
   7. Laboratory studies: sodium and potassium glucose
   8. Nutritional support: TPN
   9. Radiation therapy
   10. Antineoplastics: vincristine sulfate (Oncovin), lomustine (CeeNu), carmustine (BiCNU)
   11. Diuretics: mannitol (Osmitrol), furosemide (Lasix)
   12. Antacids: magnesium and aluminum hydroxide (Maalox), aluminum hydroxide gel (ALternaGEL)
   13. Anticovulsant: phenytoin (Dilantin)
   14. Glucocorticoid: dexamethasone (Decadron)
   15. Histamine antagonists: cimetidine (Tagamet), ranitidine (Zantac)
   16. Seizure precautions
   17. Chemotherapy
   18. Stereotactic brachytherapy
   19. Stereotaxic radiosurgery (Roentgen knife)
   20. Mucosal barrier fortifier: sucralfate (Carafate)

G. Nursing interventions and responsibilities
  1. Maintain the patient's diet
  2. Encourage the patient to drink fluids
  3. Administer I.V. fluids
  4. Administer oxygen
  5. Assess neurologic and respiratory status
  6. Keep the patient in semi-Fowler's position
  7. Monitor and record VS, UO, I/O, ICP, neurovital signs, and laboratory studies
  8. Administer TPN
  9. Administer medications, as prescribed
  10. Encourage the patient to express feelings about changes in body image and a fear of dying
  11. Assess pain
  12. Assess for increased ICP
  13. Provide oral hygiene
  14. Provide postchemotherapeutic and postradiation nursing care
    a. Provide skin, mouth, and perineal care
    b. Encourage dietary intake
    c. Administer antiemetics and antidiarrheals, as prescribed
    d. Monitor for bleeding, infection, and electrolyte imbalance
    e. Provide rest periods
  15. Maintain seizure precautions
  16. Provide information about the National Head Injury Foundation and the Association for Brain Tumor Research

H. Teaching goals (instructions to the patient and family)
  1. Keep follow-up appointments
  2. Exercise regularly
  3. Maintain a normal weight
  4. Know the action, side effects, and scheduling of medications
  5. Identify ways to reduce stress
  6. Recognize the signs and symptoms of change in level of consciousness
  7. Adhere to activity limitations
  8. Avoid exposure to people with infections
  9. Alternate rest periods with activity
  10. Monitor self for infection
  11. Follow dietary recommendations and restrictions
  12. Maintain a safe, quiet environment

I. Possible medical complications
  1. Increased ICP
  2. Brain herniation
  3. Seizures

J. Possible surgical intervention: craniotomy for surgical excision of a tumor (see page 95)

XIX. Spinal cord injury

A. Definition
   1. Traumatic injury to the spinal cord that results in sensory and motor deficits
   2. Two types of spinal cord injury
      a. Paraplegia, paralysis of the legs
      b. Quadriplegia, paralysis of all four extremities

B. Possible etiology
   1. Car accidents
   2. Falls
   3. Gunshot wounds
   4. Stab wounds
   5. Diving into shallow water
   6. Infections
   7. Tumors
   8. Congenital anomalies

C. Pathophysiology
   1. Injury may result in complete transection of the spinal cord
   2. Associated edema and hemorrhage from the injury cause ischemia
   3. Necrosis and scar tissue form in the area of the traumatized cord
   4. Injury may result in paraplegia or quadriplegia

D. Possible clinical manifestations
   1. Paralysis below the level of the injury
   2. Paresthesia below the level of the injury
   3. Neck pain
   4. Loss of bowel and bladder control
   5. Respiratory distress
   6. Numbness and tingling
   7. Flaccid muscle
   8. Absence of reflexes below the level of the injury

E. Possible diagnostic test findings
   1. Spinal X-rays: vertebral fracture
   2. CT scan: spinal cord edema, vertebral fracture, spinal cord compression
   3. MRI: spinal cord edema, vertebral fracture, spinal cord compression

F. Medical management
   1. Diet: low-calcium, high-protein
   2. I.V. therapy: heparin lock
   3. Oxygen therapy
   4. Intubation and mechanical ventilation
   5. Gastrointestinal decompression: NG tube
   6. Position: flat
   7. Activity: bed rest, passive ROM exercises

8. Monitoring: VS, UO, I/O, ECG, ICP, and neurovital signs
9. Laboratory studies: sodium, potassium, glucose, and WBC
10. Foley catheter
11. Antacids: magnesium and aluminum hydroxide (Maalox), aluminum hydroxide gel (ALternaGEL)
12. Anticonvulsant: phenytoin (Dilantin)
13. Glucocorticoid: dexamethasone (Decadron)
14. Histamine antagonists: cimetidine (Tagamet), ranitidine (Zantac)
15. Cervical collar
16. Maintenance of vertebral alignment: Stryker turning frame, Crutchfield tongs, Halo brace
17. Laxative: bisacodyl (Dulcolax)
18. Antianxiety agent: diazepam (Valium)
19. Antihypertensives: diazoxide (Hyperstat), hydralazine (Apresoline)
20. Muscle relaxant: dantrolene sodium (Dantrium)
21. Pulse oximetry
22. Specialized bed: Rotation (Rotorest, Tilt and Turn, Paragon)
23. Mucosal barrier fortifier: sucralfate (Carafate)

G. Nursing interventions and responsibilities
1. Maintain the patient's diet
2. Force fluids
3. Administer I.V. fluids
4. Administer oxygen
5. Provide suction, TCDB
6. Assess neurologic and respiratory status
7. Keep the patient flat
8. Monitor and record VS, UO, I/O, laboratory studies, and pulse oximetry
9. Administer medications, as prescribed
10. Encourage the patient to express feelings about changes in body image, changes in sexual expression and function, altered mobility
11. Turn the patient every 2 hours using the logrolling technique
12. Maintain body alignment
13. Initiate bowel and bladder retraining
14. Provide sexual counseling
15. Provide passive ROM exercises
16. Check for autonomic dysreflexia
17. Assess for spinal shock
18. Provide skin care
19. Provide heel and elbow protectors and sheepskin
20. Apply antiembolism stockings
21. Provide information about the National Spinal Cord Injury Association

H. Teaching goals (instructions to the patient and family)
1. Keep follow-up appointments
2. Exercise regularly to strengthen muscles

3. Maintain a normal weight
4. Know the action, side effects, and scheduling of medications
5. Identify ways to reduce stress
6. Recognize the signs and symptoms of autonomic dysreflexia, urinary tract infection, and upper respiratory infection
7. Monitor self for infection
8. Follow dietary recommendations and restrictions
9. Promote a safe environment
10. Seek help from community agencies and resources
11. Continue bowel and bladder program
12. Maintain acidic urine with cranberry juice
13. Consume adequate fluids: 3,000 ml/day
14. Use assistive devices for ADLs
15. Maintain skin integrity
16. Stay mobile using a wheelchair
17. Reinforce independence

I. Possible medical complications
    1. Spinal shock
    2. Autonomic dysreflexia
    3. Respiratory distress

J. Possible surgical interventions
    1. Laminectomy (see page 60)
    2. Spinal fusion (see page 61)

Points to remember

Nervous system disorders can affect the patient's body image; control over body functions; self-esteem; fears of rejection, dependence, or dying.

Before the patient has a myelogram, the nurse should check the patient for allergies to iodine, seafood, and radiopaque dyes.

Typical nursing diagnoses for a patient with a nervous system disorder include powerlessness, changes in body image, and lowered self-esteem.

Nursing assessment for a patient who has had a craniotomy should focus on changes in the level of consciousness and on signs of increasing intracranial pressure.

Alternate methods of communication need to be established for a patients with myasthenia gravis.

Glossary

The following terms are defined in Appendix A, page 354.

ataxia

decerebration

neurovital signs

papilledema

ptosis

Study questions

To evaluate your understanding of this chapter, answer the following questions in the space provided; then compare your responses with the correct answers in Appendix B, page 359.

1. Which nursing interventions are appropriate after an LP? _____

_____

_____

2. What are two key nursing interventions after a patient's craniotomy?

_____

_____

3. What is the pathophysiology in MS? _____

_____

4. How does paralysis progress in Guillain-Barré syndrome? _____

_____

_____

5. When a patient has a seizure, which activities should the nurse observe and record? _____

_____

6. How are head injuries classified? _____

_____

7. What are the signs of CVA? _____

_____

8. Which clinical manifestations would be present in a patient with a cerebellar tumor? _____

_____

9. What are two key nursing interventions for a patient with spinal cord injury?

_____

_____

CHAPTER 4

Gastrointestinal System

Learning objectives

Check off the following items once you've mastered them:

☐ Describe the psychosocial impact of gastrointestinal disorders.

☐ Differentiate between modifiable and nonmodifiable risk factors in the development of a gastrointestinal disorder.

☐ List three probable and three possible nursing diagnoses for a patient with a gastrointestinal disorder.

☐ Identify the nursing interventions and responsibilities for a patient with any of the gastrointestinal disorders.

☐ Write three goals for teaching a patient with any of the gastrointestinal disorders.

I. Anatomy and physiology

A. Mouth
1. Mechanical and chemical digestion originate here
2. Tongue and teeth are accessory organs of digestion
3. Salivary glands secrete saliva, which combines with food during mastication

B. Esophagus
1. This organ provides for the transfer of food from the oropharynx to the stomach
2. The closure of the epiglottis prevents food from entering the trachea
3. Closure of the cardiac sphincter prevents reflux of gastric contents

C. Stomach
1. Is a hollow, one-liter muscular pouch
2. Secretes pepsin, renin, lipase, mucus, hydrochloric acid, and intrinsic factor for digestion
3. Mixes and stores chyme

D. Small intestine
1. Small intestine consists of duodenum, jejunum, and ileum
   a. Chyme, in liquid or semiliquid form, enters the duodenum through the pyloric sphincter
   b. Bile and pancreatic secretions enter the duodenum through the common bile duct at the ampulla of Vater
2. Small intestine digests food
3. Small intestine absorbs nutrients
4. Small intestine is lined with villi that contain capillaries and lymphatics
5. Motor activity of the small intestine includes mixing and peristalsis

E. Large intestine
1. Large intestine consists of the cecum, colon, rectum, and anus
2. Segments of the colon are the cecum, ascending colon, transverse colon, descending colon, and sigmoid colon
3. Chyme enters the cecum through the ileocecal valve
4. Large intestine has several functions
   a. Absorption of fluid and electrolytes
   b. Synthesis of vitamin K by intestinal bacteria
   c. Storage of fecal material
5. Chyme becomes more solid as water is absorbed through the intestinal wall of the colon
6. Defecation is the movement of feces from the rectum through the anal sphincter

F. Liver
1. Is the largest organ in the body

2. Produces bile (main function) which emulsifies fats and stimulates peristalsis
3. Conveys bile to the duodenum, where it enters at the sphincter of Oddi through the common bile duct
4. Metabolizes carbohydrates, fats, and proteins
5. Synthesizes coagulation factors VII, IX, X, and prothrombin
6. Stores vitamins A, D, B_{12}, and iron
7. Detoxifies chemicals
8. Excretes bilirubin
9. Obtains dual blood supply from portal vein and hepatic artery
10. Produces and stores glycogen
11. Promotes erythropoiesis when bone marrow production is insufficient

G. Gall bladder
1. Is a hollow, pear-shaped organ that stores bile
2. Secretes bile via the cystic duct to the common bile duct

H. Pancreas
1. Accessory gland of digestion
2. Exocrine function: secretes three digestive enzymes
   a. Amylase
   b. Lipase
   c. Trypsin
3. Endocrine function: secretes hormones from the islets of Langerhans
   a. Insulin
   b. Glucagon
   c. Somatostatin
4. Main pancreatic duct joins the common bile duct and empties into the duodenum at the ampulla of Vater

II. Physical assessment findings

A. Subjective data associated with gastrointestinal (GI) disorders
1. Inadequate diet
2. Change in bowel habits
   a. Constipation
   b. Diarrhea
   c. Flatus
3. Complaints of indigestion
4. Change in weight
5. Nausea and vomiting
6. Abdominal pain
7. Difficulty in swallowing
8. Loss of appetite

B. Objective data associated with GI disorders
1. DYSPHAGIA
2. Abnormal color and consistency of stool

      a. MELENA
      b. Clay
      c. Frothy
      d. STEATORRHEA
      e. Occult blood in stool
   3. Abnormal bowel sounds
   4. Abdominal distention
   5. Rectal bleeding
   6. Jaundice
   7. Edema
   8. HEMATEMESIS
   9. Anorexia

III. Diagnostic tests and procedures

A. Upper GI series
   1. Definition and purpose
      a. Fluoroscopic procedure using barium as a contrast medium
      b. Examination of the esophagus, stomach, duodenum, and other
        portions of the small bowel after swallowing barium
   2. Nursing interventions and responsibilities before the procedure
      a. Withhold food and fluids
      b. Administer fluids, cathartics, and enemas, as prescribed
   3. Nursing interventions and responsibilities after the procedure
      a. Inform the patient that stool will be light-colored for several days
      b. Administer cathartics, fluids, and enemas, as prescribed

B. Lower GI series (barium enema)
   1. Definition and purpose
      a. Fluoroscopic procedure using barium as a contrast medium
      b. Examination of the large intestine after administration of barium
        via an enema
   2. Nursing interventions and responsibilities before the procedure
      a. Withhold food and fluids
      b. Encourage the patient to discuss feelings of embarrassment
      c. Administer bowel preparation (laxatives and enemas), as prescribed
   3. Nursing interventions and responsibilities after the procedure
      a. Determine if the patient is constipated
      b. Force fluids unless contraindicated
      c. Administer enemas and laxatives, as prescribed

C. Endoscopy
   1. Definition and purpose
      a. Procedure using an endoscope
      b. Direct visualization of the esophagus and stomach
   2. Nursing interventions and responsibilities before the procedure
      a. Withhold food and fluids

      b. Obtain written, informed consent
      c. Obtain baseline vital signs (VS)
      d. Administer sedatives, as prescribed
   3. Nursing interventions and responsibilities after the procedure
      a. Withhold food and fluids until the gag reflex returns
      b. Assess gag and cough reflexes
      c. Assess vasovagal response

D. Fecal occult blood test
   1. Definition and purpose
      a. Laboratory test using a reagent
      b. Analysis of stool for blood
   2. Nursing interventions and responsibilities before the procedure
      a. Advise the patient to avoid red meat, iron, and high fiber for 1 to 3 days
      b. Document the adminstration of aspirin, vitamin C, and anti-inflammatory drugs

E. Fecal fat
   1. Definition and purpose
      a. Laboratory test using a stain
      b. Analysis of stool for fat
   2. Nursing interventions and responsibilities before the procedure
      a. Advise the patient to restrict alcohol intake and maintain a high-fat diet 72 hours before the exam
      b. Refrigerate specimen
      c. Document current medications

F. Proctosigmoidoscopy
   1. Definition and purpose
      a. Procedure using a lighted scope
      b. Direct visualization of the sigmoid colon, rectum, and anal canal
   2. Nursing interventions and responsibilities before the procedure
      a. Encourage the patient to discuss feelings of embarrassment
      b. Inform the patient that the procedure requires a knee-chest position
      c. Administer bowel preparation, as prescribed
      d. Obtain written, informed consent
      e. Document iron intake
   3. Nursing interventions and responsibilities after the procedure
      a. Check the patient for bleeding
      b. Monitor the patient's VS

G. Barium swallow
   1. Definition and purpose
      a. Procedure using barium as a contrast medium
      b. Fluoroscopic examination of the pharynx and esophagus after administration of barium

   2. Nursing interventions and responsibilities before the procedure
      a. Withhold food and fluids
      b. Explain the procedure to the patient
   3. Nursing interventions and responsibilities after the procedure
      a. Determine if the patient is constipated
      b. Force fluids unless contraindicated
      c. Administer laxatives, as prescribed

H. Cholangiography
   1. Definition and purpose
      a. Procedure using an injection of a radiopaque dye through a
         catheter
      b. Radiographic examination of the biliary duct system
   2. Nursing interventions and responsibilities before the procedure
      a. Encourage a low-residue, high-simple fat diet 1 day before the exam
      b. Withhold food and fluid after midnight
      c. Note the patient's allergies to iodine, seafood, and radiopaque dyes
      d. Inform the patient about possible throat irritation and flushing of
         the face
   3. Nursing interventions and responsibilities after the procedure
      a. Check the injection site for bleeding
      b. Monitor VS

I. Liver scan
   1. Definition and purpose
      a. Procedure using an I.V. injection of a radioisotope
      b. Visual imaging of the distribution of blood flow in the liver
   2. Nursing interventions and responsibilities before the procedure
      a. Determine the patient's ability to lie still during the procedure
      b. Check the patient for possible allergies
   3. Nursing interventions and responsibilities after the procedure
      a. Assess the I.V. insertion site for bleeding, bruising, or hematoma
      b. Assess the patient for signs of delayed allergic reaction to the
         radioisotope, such as itching and hives

J. Gastric analysis
   1. Definition and purpose
      a. Procedure that aspirates the contents of the stomach through a
         nasogastric (NG) tube
      b. Fasting analysis to measure the acidity of gastric secretions
   2. Nursing interventions and responsibilities before the procedure
      a. Withhold food and fluids after midnight
      b. Instruct the patient not to smoke for 8 to 12 hours before the test
      c. Withhold medications that can affect gastric secretions for 24 hours
         before the procedure
   3. Nursing interventions and responsibilities after the procedure
      a. Obtain VS

       b. Note reactions to gastric acid stimulant, if used

K. Ultrasonography
  1. Definition and purpose
    a. Noninvasive procedure examination that uses echoes from sound waves
    b. Visualization of body organs
  2. Nursing interventions and responsibilities before the procedure
    a. Withhold food and fluids for 8 to 12 hours
    b. Determine the patient's ability to lie still during the procedure
    c. Ask the patient not to smoke or chew gum for 8 to 12 hours before the test
    d. Administer enemas, as prescribed
    e. Remove abdominal dressings

L. Blood chemistry
  1. Definition and purpose
    a. Laboratory test of a blood sample
    b. Analysis for potassium, sodium, calcium, phosphorus, glucose, bicarbonate, blood urea nitrogen (BUN), creatinine, protein, albumin, osmolality, amylase, lipase, alkaline phosphatase, ammonia, bilirubin, lactic dehydrogenase (LDH), bromsulphalein (BSP) test, serum aspartate aminotransferase (AST, formerly serum glutamic oxaloacetic transaminase [SGOT]), serum alanine aminotransferase (ALT, formerly serum glutamic pyruvic transaminase [SGPT]), hepatitis-associated antigens, carcinoembryonic antigen (CEA), and alpha-fetoprotein (AFP)
  2. Nursing interventions and responsibilities
    a. Withhold food and fluid, as directed, before the procedure
    b. Check the site for bleeding after the procedure

M. Hematologic studies
  1. Definition and purpose
    a. Laboratory test of a blood sample
    b. Analysis for red blood cells (RBCs), white blood cells (WBCs), platelets, prothrombin time (PT), partial thromboplastin time (PTT), hemoglobin (Hgb), hematocrit (Hct)
  2. Nursing interventions and responsibilities
    a. Note current drug therapy before the procedure
    b. Check the site for bleeding after the procedure

N. Liver biopsy
  1. Definition and purpose
    a. Procedure using a needle for the percutaneous removal of a small amount of liver tissue
    b. Histologic evaluation of liver tissue
  2. Nursing interventions and responsibilities before the procedure
    a. Withhold food and fluids after midnight

　　b. Obtain written, informed consent
　　c. Assess baseline clotting studies and VS
　3. Nursing interventions and responsibilities after the procedure
　　a. Check the insertion site for bleeding
　　b. Monitor VS
　　c. Observe the patient for signs of shock and pneumothorax

IV. Psychosocial impact of GI disorders

A. Developmental impact
　1. Changes in body image
　2. Feeling of lack of control over body function
　3. Fear of rejection
　4. Embarrassment from changes in body function and structure
　5. Decreased self-esteem

B. Economic impact
　1. Disruption of employment
　2. Cost of special diet
　3. Cost of special diversion appliances
　4. Cost of medications

C. Occupational and recreational impact
　1. Change of occupation
　2. Changes in leisure activity
　3. Restrictions in physical activity

D. Social impact
　1. Changes in eating patterns and modes
　2. Changes in elimination patterns and modes
　3. Social withdrawal and isolation
　4. Changes in sexual function

V. Risk factors for developing GI disorders

A. Modifiable risk factors
　1. Diet: low-fiber
　2. Smoking
　3. Alcohol consumption
　4. Inactivity
　5. Stress
　6. Contaminated water and food
　7. Anger, fear, or anxiety

B. Nonmodifiable risk factors
　1. Family history of GI disorders
　2. History of previous GI dysfunction
　3. Culturally based reluctance to discuss personal hygiene and health
　　habits

VI. Nursing diagnostic categories for a patient with a GI disorder

A. Probable nursing diagnostic categories
   1. Constipation
   2. Diarrhea
   3. Pain
   4. Altered nutrition: less than body requirements
   5. Fluid volume deficit

B. Possible nursing diagnostic categories
   1. Body image disturbance
   2. Self-esteem disturbance
   3. Impaired skin integrity
   4. Noncompliance
   5. Knowledge deficit
   6. Anxiety
   7. Sexual dysfunction

VII. Gall bladder and pancreatic surgeries

A. Definition
   1. Cholecystostomy: surgical incision into the gallbladder to drain bile
   2. Choledochotomy: surgical incision into the common bile duct to remove stones
   3. Cholecystotomy: surgical incision into the gallbladder to remove gallstones
   4. Choledochostomy: surgical opening of the common bile duct to insert a T tube or catheter for drainage
   5. Cholecystectomy: surgical removal of the gallbladder
   6. Pancreatectomy: surgical removal of part or all of the pancreas

B. Preoperative nursing interventions and responsibilities
   1. Complete patient and family preoperative teaching
      a. Determine the patient's understanding of the procedure
      b. Describe the operating room (OR), postanesthesia care unit (PACU), and preoperative and postoperative routines
      c. Demonstrate postoperative turning, coughing, and deep breathing (TCDB), splinting, leg exercises, and range-of-motion (ROM) exercises
      d. Explain the postoperative need for drainage tubes, surgical dressings, oxygen therapy, I.V. therapy, and pain control
   2. Complete a preoperative checklist
   3. Administer preoperative medications, as prescribed
   4. Allay the patient's and family's anxiety about surgery
   5. Document the patient's history and physical assessment data base

C. Postoperative nursing interventions and responsibilities
   1. Check respiratory status and fluid balance

2. Assess pain and administer postoperative analgesics, as prescribed
3. Assess for return of peristalsis; give solid foods and liquids, as tolerated
4. Administer I.V. fluids and transfusion therapy, as prescribed
5. Allay the patient's anxiety
6. Inspect the surgical dressing and change, as directed
7. Reinforce TCDB and splinting of incision
8. Keep the patient in semi-Fowler's position
9. Provide incentive spirometry
10. Maintain activity, as tolerated
11. Monitor VS, urine output (UO), intake and output (I/O), and laboratory studies
12. Monitor and maintain position and patency of drainage tubes: NG, wound drainage, T tube
13. Administer antibiotics, as prescribed
14. Provide care for pancreatic surgery
    a. Monitor urine glucose
    b. Monitor ketones

D. Possible surgical complications
    1. Pneumonia
    2. Atelectasis
    3. Peritonitis
    4. Hemorrhage

E. Postoperative teaching goals (instructions to the patient and family)
    1. Keep follow-up appointments
    2. Exercise regularly
    3. Stop smoking
    4. Maintain a normal weight
    5. Know the action, side effects, and scheduling of medications
    6. Recognize the signs and symptoms of infection
    7. Avoid lifting for 6 weeks
    8. Complete incision care daily
    9. Continue care of the T tube
    10. Adhere to a low-fat diet for 6 weeks
    11. Follow instructions specific to gall bladder surgeries
        a. Monitor and report color of stool
        b. Monitor and report amount and consistency of stool
    12. Follow instructions specific to pancreatic surgery
        a. Monitor urine glucose and ketones
        b. Recognize the signs of hyperglycemia

VIII. Portal-systemic shunts

A. Definition
  1. Portacaval shunt: surgical anastomosis of the portal vein to the inferior vena cava to divert blood from the portal system to decrease pressure
  2. Splenorenal shunt: surgical anastomosis of the splenic vein to the left renal vein to divert blood from the portal system to decrease pressure
  3. Mesocaval shunt: surgical anastomosis of the inferior vena cava to the side of the superior mesenteric vein to divert blood from the portal system to decrease pressure

B. Preoperative nursing interventions and responsibilities
  1. Complete patient and family preoperative teaching
     a. Determine the patient's understanding of the procedure
     b. Describe the OR, PACU, and preoperative and postoperative routines; demonstrate postoperative TCDB, splinting, and leg and ROM exercises
     c. Explain the postoperative need for drainage tubes, surgical dressings, oxygen therapy, I.V. therapy, and pain control
  2. Complete a preoperative checklist
  3. Administer preoperative medications, as prescribed
  4. Allay the patient's and family's anxiety about surgery
  5. Document the patient's history and physical assessment data base
  6. Administer antibiotics, as prescribed
  7. Administer vitamin K, as prescribed
  8. Administer I.V. and transfusion therapy, as prescribed
  9. Administer lactulose, as prescribed
  10. Maintain patency of NG tube
  11. Monitor central venous pressure (CVP)

C. Postoperative nursing interventions and responsibilities
  1. Assess cardiac, respiratory, and neurologic status and fluid balance
  2. Assess pain and administer postoperative analgesics, as prescribed
  3. Administer I.V. fluids, total parental nutrition (TPN), and transfusion therapy, as prescribed
  4. Allay the patient's anxiety
  5. Inspect the surgical dressing
  6. Reinforce TCDB and splinting of the incision
  7. Keep the patient in semi-Fowler's position
  8. Assess for return of peristalsis
  9. Provide suction
  10. Maintain activity: bed rest; active and passive ROM and isometric exercises
  11. Administer oxygen and maintain endotracheal tube to ventilator
  12. Monitor VS, UO, I/O, CVP, laboratory studies, ECG, neurovital signs, and pulse oximetry

13. Monitor and maintain position and patency of drainage tubes: NG, Foley, wound drainage
14. Allay the patient's anxiety
15. Measure and record the patient's abdominal girth
16. Monitor stool and NG drainage for occult blood
17. Monitor for hemorrhage
18. Check for peripheral edema
19. Provide skin, nares, and mouth care
20. Reorient frequently
21. Administer antibiotics, as prescribed
22. Administer vitamin K, as prescribed
23. Elevate extremities

D. Possible surgical complications
    1. Acute hepatic failure
    2. Chronic portal systemic encephalopathy
    3. Coagulopathy
    4. Shunt malfunction

E. Postoperative teaching goals (instructions to the patient and family)
    1. Keep follow-up appointments
    2. Exercise regularly
    3. Stop smoking
    4. Maintain a normal weight
    5. Know the action, side effects, and scheduling of medications
    6. Recognize the signs and symptoms of infection
    7. Adhere to activity limitations
    8. Complete incision care daily
    9. Avoid using alcohol
    10. Adhere indefinitely to a protein-restricted diet
    11. Avoid using over-the-counter medications

IX. Gastric surgery

A. Definition
    1. Vagotomy: surgical ligation of the vagus nerve to decrease the secretion of gastric acid
    2. Antrectomy: surgical removal of the antrum of the stomach
    3. Pyloroplasty: surgical dilatation of the pyloric sphincter to increase the rate of gastric emptying
    4. Gastroduodenostomy (Bilroth I): surgical removal of the lower portion of the stomach with anastomosis of the remaining portion of the stomach to the duodenum
    5. Gastrojejunostomy (Bilroth II): surgical removal of the antrum and distal portion of the stomach and duodenum with anastomosis of the stomach to the jejunum
    6. Subtotal gastrectomy: surgical removal of 60% to 80% of the stomach

7. Esophagojejunostomy (total gastrectomy): surgical removal of the entire stomach with a loop of the jejunum anastomosed to the esophagus

B. Preoperative nursing interventions and responsibilities
  1. Complete patient and family preoperative teaching
    a. Determine the patient's understanding of the procedure
    b. Describe the OR, PACU, and preoperative and postoperative routines
    c. Demonstrate postoperative TCDB, splinting, and leg and ROM exercises
    d. Explain the postoperative need for drainage tubes, surgical dressings, oxygen therapy, I.V. therapy, and pain control
  2. Complete a preoperative checklist
  3. Administer preoperative medications, as prescribed
  4. Allay the patient's and family's anxiety about surgery
  5. Document the patient's history and physical assessment data base
  6. Administer bowel preparation, as prescribed

C. Postoperative nursing interventions and responsibilities
  1. Assess respiratory status and fluid balance
  2. Assess pain and administer postoperative analgesics, as prescribed
  3. Administer I.V. fluids, NG tube feedings, and transfusion therapy, as prescribed
  4. Allay the patient's anxiety
  5. Inspect the surgical dressing and change, as directed
  6. Reinforce TCDB and splinting of incision
  7. Keep the patient in semi-Fowler's position
  8. Apply antiembolism or pneumatic stockings
  9. Assess for return of peristalsis
  10. Provide incentive spirometry
  11. Maintain activity, as tolerated
  12. Administer oxygen
  13. Monitor VS, UO, I/O, laboratory studies, and pulse oximetry
  14. Monitor and maintain position and patency of drainage tubes: NG, Foley, wound drainage
  15. Monitor NG drainage for overt bleeding
  16. Irrigate NG tube gently; do not reposition NG tube
  17. Weigh the patient daily
  18. Monitor gastric pH

D. Possible surgical complications
  1. Dumping syndrome after a partial gastrectomy
  2. Hemorrhage
  3. Dehydration
  4. Infection
  5. Dehiscence

E. Postoperative teaching goals (instructions to the patient and family)
  1. Keep follow-up appointments

2. Exercise regularly
3. Stop smoking
4. Maintain a normal weight
5. Know the action, side effects, and scheduling of medications
6. Recognize the signs and symptoms of infection and dehydration
7. Complete incision care daily
8. Identify ways to reduce stress
9. Maintain a normal weight
10. Increase food intake gradually
11. Eat six small meals a day
12. Limit fluids with meals

X. Hemorrhoidectomy

A. Definition — surgical removal of hemorrhoids by clamp, excision, or cautery

B. Preoperative nursing interventions and responsibilities
   1. Complete patient and family preoperative teaching
      a. Determine the patient's understanding of the procedure
      b. Describe the OR, PACU, and preoperative and postoperative routines; demonstrate postoperative TCDB, splinting, and leg and ROM exercises
      c. Explain the postoperative need for drainage tubes, surgical dressings, oxygen therapy, I.V. therapy, and pain control
   2. Complete a preoperative checklist
   3. Administer preoperative medications, as prescribed
   4. Allay the patient's and family's anxiety about surgery
   5. Document the patient's history and physical assessment data base
   6. Administer bowel preparation, as prescribed
      a. Cleansing enemas
      b. Laxatives

C. Postoperative nursing interventions and responsibilities
   1. Assess pain and administer postoperative analgesics, as prescribed
   2. Assess for return of peristalsis; give solid foods and liquids, as tolerated
   3. Administer I.V. fluids
   4. Allay the patient's anxiety
   5. Inspect the surgical dressing and remove anal packing, as directed
   6. Reinforce TCDB
   7. Keep the patient prone or on the side
   8. Provide incentive spirometry
   9. Maintain activity: as tolerated
   10. Monitor VS, UO, I/O, and laboratory studies
   11. Encourage the patient to discuss feelings of embarrassment and fear of defecation
   12. Administer analgesics, as prescribed, before the first bowel movement

13. Provide sitz baths
14. Provide a flotation pad when sitting
15. Administer stool softeners, as prescribed

D. Possible surgical complications
1. Rectal hemorrhage
2. Urine retention

E. Postoperative teaching goals (instructions to the patient and family)
1. Keep follow-up appointments
2. Exercise regularly
3. Maintain a normal weight
4. Know the action, side effects, and scheduling of medications
5. Recognize the signs and symptoms of bleeding and infection
6. Avoid heavy lifting and prolonged standing or sitting
7. Avoid constipation
8. Defecate when urge is felt
9. Provide perineal care daily
10. Anticipate a small amount of bleeding postoperatively with bowel movements
11. Increase fluid intake
12. Follow dietary recommendations and restrictions
13. Avoid Valsalva's maneuver

XI. Bowel surgery

A. Definition
1. Abdominoperineal resection: removal of distal sigmoid colon, rectum, and anus with the creation of a permanent colostomy
2. Colectomy: surgical excision of the right colon (right hemicolectomy) or left colon (left hemicolectomy)
3. Ileostomy: surgical opening of the ileum to the abdominal surface to form a stoma
4. Continent ileostomy (Koch's pouch): surgical creation of an intraabdominal reservoir for stool
5. Bowel resection: surgical excision of a portion of the bowel
6. Permanent colostomy: surgical opening of the colon to the abdominal surface to form a single stoma after the distal portion of the bowel is removed
7. Double-barrel colostomy: surgical opening of the colon to the abdominal surface to form two stomas to prevent passage of stool into the distal bowel

B. Preoperative nursing interventions and responsibilities
1. Complete patient and family preoperative teaching
   a. Determine the patient's understanding of the procedure

       b. Describe the OR, PACU, and preoperative and postoperative routines; demonstrate postoperative TCDB, splinting, and leg and ROM exercises

       c. Explain the postoperative need for drainage tubes, gastrostomy feeding tube, surgical dressings, oxygen therapy, I.V. therapy, and pain control

2. Complete a preoperative checklist
3. Administer preoperative medications, as prescribed
4. Allay the patient's and family's anxiety about surgery
5. Document the patient's history and physical assessment data base
6. Administer bowel preparation, as prescribed
   a. Antibiotics
   b. Cleansing enemas
7. Arrange a preoperative visit with an enterostomal therapist
8. Encourage the patient to express feelings about changes in body image

C. Postoperative nursing interventions and responsibilities
1. Assess cardiac status and fluid balance
2. Assess pain and administer postoperative analgesics, as prescribed
3. Assess for return of peristalsis; give solid foods and liquids, as tolerated
4. Administer I.V. fluids, TPN, and transfusion therapy, as prescribed
5. Allay the patient's anxiety
6. Inspect the surgical dressing and change, as directed
7. Reinforce TCDB and splinting of incision
8. Keep the patient in semi-Fowler's position
9. Provide incentive spirometry
10. Maintain activity, as tolerated
11. Apply antiembolism or pneumatic stockings
12. Monitor VS, UO, I/O, laboratory studies, and pulse oximetry
13. Monitor and maintain position and patency of drainage tubes: NG, Foley, wound drainage
14. Encourage the patient to express feelings about changes in body image
15. Monitor and record the color, consistency, and amount of the patient's stool
16. Provide routine colostomy care
   a. Prevent skin breakdown by thorough cleaning of skin around the stoma
   b. Check stoma
   c. Control odor
   d. Change ostomy bag as needed
   e. Irrigate
17. Increase fluid intake to 3,000 ml/day

D. Possible surgical complications
1. Infection
2. Hemorrhage

3. Dehiscence
4. Evisceration
5. Paralytic ileus
6. Prolapsed stoma
7. Abscess

E. Postoperative teaching goals (instructions to the patient and family)
1. Keep follow-up appointments
2. Exercise regularly
3. Stop smoking
4. Maintain a normal weight
5. Know the action, side effects, and scheduling of medications
6. Recognize the signs and symptoms of infection and intestinal obstruction
7. Adhere to activity limitations
8. Complete incision care daily
9. Use ostomy bags
10. Check the condition of the stoma daily and report bleeding and changes
11. Report changes in the color and consistency of stools
12. Perform colostomy care daily
13. Identify foods that cause flatus and irritability of the colon
14. Discuss concerns about sexual activities

XII. Hiatal hernia (esophageal hernia)

A. Definition — protrusion of the stomach through the diaphragm into the thoracic cavity

B. Possible etiology
1. Congenital weakness
2. Obesity
3. Pregnancy
4. Trauma
5. Increased abdominal pressure
6. Aging

C. Pathophysiology
1. The opening (hiatus) in the diaphragm where the esophagus enters the stomach becomes enlarged and weakened
2. The upper portion of the stomach enters the lower thorax
3. Sliding of the esophagus and stomach into the chest results in reflux of gastric acid

D. Possible clinical manifestations
1. Pyrosis
2. Dysphagia
3. Regurgitation

   4. Sternal pain after eating
   5. Vomiting
   6. Feeling of fullness
   7. Dyspnea
   8. Cough
   9. Tachycardia

E. Possible diagnostic test findings
   1. Esophagoscopy: incompetent cardiac sphincter
   2. Barium swallow: protrusion of the hernia
   3. Chest X-ray: protrusion of abdominal organs into thorax
   4. Gastric analysis: increased pH

F. Medical management
   1. Diet: bland diet with decreased intake of caffeine and spicy foods
   2. Oxygen therapy
   3. GI decompression: NG tube
   4. Position: semi-Fowler's
   5. Activity: as tolerated
   6. Monitoring: VS, UO, and I/O
   7. Anticholinergic: propantheline bromide (Pro-Banthine)
   8. Antacids: magnesium and aluminum hydroxide (Maalox), aluminum hydroxide gel (ALternaGEL)
   9. Histamine antagonists: cimetidine (Tagamet), ranitidine (Zantac)
  10. Weight loss

G. Nursing interventions and responsibilities
   1. Maintain the patient's diet
   2. Administer oxygen
   3. Assess respiratory status
   4. Maintain position, patency, and low suction of NG tube
   5. Keep the patient in semi-Fowler's position
   6. Monitor and record VS, UO, I/O, and daily weight
   7. Administer medications, as prescribed
   8. Allay the patient's anxiety
   9. Avoid flexion at the waist in positioning the patient

H. Teaching goals (instructions to the patient and family)
   1. Keep follow-up appointments
   2. Exercise regularly
   3. Stop smoking
   4. Maintain a normal weight
   5. Know the action, side effects, and scheduling of medications
   6. Follow dietary recommendations and restrictions
   7. Eat small, frequent meals
   8. Stop drinking carbonated beverages and alcohol
   9. Stay upright for 2 hours after eating
  10. Avoid wearing constrictive clothing

11. Avoid lifting, bending, straining, and coughing

I. Possible medical complications
    1. Hemorrhage
    2. Ulceration
    3. Aspiration
    4. Incarceration of stomach in chest

J. Possible surgical interventions
    1. Reduction of hiatal hernia
    2. Fundoplication

XIII. Gastric ulcer (peptic ulcer)

A. Definition—erosion of mucosal lining of the stomach

B. Possible etiology
    1. Alcohol abuse
    2. Stress
    3. Drug-induced: salicylates, steroids, indomethacin, reserpine
    4. Smoking
    5. Gastritis
    6. Zollinger-Ellison syndrome

C. Pathophysiology
    1. Increased emptying time of gastric acid from the gastric lumen into the gastric mucosa causes an inflammatory reaction with tissue breakdown
    2. Bile refluxes into the stomach if the pyloric valve is involved
    3. Combination of hydrochloric acid and pepsin destroys gastric mucosa

D. Possible clinical manifestations
    1. Left epigastric pain 1 to 2 hours after eating
    2. Weight loss
    3. Nausea and vomiting
    4. Hematemesis
    5. Melena
    6. Anorexia
    7. Relief of pain after administration of antacids

E. Possible diagnostic test findings
    1. Hematology: decreased Hgb, Hct, PT, PTT
    2. Blood chemistry: increased sodium
    3. Gastric analysis: normal for gastric ulcer
    4. Upper GI: location of ulcer
    5. Barium swallow: ulceration of gastric mucosa
    6. Fecal occult blood: positive
    7. Serum gastrin: normal or increased

F. Medical management
   1. Diet: low-fiber in small, frequent feedings
   2. GI decompression: NG tube
   3. Position: semi-Fowler's
   4. Activity: bed rest
   5. Monitoring: VS, UO, and I/O
   6. Laboratory studies: Hgb, Hct
   7. Treatments: saline lavage by NG tube
   8. Transfusion therapy: packed RBCs
   9. Anticholinergics: propantheline bromide (Pro-Banthine), dicyclomine hydrochloride (Bentyl)
  10. Antacids: magnesium and aluminum hydroxide (Maalox), aluminum hydroxide gel (ALternaGEL)
  11. Histamine antagonists: cimetidine (Tagamet), ranitidine (Zantac), nizatidine (Axid)
  12. Prostaglandin: misoprostol (Cytotec)
  13. Mucosal barrier fortifier: sucralfate (Carafate)
  14. Endoscopic laser
  15. Photocoagulation
  16. Hormone: vasopressin (Pitressin)

G. Nursing interventions and responsibilities
   1. Maintain the patient's diet with small frequent feedings
   2. Assess respiratory and cardiovascular status
   3. Maintain position, patency, and low suction of NG tube if gastric decompression is ordered
   4. Keep the patient in semi-Fowler's position
   5. Monitor and record VS, UO, I/O, laboratory studies, fecal occult blood, and gastric pH
   6. Administer medications, as prescribed
   7. Allay the patient's anxiety
   8. Provide nares and mouth care
   9. Minimize environmental stress
  10. Maintain a quiet environment
  11. Irrigate the NG tube
  12. Monitor the consistency, color, amount, and frequency of stools

H. Teaching goals (instructions to the patient and family)
   1. Keep follow-up appointments
   2. Exercise regularly
   3. Stop smoking
   4. Maintain a normal weight
   5. Know the action, side effects, and scheduling of medications
   6. Identify ways to reduce stress
   7. Follow dietary recommendations and restrictions; avoid caffeine, alcohol, and spicy and fried foods
   8. Maintain a quiet environment

I. Possible medical complications
    1. Hemorrhage
    2. Perforation
    3. Chemical peritonitis
    4. Intestinal obstruction

J. Possible surgical interventions
    1. Bilroth I (see page 137)
    2. Bilroth II (see page 137)
    3. Pyloroplasty and vagotomy (see page 137)

XIV. Gastric cancer

A. Definition—malignant stomach tumor that is primary or metastatic

B. Possible etiology
    1. High intake of salted and smoked foods
    2. Low intake of vegetables and fruits
    3. Chronic gastritis
    4. Achlorhydria
    5. Pernicious anemia
    6. Gastric ulcer

C. Pathophysiology
    1. Unregulated cell growth and uncontrolled cell division result in the development of a neoplasm
    2. Tumor usually develops in the distal third of stomach and metastasizes to the abdominal organs, lungs, and bones
    3. Most common neoplasm is adenocarcinoma

D. Possible clinical manifestations
    1. Fatigue
    2. Weakness
    3. Syncope
    4. Shortness of breath
    5. Nausea and vomiting
    6. Weight loss
    7. Hematemesis
    8. Indigestion
    9. Epigastric fullness and pain
    10. Malaise
    11. Melena
    12. Regurgitation
    13. Anorexia

E. Possible diagnostic test findings
    1. Fecal occult blood: positive
    2. CEA: positive
    3. Hematology: decreased Hgb, Hct

4. Blood chemistry: increased AST, LDH, and amylase
5. Gastric analysis: positive cancer cells, achlorhydria
6. GI series: gastric mass
7. Gastroscopy: biopsy positive for cancer cells

F. Medical management
1. Diet: high-protein, high-calorie, high-fat, and low-carbohydrate
2. I.V. therapy: heparin lock
3. GI decompression: NG tube
4. Position: semi-Fowler's
5. Activity: as tolerated
6. Monitoring: VS, UO, and I/O
7. Laboratory studies: Hgb, Hct, and fecal occult blood
8. Nutritional support: TPN
9. Radiation therapy
10. Antineoplastics: carmustine (BiCNU), 5-fluorouracil (Adrucil)
11. Vitamin supplements: folic acid (Folvite), cyanocobalamin (vitamin B_{12})
12. Chemotherapy
13. Analgesics: meperidine (Demerol), morphine sulfate (Roxanol)
14. Antiemetic: nabilone (Cesamet)

G. Nursing interventions and responsibilities
1. Maintain the patient's diet
2. Assess GI status
3. Maintain position, patency, and low suction of NG tube
4. Keep the patient in semi-Fowler's position
5. Monitor and record VS, UO, I/O, laboratory studies, and daily weight
6. Administer TPN
7. Administer medications, as prescribed
8. Encourage the patient to express feelings about a fear of dying
9. Provide skin and mouth care
10. Provide rest periods
11. Monitor the consistency, amount, and frequency of stool
12. Monitor the color of stool for blood
13. Provide postchemotherapeutic and postradiation nursing care
    a. Provide skin, mouth, and perineal care
    b. Encourage dietary intake
    c. Administer antiemetics and antidiarrheals, as prescribed
    d. Monitor for bleeding, infection, and electrolyte imbalance
    e. Provide rest periods
14. Provide information about the American Cancer Society

H. Teaching goals (instructions to the patient and family)
1. Keep follow-up appointments
2. Maintain a normal weight
3. Know the action, side effects, and scheduling of medications

    4. Recognize the signs and symptoms of infection and ulceration
    5. Avoid exposure to people with infections
    6. Alternate rest periods with activity
    7. Monitor self for infection
    8. Follow dietary recommendations and restrictions
    9. Seek help from community agencies and resources
  10. Complete skin care daily

I. Possible medical complications
    1. Obstruction
    2. Ulceration
    3. Metastasis

J. Possible surgical interventions
    1. Subtotal gastrectomy (see page 137)
    2. Total gastrectomy (see page 138)
    3. Bilroth I (see page 137)
    4. Bilroth II (see page 137)

XV. Ulcerative colitis

A. Definition – inflammatory disorder of the large bowel

B. Possible etiology
    1. Emotional stress
    2. Autoimmune disease
    3. Genetics
    4. Idiopathic cause
    5. Allergies
    6. Viral and bacterial infections

C. Pathophysiology
    1. Inflammatory edema of the mucous membrane of the colon and rectum leads to bleeding and shallow ulcerations
    2. Abscess formation causes bowel-wall shortening, thinning, fragility, hypermotility, and decreased absorption
    3. Mucosal ulcerations begin in the distal end of the colon and ascend the large intestine

D. Possible clinical manifestations
    1. Abdominal tenderness
    2. Weakness
    3. Debilitation
    4. Anorexia
    5. Nausea and vomiting
    6. Dehydration
    7. Bloody, purulent, mucoid, watery stools (15 to 20/day)
    8. Elevated temperature
    9. Cachexia

10. Weight loss
11. Abdominal cramping
12. Tenesmus
13. Hyperactive bowel sounds
14. Abdominal distention

E. Possible diagnostic test findings
  1. Sigmoidoscopy: ulceration and hyperemia
  2. Barium enema: ulcerations
  3. Blood chemistry: decreased potassium; increased osmolality
  4. Hematology: decreased Hgb, Hct
  5. Urine chemistry: increased specific gravity
  6. Stool specimen: positive for blood and mucus

F. Medical management
  1. Diet: two types
     a. High-protein, high-calorie, low-residue; bland foods in small, frequent feedings with restricted intake of milk and gas-forming foods
     b. No food and fluids
  2. I.V. therapy: hydration, electrolyte replacement, and heparin lock
  3. GI decompession: NG tube
  4. Position: semi-Fowler's
  5. Activity: bed rest with bedside commode
  6. Monitoring: VS, UO, I/O, daily weight, specific gravity, calorie count, and stools for occult blood
  7. Laboratory studies: potassium, Hgb, Hct, and osmolality
  8. Nutritional support: TPN
  9. Treatments: Foley catheter, sitz baths
  10. Antibiotic: sulfasalazine (Azulfidine)
  11. Analgesic: meperidine hydrochloride (Demerol)
  12. Sedative: phenobarbital (Luminal)
  13. Anticholinergic: propantheline bromide (Pro-Banthine), dicyclomine hydrochloride (Bentyl)
  14. Antacids: magnesium and aluminum hydroxide (Maalox), aluminum hydroxide gel (ALternaGEL)
  15. Corticosteroid: hydrocortisone (Solu-Cortef)
  16. Antiemetic: prochlorperazine (Compazine)
  17. Antidiarrheals: diphenoxylate (Lomotil), loperamide (Imodium)
  18. Transfusion therapy: packed RBCs
  19. Antianemics: ferrous sulfate (Feosol), ferrous gluconate (Fergon)
  20. Immunosuppressive agents: azathioprine (Imuran), cyclophosphamide (Cytoxan)
  21. Vitamins and minerals
  22. Tranquilizers: diazepam (Valium)
  23. Potassium supplement: potassium chloride (K-Lor), potassium gluconate (Kaon)

24. Anti-inflammatory: olsalazine sodium (Dipentum)

G. Nursing interventions and responsibilities
1. Maintain the patient's diet; withhold food and fluids as necessary
2. Administer I.V. fluids
3. Assess GI status and fluid balance
4. Maintain position, patency, and low suction of NG tube
5. Keep the patient in semi-Fowler's position
6. Monitor and record VS, UO, I/O, laboratory studies, daily weight, specific gravity, calorie count, and fecal occult blood
7. Administer TPN and transfusion therapy
8. Administer medications, as prescribed
9. Allay the patient's anxiety
10. Provide skin, mouth, nares, perianal care
11. Maintain bed rest with bedside commode
12. Turn the patient every 2 hours
13. Minimize environmental stress
14. Provide rest periods
15. Maintain a quiet environment
16. Promote independence in activities of daily living (ADLs)
17. Assess bowel sounds
18. Administer sitz baths
19. Monitor the number, amount, and character of stools
20. Assess perineal excoriation
21. Provide information about the United Ostomy Association and the National Foundation of Ileitis and Colitis

H. Teaching goals (instructions to the patient and family)
1. Keep follow-up appointments
2. Exercise regularly
3. Stop smoking
4. Maintain a normal weight
5. Know the action, side effects, and scheduling of medications
6. Identify ways to reduce stress
7. Recognize the signs and symptoms of rectal hemorrhage and intestinal obstructions
8. Alternate rest periods with activity
9. Follow dietary recommendations and restrictions
10. Maintain a quiet environment
11. Seek help from community agencies and resources
12. Complete sitz baths and perianal care daily

I. Possible medical complications
1. Anemia
2. Malnutrition
3. GI perforation
4. Megacolon

5. Dehydration
6. GI obstruction
7. Hypokalemia
8. Massive rectal hemorrhage
9. Amyloidosis

J. Possible surgical interventions
1. Ileostomy (see page 140)
2. Colectomy (see page 140)

XVI. Regional enteritis (Crohn's disease)

A. Definition
1. Chronic inflammatory disease of the small intestine, usually affecting the terminal ileum and ascending colon
2. Slowly progressive with exacerbations and remissions

B. Possible etiology
1. Unknown
2. Emotional upsets
3. Milk and milk products
4. Fried foods

C. Pathophysiology
1. Ulcerations of intestinal mucosa are accompanied by congestion, thickening of the small bowel, and fissure formations
2. Enlarged regional mesenteric lymph nodes accompany fibrosis and narrowing of intestinal wall

D. Possible clinical manifestations
1. Pain in lower right quadrant
2. Mesenteric lymphadenitis
3. Abdominal cramps and spasms after meals
4. Nausea
5. Flatulence
6. Weight loss
7. Elevated temperature
8. Chronic diarrhea with blood
9. Borborygmus

E. Possible diagnostic test findings
1. Abdominal X-ray: congested, thickened, fibrosed, and narrowed intestinal wall
2. Proctosigmoidoscopy: ulceration
3. Fecal occult blood: positive
4. Fecal fat test: increased
5. Upper GI: classic "string sign" at terminal ileum
6. Barium enema: lesions in terminal ileum

F. Medical management
1. Diet: two types
   a. High-protein, high-calorie, low-residue, low-fat, low-fiber, high-carbohydrate; bland foods in small, frequent feedings with restricted intake of milk and gas-forming foods
   b. No food and fluids
2. I.V. therapy: heparin lock
3. Activity: as tolerated
4. Monitoring: VS, I/O, daily weights, stools for occult blood, and specific gravity
5. Laboratory studies: potassium, Hgb, Hct, and osmolality
6. Nutritional support: TPN
7. Antibiotic: sulfasalazine (Azulfidine)
8. Analgesic: meperidine hydrochloride (Demerol)
9. Anticholinergics: propantheline bromide (Pro-Banthine), dicyclomine hydrochloride (Bentyl)
10. Antacids: magnesium and aluminum hydroxide (Maalox), aluminum hydroxide gel (ALternaGEL)
11. Corticosteroid: prednisone (Deltasone)
12. Antiemetic: prochlorperazine (Compazine)
13. Antidiarrheals: diphenoxylate (Lomotil)
14. Antianemics: ferrous sulfate (Feosol), ferrous gluconate (Fergon)
15. Vitamins and minerals
16. Potassium supplement: potassium chloride (K-Lor), potassium gluconate (Kaon)
17. Anti-inflammatory: olsalazine sodium (Dipentum)
18. Antibacterial: metronidazole (Flagyl)
19. Immunosuppressants: mercaptopurine (Purinethol), azathioprine (Imuran)

G. Nursing interventions and responsibilities
1. Maintain the patient's diet; withhold food and fluids as necessary
2. Assess GI status and fluid balance
3. Monitor and record VS, I/O, laboratory studies, daily weight, specific gravity, and fecal occult blood
4. Administer TPN
5. Administer medications, as prescribed
6. Allay the patient's anxiety
7. Provide skin and perianal care
8. Minimize environmental stress
9. Maintain a quiet environment
10. Promote independence in ADLs
11. Monitor the number, amount, and character of stools
12. Assess abdominal distention

H. Teaching goals (instructions to the patient and family)
1. Keep follow-up appointments

2. Exercise regularly
3. Stop smoking
4. Maintain a normal weight
5. Know the action, side effects, and scheduling of medications
6. Identify ways to reduce stress
7. Recognize the signs and symptoms of rectal hemorrhage and intestinal obstructions
8. Alternate rest periods with activity
9. Follow dietary recommendations and restrictions
10. Maintain a quiet environment
11. Seek help from community agencies and resources
12. Complete perianal care daily
13. Avoid laxatives and aspirin

I. Possible medical complications
    1. Intestinal obstruction
    2. Intestinal fistulas
    3. Intestinal perforation
    4. Hemorrhage
    5. Malnutrition
    6. Anemia

J. Possible surgical interventions
    1. Bowel resection with anastomosis (see page 140)
    2. Gastrojejunostomy with vagotomy (see page 137)
    3. Ileoanal reservoir

XVII. Diverticulosis and diverticulitis

A. Definition
    1. Diverticulum: outpouching of intestinal mucosa through the muscular wall of the intestine
    2. Diverticulosis: multiple diverticula
    3. Diverticulitis: inflammation of diverticula

B. Possible etiology
    1. Stress
    2. Congenital weakening of the intestinal wall
    3. Low intake of roughage and fiber
    4. Straining at the stool
    5. Chronic constipation

C. Pathophysiology
    1. Muscle tone is weakened in the intestinal wall, resulting in a saclike outpouching (diverticulum)
    2. Inflammation (diverculitis) is caused by bacteria and fecal material trapped in the diverticula
    3. Intestinal wall thickens and narrows

    4. Common site is sigmoid colon

D. Possible clinical manifestations
    1. Left lower quadrant pain
    2. Constipation and diarrhea
    3. Bloody stools
    4. Elevated temperature
    5. Rectal bleeding
    6. Change in bowel habits
    7. Flatulence
    8. Nausea

E. Possible diagnostic test findings
    1. Sigmoidoscopy: diverticula, thickened wall
    2. Barium enema, contraindicated in acute diverticulitis: inflammation, narrow lumen of the bowel, diverticula
    3. Hematology: increased WBCs, erythrocyte sedimentation rate (ESR)

F. Medical management
    1. Diet: high-fiber, high-residue
    2. I.V. therapy: hydration, heparin lock
    3. GI decompression: NG tube
    4. Position: semi-Fowler's
    5. Activity: bed rest; active ROM and isometric exercises
    6. Monitoring: VS, UO, and I/O
    7. Laboratory studies: Hgb, Hct, and WBCs
    8. Nutritional support: TPN
    9. Antibiotics: gentamicin (Garamycin), tobramycin sulfate (Nebcin), clindamycin (Cleocin)
   10. Anticholinergic: propantheline bromide (Pro-Banthine)
   11. Stool softeners: docusate sodium (Colace)

G. Nursing interventions and responsibilities
    1. Maintain the patient's diet
    2. Assess abdominal distention
    3. Maintain position, patency, and low suction of NG tube
    4. Keep the patient in semi-Fowler's position
    5. Monitor and record VS, UO, I/O, and laboratory studies
    6. Administer TPN
    7. Administer medications, as prescribed
    8. Allay the patient's anxiety
    9. Provide nares and mouth care
   10. Provide rest periods
   11. Administer cleansing enemas
   12. Monitor stools for occult blood
   13. Assess bowel sounds

H. Teaching goals (instructions to the patient and family)
1. Keep follow-up appointments
2. Know the action, side effects, and scheduling of medications
3. Identify ways to reduce stress
4. List measures to decrease constipation
5. Follow dietary recommendations and restrictions; avoid corn, nuts, and fruits and vegetables with seeds
6. Monitor stools for bleeding

I. Possible medical complications
1. Bowel perforation
2. Peritonitis
3. Abscess
4. Fistula
5. Hemorrhage

J. Possible surgical interventions: resection of the bowel (see page 140)

XVIII. Intestinal obstruction

A. Definition—blockage of intestinal lumen

B. Possible etiology
1. Adhesions
2. Hernias
3. Tumors
4. Fecal impaction
5. Mesenteric thrombosis
6. Paralytic ileus
7. Diverticulitis
8. Inflammation (Crohn's disease)
9. Volvulus

C. Pathophysiology
1. Gas, fluid, and digested substances accumulate proximal to the obstruction
2. Fluids and gases cause bowel distention
3. Peristalsis increases proximal to the obstruction
4. Water and electrolytes are secreted into the blocked bowel
5. Bowel inflammation increases and absorption by bowel mucosa is inhibited
6. Fluid loss results in dehydration

D. Possible clinical manifestations
1. Cramping pain
2. Nausea
3. Abdominal distention
4. Vomiting fecal material
5. Constipation

6. Singultus
7. Elevated temperature
8. Diminished or absent bowel sounds
9. Weight loss

E. Possible diagnostic test findings
   1. Blood chemistry: decreased sodium, potassium
   2. Hematology: increased WBCs
   3. Barium enema: stops at obstruction
   4. Abdominal X-rays: increased amount of gas in bowel

F. Medical management
   1. Diet: withhold food and fluids
   2. I.V. therapy: hydration, electrolyte replacement; heparin lock
   3. GI decompression: NG tube, Miller-Abbott tube, Cantor tube
   4. Position: semi-Fowler's
   5. Activity: bed rest
   6. Monitoring: VS, UO, and I/O
   7. Laboratory studies: sodium, potassium, and WBCs
   8. Treatments: Foley catheter, NG irrigation
   9. Antibiotic: gentamicin (Garamycin)
   10. Analgesic: meperidine hydrochloride (Demerol)

G. Nursing interventions and responsibilities
   1. Withhold food and fluids
   2. Administer I.V. fluids
   3. Assess bowel sounds
   4. Measure and record the patient's abdominal girth
   5. Monitor and record the frequency, color, and amount of stools
   6. Maintain position, patency, and low suction of NG tube and Miller-Abbott tube
   7. Keep the patient in semi-Fowler's position
   8. Monitor and record VS, UO, I/O, and laboratory studies
   9. Administer medications, as prescribed
   10. Allay the patient's anxiety
   11. Provide nares and mouth care
   12. Provide information about the American Ostomy Association

H. Teaching goals (instructions to the patient and family)
   1. Keep follow-up appointments
   2. Know the action, side effects, and scheduling of medications
   3. Recognize the signs and symptoms of diverticulitis
   4. Monitor the frequency and color of stools
   5. Avoid constipating foods

I. Possible medical complications
   1. Peritonitis
   2. Strangulation of bowel

3. Infection
4. Sepsis
5. Bowel necrosis

J. Possible surgical interventions
   1. Resection of the bowel (see page 140)
   2. Colostomy (see page 140)

XIX. Peritonitis

A. Definition — localized or generalized inflammation of peritoneal cavity

B. Possible etiology
   1. Bacterial infection
   2. Pancreatitis
   3. Blunt or penetrating trauma
   4. Inflammation of colon or kidneys
   5. Volvulus
   6. Intestinal ischemia
   7. Intestinal obstruction
   8. Peptic ulceration
   9. Biliary tract disease
   10. Neoplasms
   11. Nephrosis
   12. Cirrhosis
   13. Intestinal perforation

C. Pathophysiology
   1. Peritoneal irritants cause inflammatory edema, vascular congestion, and hypermotility of the bowel
   2. Movement of extracellular fluid into the peritoneal cavity leads to hypovolemia and decreased urine output

D. Possible clinical manifestations
   1. Constant, diffuse, and intense abdominal pain
   2. Rebound tenderness
   3. Malaise
   4. Nausea
   5. Elevated temperature
   6. Abdominal rigidity and distention
   7. Anorexia
   8. Decreased urine output
   9. Shallow respirations
   10. Weak, rapid pulse
   11. Decreased peristalsis
   12. Decreased or absent bowel sounds
   13. Abdominal resonance and tympany on percussion

E. Possible diagnostic test findings
   1. Hematology: increased WBCs, Hct
   2. Peritoneal aspiration: positive for blood, pus, bile, bacteria, or amylase
   3. Abdominal X-ray: free air in abdomen under diaphragm

F. Medical management
   1. Diet: withhold food or fluid
   2. I.V. therapy: hydration, electrolyte replacement; heparin lock
   3. GI decompression: NG tube
   4. Position: semi-Fowler's
   5. Activity: bed rest
   6. Monitoring: VS, UO, I/O, CVP, and specific gravity
   7. Laboratory studies: Hgb, Hct, potassium, sodium, calcium, osmolality, and WBCs
   8. Nutritional support: TPN
   9. Treatments: Foley catheter, incentive spirometry
   10. Antibiotics: gentamicin (Garamycin), clindamycin (Cleocin), cephalothin (Keflin), ampicillin sodium/sulbactam sodium (Unasyn)
   11. Analgesic: meperidine hydrochloride (Demerol)

G. Nursing interventions and responsibilities
   1. Withhold food and fluids
   2. Administer I.V. fluids
   3. Provide TCDB
   4. Assess respiratory status and fluid balance
   5. Maintain position, patency, and low suction of NG tube
   6. Keep the patient in semi-Fowler's position
   7. Monitor and record VS, UO, I/O, laboratory studies, CVP, daily weight, and specific gravity
   8. Administer TPN
   9. Administer medications, as prescribed
   10. Allay the patient's anxiety
   11. Provide nares and mouth care
   12. Turn the patient every 2 hours
   13. Maintain bed rest
   14. Assess pain
   15. Assess bowel sounds
   16. Measure and record the patient's abdominal girth
   17. Avoid giving the patient laxatives
   18. Do not apply heat to the patient's abdomen

H. Teaching goals (instructions to the patient and family)
   1. Keep follow-up appointments
   2. Know the action, side effects, and scheduling of medications
   3. Recognize the signs and symptoms of GI obstruction
   4. Follow nutritional support measures

I. Possible medical complications
   1. Adhesions
   2. Abscesses
   3. Obstructions
   4. Septic shock
   5. Paralytic ileus

J. Possible surgical interventions
   1. Exploratory laparotomy
   2. Bowel resection (see page 140)
   3. Incision and drainage of abscess
   4. Closure of perforation

XX. Hemorrhoids

A. Definition—congested and dilated internal or external vessels of the rectum and anus

B. Possible etiology
   1. Chronic constipation
   2. Prolonged sitting or standing
   3. Straining at the stool
   4. Pregnancy
   5. Heavy lifting
   6. Portal hypertension
   7. Heredity
   8. Obesity
   9. Anal infection

C. Pathophysiology
   1. Increased abdominal pressure impairs the flow of blood through the hemorrhoidal venous plexus
   2. Decreased blood flow causes dilation and congestion of the vessels of the rectum and anus

D. Possible clinical manifestations
   1. Anal pain with defecation, sitting, or walking
   2. Anal pruritus
   3. Protrusion of hemorrhoids
   4. Rectal bleeding
   5. Rectal mucus discharge
   6. Bleeding during defecation
   7. Sensation of incomplete fecal evacuation

E. Possible diagnostic test findings
   1. Digital exam: hemorrhoids
   2. Barium enema: hemorrhoids
   3. Proctoscopy: internal hemorrhoids
   4. Hematology: decreased Hgb, Hct

F. Medical management
1. Diet: high-fiber, low-roughage with increased fluid intake
2. Position: side-lying or prone
3. Activity: as tolerated
4. Monitoring: VS, frequency of stools
5. Laboratory studies: Hgb, Hct
6. Treatments: witch hazel compresses, sitz baths
7. Corticosteroids: hydrocortisone (Hydrocortisone cream)
8. Analgesic: acetaminophen (Tylenol)
9. Antipruritic: diphenhydramine (Benadryl)
10. Stool softeners: docusate sodium (Colace)
11. Anesthetic: lidocaine hydrochloride (Xylocaine)
12. Laxative: magnesium hydroxide (Milk of Magnesia)
13. Cryodestruction

G. Nursing interventions and responsibilities
1. Maintain the patient's diet with increased fluids
2. Assess bowel elimination and rectal bleeding
3. Keep the patient on the side or prone
4. Monitor and record VS, I/O, and laboratory studies
5. Administer medications, as prescribed
6. Allay the patient's anxiety
7. Provide perineal care
8. Administer sitz baths and witch hazel compresses
9. Provide privacy and time for defecation

H. Teaching goals (instructions to the patient and family)
1. Keep follow-up appointments
2. Exercise regularly
3. Maintain a normal weight
4. Know the action, side effects, and scheduling of medications
5. Recognize the signs and symptoms of rectal bleeding
6. Avoid heavy lifting
7. Avoid prolonged sitting or standing
8. Follow dietary recommendations and restrictions
9. Complete perineal care daily
10. Avoid constipation
11. Defecate when urge is felt
12. Use sitz baths and witch hazel compresses

I. Possible medical complications
1. Megacolon
2. Diverticulitis
3. Hemorrhage

J. Possible surgical interventions
1. Hemorrhoidectomy (see page 139)
2. Barron rubber-band ligation

XXI. Colorectal cancer

A. Definition — malignant tumor of the colon or rectum that is primary or metastatic

B. Possible etiology
1. Diverticulosis
2. Chronic ulcerative colitis
3. Familial polyposis
4. Aging
5. Low-fiber, high-carbohydrate diet
6. Chronic constipation

C. Pathophysiology
1. Unregulated cell growth and uncontrolled cell division result in the development of a neoplasm
2. Metastasis often occurs in the liver
3. Adenocarcinomas occur in the colon, rectum, jejunum, and duodenum
4. Adenocarcinomas infiltrate and cause obstruction, ulcerations, and hemorrhage

D. Possible clinical manifestations
1. Abdominal cramps
2. Abdominal distention
3. Diarrhea and constipation
4. Weakness
5. Pallor
6. Weight loss
7. Anorexia
8. Change in shape of stool
9. Rectal bleeding
10. Palpable mass
11. Fecal oozing
12. Change in bowel habits
13. Melena
14. Vomiting

E. Possible diagnostic test findings
1. Fecal occult blood: positive
2. Hematology: decreased Hgb, Hct
3. Sigmoidoscopy: identification and location of mass
4. Barium enema: location of mass
5. Biopsy: cytology positive for cancer cells
6. CEA: positive
7. GI series: location of mass

F. Medical management
1. Diet: high-fiber, low-fat, low-refined carbohydrate

 2. I.V. therapy: heparin lock
 3. Position: semi-Fowler's
 4. Activity: as tolerated
 5. Monitoring: VS, U/O, and I/O
 6. Laboratory studies: Hgb, Hct
 7. Nutritional support: TPN
 8. Radiation therapy
 9. Antineoplastics: doxorubicin hydrochloride (Adriamycin), 5-fluorouracil (Adrucil)
10. Chemotherapy
11. Immunomodulator: levamisole hydrochloride (Ergamisol)
12. Folic acid derivative: leucovorin (Citrovorum factor)
13. Antiemetic: nabilone (Cesamet)

G. Nursing interventions and responsibilities
 1. Maintain the patient's diet
 2. Keep the patient in semi-Fowler's position
 3. Monitor and record VS, UO, I/O, laboratory studies, and daily weight
 4. Administer TPN
 5. Administer medications, as prescribed
 6. Encourage the patient to express feelings about changes in body image and a fear of dying
 7. Provide skin and mouth care
 8. Provide rest periods
 9. Monitor and record the color, consistency, amount, and frequency of stools
10. Assess for signs of intestinal obstruction and rectal bleeding
11. Provide postchemotherapeutic and postradiation nursing care
     a. Provide skin, mouth, and perineal care
     b. Encourage dietary intake
     c. Administer antiemetics and antidiarrheals, as prescribed
     d. Monitor for bleeding, infection, and electrolyte imbalance
     e. Provide rest periods
12. Provide information about the United Ostomy Association and the American Cancer Society

H. Teaching goals (instructions to the patient and family)
 1. Keep follow-up appointments
 2. Maintain a normal weight
 3. Know the action, side effects, and scheduling of medications
 4. Recognize the signs and symptoms of infection
 5. Alternate rest periods with activity
 6. Monitor self for infection
 7. Follow dietary recommendations and restrictions
 8. Seek help from community agencies and resources
 9. Monitor changes in bowel elimination

I. Possible medical complications
   1. Anemia
   2. Hemorrhage
   3. Intestinal obstruction

J. Possible surgical interventions
   1. Abdominoperineal resection (see page 140)
   2. Colostomy (see page 140)

XXII. Cholecystitis

A. Definition — acute or chronic inflammation of the gall bladder; most commonly associated with cholelithiasis

B. Possible etiology
   1. Cholelithiasis: cholesterol, bile pigment, calcium stones
   2. Obesity
   3. Infection of the gall bladder
   4. Estrogen therapy

C. Pathophysiology
   1. Inflamed gall bladder cannot contract in response to fatty foods entering the duodenum because of obstruction by calculi or edema
   2. Inability to constrict causes pain
   3. Accumulated bile is absorbed into the blood

D. Possible clinical manifestations
   1. Indigestion or chest pain after eating fatty or fried foods
   2. Episodic colicky pain in epigastric area, which radiates to back and shoulder
   3. Nausea and vomiting
   4. Elevated temperature
   5. Jaundice
   6. Flatulence
   7. Belching
   8. Clay-colored stools
   9. Dark amber urine
   10. Pruritus
   11. Ecchymosis
   12. Steatorrhea

E. Possible diagnostic test findings
   1. Cholangiogram: stones in biliary tree
   2. Gall bladder series: stones in biliary tree
   3. Ultrasound: bile duct distention and calculi
   4. Liver scan: obstruction of biliary tree
   5. Blood chemistry: increased alkaline phosphatase, bilirubin, direct bilirubin transaminase, amylase, lipase, AST, and LDH
   6. Hematology: increased WBCs

F. Medical management
   1. Diet: two types
      a. Low-fat, high-carbohydrate, high-protein, high-fiber, low-calorie in small, frequent feedings with restricted intake of gas-forming foods
      b. No foods and fluids, as directed
   2. I.V. therapy: hydration, electrolyte replacement; heparin lock
   3. GI decompression: NG tube, Miller-Abbott tube
   4. Position: semi-Fowler's
   5. Activity: bed rest
   6. Monitoring: VS, U/O, I/O, and specific gravity
   7. Laboratory studies: amylase, lipase, bilirubin, alkaline phosphatase, and WBCs
   8. Treatments: incentive spirometry, tepid baths without soap
   9. Antilithic: chenodiol (Chenix)
  10. Antibiotic: cephalothin (Keflin)
  11. Analgesic: meperidine hydrochloride (Demerol)
  12. Anticholinergics: propantheline bromide (Pro-Banthine), dicyclomine hydrochloride (Bentyl)
  13. Antiemetics: prochlorperazine (Compazine)
  14. Antipruritics: diphenhydramine (Benadryl)
  15. Vitamins: phytonadione (AquaMEPHYTON), cyanocobalamin (vitamin B_{12})
  16. Extracorporeal shock wave lithotripsy
  17. Endoscopic sphincterotomy

G. Nursing interventions and responsibilities
   1. Maintain the patient's diet; withhold food and fluids
   2. Administer I.V. fluids
   3. Provide TCDB
   4. Assess pain
   5. Maintain position, patency, and low suction of NG tube
   6. Keep the patient in semi-Fowler's position
   7. Monitor and record VS, U/O, I/O, laboratory studies, and specific gravity
   8. Administer medications, as prescribed
   9. Allay the patient's anxiety
  10. Provide skin, nares, and mouth care
  11. Maintain bed rest
  12. Maintain a quiet environment
  13. Administer tepid baths without soap
  14. Prevent scratching if pruritus occurs

H. Teaching goals (instructions to the patient and family)
   1. Keep follow-up appointments
   2. Exercise regularly
   3. Stop smoking
   4. Maintain a normal weight

5. Know the action, side effects, and scheduling of medications
6. Recognize the signs and symptoms of renal colic
7. Follow dietary recommendations and restrictions
8. Complete skin care daily

I. Possible medical complications
   1. Hemorrhage
   2. Cirrhosis
   3. Intestinal perforation
   4. Peritonitis
   5. Pancreatitis

J. Possible surgical interventions
   1. Cholecystectomy (see page 134)
   2. Choledochostomy (see page 134)
   3. Cholecystostomy (see page 134)
   4. Laparoscopic laser cholecystectomy (endoscopic cholecystectomy)

XXIII. Pancreatitis

A. Definition — acute or chronic inflammation of the pancreas with varying degrees of pancreatic edema, fat necrosis, and hemorrhage

B. Possible etiology
   1. Biliary tract disease
   2. Alcoholism
   3. Hyperparathyroidism
   4. Hyperlipidemia
   5. Blunt trauma to pancreas or abdomen
   6. Bacterial or viral infection
   7. Duodenal ulcer
   8. Drug induced: steroids, thiazide diuretics, oral contraceptives

C. Pathophysiology
   1. Acute: pancreatic enzymes are activated in the pancreas rather than the duodenum, resulting in tissue damage and autodigestion of the pancreas
   2. Chronic: chronic inflammation results in fibrosis and calcification of the pancreas, obstruction of the ducts, and destruction of the secreting acinar cells

D. Possible clinical manifestations
   1. Nausea and vomiting
   2. Tachycardia
   3. Abrupt onset of pain in epigastric area that radiates to the shoulder, substernal area, back, and flank
   4. Aching, burning, stabbing, pressing pain
   5. Abdominal tenderness and distention
   6. Elevated temperature

7. Steatorrhea
8. Weight loss
9. Jaundice
10. Hypotension
11. Pain upon eating
12. Dyspnea
13. Decreased or absent bowel sounds

E. Possible diagnostic test findings
1. CT scan: enlarged pancreas
2. Blood chemistry: increased amylase, lipase, lactic dehydrogenase, glucose, aspartate aminotransferase (AST), lipids; decreased calcium and potassium
3. Hematology: increased WBCs, RBCs
4. Grey Turner's sign: positive
5. Ultrasonography: cysts; bile duct inflammation and dilation
6. Cullen's sign: positive
7. Urine chemistry: increased amylase
8. Fecal fat: positive
9. Arteriography: fibrous tissue and calcification of pancreas
10. Glucose tolerance test: increased
11. ERCP: biliary obstruction

F. Medical management
1. Diet: low-fat, low-protein, high-carbohydrate, in small, frequent feedings with restricted intake of caffeine, alcohol, and gas-forming foods
2. I.V. therapy: hydration, electrolyte replacement; heparin lock
3. GI decompression: NG tube
4. Position: semi-Fowler's
5. Activity: bed rest
6. Monitoring: VS, UO, I/O, CVP, specific gravity, and urine glucose and ketones
7. Laboratory studies: glucose, potassium, amylase, lipase, calcium, and lipids
8. Nutritional support: TPN
9. Transfusion therapy: packed RBCs
10. Antibiotic: cephalothin (Keflin)
11. Analgesic: meperidine hydrochloride (Demerol)
12. Anticholinergics: propantheline bromide (Pro-Banthine), dicyclomine hydrochloride (Bentyl)
13. Antacids: magnesium and aluminum hydroxide (Maalox), aluminum hydroxide gel (ALternaGEL)
14. Corticosteroid: hydrocortisone (Solu-Cortef)
15. Antiemetic: prochlorperazine (Compazine)
16. Histamine antagonists: cimetidine (Tagamet), ranitidine (Zantac)
17. Vitamins and minerals

18. Tranquilizer: diazepam (Valium)
19. Digestants: pancrelipase (Viokase, Cotazym)
20. Potassium supplement: potassium chloride (K-Lor), potassium gluconate (Kaon)
21. Peritoneal lavage
22. Dialysis
23. Calcium supplement: calcium gluconate (Kalcinate), calcium carbonate (OsCal)
24. Antidiabetic agent: insulin
25. Muscosal barrier fortifier: sucralfate (Carafate)

G. Nursing interventions and responsibilities
   1. Maintain the patient's diet; withhold food and fluids as necessary
   2. Administer I.V. fluids
   3. Assess fluid balance
   4. Maintain position, patency, and low suction of NG tube
   5. Keep the patient in semi-Fowler's position
   6. Monitor and record VS, UO, I/O, laboratory studies, CVP, daily weight, specific gravity, and urine glucose and ketones
   7. Administer TPN
   8. Administer medications, as prescribed
   9. Allay the patient's anxiety
   10. Provide skin, nares, and mouth care
   11. Keep the patient in bed and turn every 2 hours
   12. Provide a quiet, restful environment
   13. Monitor urine and stool for color, character, and amount

H. Teaching goals (instructions to the patient and family)
   1. Keep follow-up appointments
   2. Stop smoking
   3. Maintain a normal weight
   4. Know the action, side effects, and scheduling of medications
   5. Recognize the signs and symptoms of infection and increased blood glucose
   6. Adhere to activity limitations
   7. Alternate rest periods with activity
   8. Monitor self for infection
   9. Follow dietary recommendations and restrictions
   10. Maintain a quiet environment
   11. Monitor self for steatorrhea
   12. Monitor urine for glucose and ketones

I. Possible medical complications
   1. Ileus
   2. Hypovolemic shock
   3. Diabetes mellitus

4. Infection
5. Jaundice
6. Pancreatic fistula
7. Pancreatic abscess
8. Hypocalcemia
9. Septic shock
10. Disseminated intravascular coagulation (DIC)
11. Adult respiratory distress syndrome (ARDS)

J. Possible surgical interventions: pancreatectomy (see page 134)

XXIV. Hepatic cirrhosis

A. Definition
1. Chronic, progressive disease characterized by inflammation, fibrosis, and degeneration of liver parenchymal cells
2. Three types of hepatic cirrhosis
   a. Laënnec's (micronodular)
   b. Postnecrotic (macronodular)
   c. Biliary

B. Possible etiology
1. Alcohol use or abuse
2. Malnutrition
3. Viral hepatitis
4. Cholecystitis

C. Pathophysiology
1. Inflammation causes liver parenchymal cell destruction, with subsequent fibrosis
2. Fibrotic changes cause obstruction of hepatic blood flow and normal liver function
3. Obstruction causes portal hypertension
4. Decreased liver function results in changes in body chemistry
   a. Decreased absorption and utilization of fat-soluble vitamins (A, D, E, K)
   b. Increased secretion of aldosterone
   c. Ineffective detoxification of protein wastes

D. Possible clinical manifestations
1. Nausea and vomiting
2. Weakness and fatigue
3. Anorexia and weight loss
4. Jaundice
5. Ecchymosis
6. Palmar erythema
7. Indigestion
8. Pruritus

9. Irregular bowel habits
10. Pain in right upper quadrant
11. Peripheral edema
12. Petechiae
13. Epistaxis
14. Hematemesis
15. Telangiectasis
16. Gynecomastia and impotence
17. Amenorrhea
18. Hemorrhoids
19. Hepatomegaly

E. Possible diagnostic test findings
   1. Blood chemistry: increased AST, ALT, LDH, alkaline phosphatase, ammonia, bilirubin, BSP; decreased albumin, total protein
   2. Hematology: decreased Hgb, Hct, WBCs; increased PT
   3. Liver scan: fibrotic liver, increased uptake
   4. Liver biopsy: destruction of parenchymal cells
   5. Esophagoscopy: esophageal varices
   6. ABGs: metabolic acidosis
   7. Urine chemistry: proteinuria
   8. CT scan: ASCITES

F. Medical management
   1. Diet: high-calorie, high-carbohydrate, low-fat, low-sodium in small, frequent feedings with restricted intake of alcohol, fluids, and protein
   2. I.V. therapy: hydration, electrolyte replacement; heparin lock
   3. Oxygen therapy
   4. GI decompression: NG tube, Sengstaken-Blakemore tube
   5. Position: semi-Fowler's
   6. Activity: bed rest
   7. Monitoring: VS, U/O, I/O, neurovital signs, ECG, hemodynamic variables, and stools for occult blood
   8. Laboratory studies: AST, ALT, LDH, PT, amylase, lipase, Hgb, Hct, bilirubin, albumin, WBCs, and ABGs
   9. Nutritional support: TPN, NG feedings
  10. Treatments: Foley catheter; incentive spirometry; tepid bath; cool, moist compresses
  11. Precautions: enteric and protective
  12. Transfusion therapy: platelets, packed RBCs, fresh frozen plasma (FFP)
  13. Antibiotics: neomycin sulfate (Neobiotic)
  14. Diuretics: spironolactone (Aldactone), furosemide (Lasix)
  15. Sedative: phenobarbital (Luminal)
  16. Stool softeners: docusate sodium (Colace)
  17. Ammonia detoxicant: lactulose (Cephulac)
  18. Vitamins: phytonadione (AquaMEPHYTON), cyanocobalamin (vitamin B_{12})

19. Antacids: magnesium and aluminum hydroxide (Maalox), aluminum hydroxide gel (ALternaGEL)
20. Analgesic: oxycodone hydrochloride (Tylox)
21. Enzyme replacement: pancrelipase (Viokase)
22. Sclerosing agent: ethanolamine oleate (Ethamolin)
23. Abdominal paracentesis

G. Nursing interventions and responsibilities
1. Maintain the patient's diet; or withhold food and fluids as necssary
2. Administer I.V. fluids
3. Administer oxygen
4. Provide TCDB, incentive spirometry
5. Assess respiratory status, GI bleeding, and fluid balance
6. Maintain position, patency, and low suction of NG tube
7. Keep the patient in semi-Fowler's position
8. Monitor and record VS, UO, I/O, laboratory studies, hemodynamic variables, daily weight, specific gravity, fecal occult blood, and neurovital signs
9. Measure and record the patient's abdominal girth
10. Monitor for infection
11. Administer TPN
12. Administer medications, as prescribed
13. Allay the patient's anxiety
14. Provide skin, nares, and mouth care
15. Maintain enteric and protective precautions
16. Maintain bed rest
17. Maintain a quiet environment
18. Administer tepid baths without soap; apply cool, moist compresses
19. Prevent scratching
20. Use small-gauge needles for intramuscular injections
21. Apply prolonged pressure after venipuncture
22. Monitor stool for color, consistency, and amount
23. Provide information on Alcoholics Anonymous (AA)

H. Teaching goals (instructions to the patient and family)
1. Keep follow-up appointments
2. Stop smoking
3. Maintain a normal weight
4. Know the action, side effects, and scheduling of medications
5. Avoid using alcohol
6. Recognize the signs and symptoms of GI bleeding
7. Avoid exposure to people with infections
8. Alternate rest periods with activity
9. Monitor self for infection
10. Follow dietary recommendations and restrictions
11. Complete skin care daily

12. Avoid straining at stool, vigorous blowing of nose, coughing, and using a hard toothbrush
13. Avoid using over-the-counter medications

I. Possible medical complications
   1. Ascites
   2. Esophageal varices
   3. Hemorrhoids
   4. Hemorrhage
   5. Estrogen and androgen imbalance
   6. Portal hypertension
   7. Hepatic coma
   8. Pancytopenia

J. Possible surgical interventions
   1. Portacaval shunt (see page 136)
   2. LeVeen peritoneovenous shunt

XXV. Hepatitis

A. Definition
   1. Inflammation of the liver
   2. Three types of hepatitis
      a. Hepatitis A (infectious)
      b. Hepatitis B (serum)
      c. Non-A, non-B hepatitis

B. Possible etiology
   1. Contaminated food, milk, water (hepatitis A)
   2. Contaminated needles (hepatitis A, hepatitis B)
   3. RNA virus (hepatitis A)
   4. DNA virus (hepatitis B)
   5. Blood transfusions (non-A, non-B hepatitis)
   6. Blood, saliva, semen (hepatitis B)

C. Pathophysiology
   1. Inflammation of liver tissue causes inflammation of hepatic cells, hypertrophy, and proliferation of Kupffer's cells and bile stasis
   2. Type A virus (HAV) is transmitted by fecal or oral route and causes hepatitis A
   3. Type B virus (HBV) is transmitted by blood and body fluids and causes hepatitis B

D. Possible clinical manifestations
   1. Preicteric
      a. Anorexia
      b. Nausea and vomiting
      c. Fatigue
      d. Constipation and diarrhea

   e. Weight loss
   f. Right upper quadrant pain
   g. Hepatomegaly
   h. Splenomegaly
   i. Malaise
   j. Elevated temperature
   k. Pharyngitis
   l. Nasal discharge
   m. Headache
   n. Pruritus
2. Icteric
   a. Fatigue
   b. Weight loss
   c. Clay-colored stools
   d. Dark urine
   e. Hepatomegaly
   f. Jaundice
   g. Splenomegaly
   h. Pruritus
3. Posticteric
   a. Fatigue
   b. Decreasing hepatomegaly
   c. Decreasing jaundice
   d. Improved appetite

E. Possible diagnostic test findings
   1. Blood chemistry: increased ALT, AST, alkaline phosphatase, LDH, bilirubin, ESR, positive anti-HAV (IgM) or positive HBsAg (surface antigen)
   2. Hematology: increased PT
   3. BSP: increased
   4. Urine chemistry: increased urobilinogen
   5. Stool: hepatitis A virus

F. Medical management
   1. Diet: high-calorie, moderate-protein, and low-fat
   2. Activity: bed rest
   3. Monitoring: VS, UO, and I/O
   4. Laboratory studies: ALT, AST, LDH, bilirubin, PT, and PTT
   5. Precautions: enteric (hepatitis A); body/fluid (hepatitis B and non-A, non-B)
   6. Antiemetic: prochlorperazine (Compazine)
   7. Vitamins and minerals: vitamin K (AquaMEPHYTON)

G. Nursing interventions and responsibilities
   1. Maintain the patient's diet

2. Monitor and record VS, UO, I/O, and laboratory studies
3. Administer medications, as prescribed
4. Allay the patient's anxiety
5. Maintain body fluid and enteric precautions
6. Provide rest periods
7. Encourage small, frequent meals

H. Teaching goals (instructions to the patient and family)
  1. Keep follow-up appointments
  2. Know the action, side effects, and scheduling of medications
  3. Avoid exposure to people with infections
  4. Alternate rest periods with activity
  5. Monitor self for infection
  6. Follow dietary recommendations and restrictions
  7. Avoid alcohol
  8. Maintain good personal hygiene
  9. Refrain from donating blood
  10. Increase fluid intake to 3,000 ml/day
  11. Abstain from sexual intercourse until serum liver studies are within normal limits

I. Possible medical complications
  1. Pancreatitis
  2. Aplastic anemia
  3. Glomerulonephritis
  4. Vasculitis

J. Possible surgical interventions: none

XXVI. Esophageal varices

A. Definition — dilation of esophageal veins in the lower part of the esophagus

B. Possible etiology
  1. Portal hypertension
  2. Increased intra-abdominal pressure
  3. Alcohol abuse
  4. Cirrhosis

C. Pathophysiology
  1. Venous drainage from the liver into the portal vein is decreased
  2. Drainage obstruction results in portal hypertension
  3. Return of venous blood from the intestinal tract and spleen to the right atrium via the collateral circulation is obstructed
  4. The increased pressure dilates the esophageal veins, which then protrude into the esophageal lumen

D. Possible clinical manifestations
  1. Anorexia

2. Nausea and vomiting
3. Hematemesis
4. Fatigue and weakness
5. Splenomegaly
6. Ascites
7. Peripheral edema
8. Melena
9. Dysphagia
10. Pallor

E. Possible diagnostic test findings
   1. Hematology: increased PT; decreased RBCs, Hgb, Hct
   2. Blood chemistry: increased BUN, LDH, AST; decreased albumin
   3. Barium swallow: narrowed and irregular esophagus
   4. Esophagoscopy: varices

F. Medical management
   1. Diet: withhold food and fluids
   2. I.V. therapy: hydration; heparin lock
   3. Oxygen therapy
   4. GI decompression: NG tube
   5. Position: semi-Fowler's
   6. Activity: bed rest
   7. Monitoring: VS, UO, and I/O
   8. Laboratory studies: Hgb, Hct, PT, and PTT
   9. Treatments: Foley catheter
   10. Transfusion therapy: packed RBCs
   11. Sengstaken-Blakemore tube
   12. Paracentesis
   13. Injection sclerotherapy: 5% morrhuate sodium
   14. Diuretic: furosemide (Lasix)
   15. Hormones: I.V. vasopressin (Pitressin) with nitroglycerin therapy (VP and NTG therapy)
   16. Antacids: magnesium and aluminum hydroxide (Maalox), aluminum hydroxide gel (ALternaGEL)
   17. Histamine antagonists: cimetidine (Tagamet), ranitidine (Zantac)
   18. Vitamins: vitamin K (AquaMEPHYTON)
   19. Iced saline lavage by NG tube
   20. Stool softeners: docusate sodium (Colace)
   21. Sclerosing agent: ethanolamine oleate (Ethamolin)
   22. Epdoscopy injection sclerotherapy (EIS)
   23. Mucosal barrier fortifier: sucralfate (Carafate)

G. Nursing interventions and responsibilities
   1. Withhold food and fluids
   2. Administer I.V. fluids
   3. Administer oxygen

   4. Assess cardiovascular and respiratory status
   5. Maintain position, patency, and low suction of NG tube and Sengstaken-Blakemore tube
   6. Keep the patient in semi-Fowler's position
   7. Monitor and record VS, UO, I/O, laboratory studies, CVP, and daily weight
   8. Administer medications, as prescribed
   9. Allay the patient's anxiety
  10. Provide nares and mouth care
  11. Minimize environmental stress
  12. Check for signs of bleeding
  13. Avoid activities that increase intra-abdominal pressure
  14. Monitor and record amount, color, frequency, and consistency of stools
  15. Assess level of consciousness
  16. Provide information about Alcoholics Anonymous

H. Teaching goals (instructions to the patient and family)
   1. Keep follow-up appointments
   2. Stop smoking
   3. Know the action, side effects, and scheduling of medications
   4. Identify ways to reduce stress
   5. Monitor stools for occult blood
   6. Avoid lifting and straining
   7. Avoid using alcohol

I. Possible medical complications
   1. Hemorrhage
   2. Shock
   3. Metabolic imbalance

J. Possible surgical interventions
   1. Ligation of varices
   2. Portacaval shunt (see page 136)
   3. Splenorenal shunt (see page 136)
   4. Mesocaval shunt (see page 136)

Points to remember

Occult blood in stool and emesis is a common finding in gastrointestinal disorders.

Imposed changes in eating and bowel habits may result in social isolation.

Peritonitis, pneumonia, atelectasis, and hemorrhage are potential complications of gallbladder surgeries.

Glossary

The following terms are defined in Appendix A, page 354.

ascites

dysphagia

hematemesis

melena

steatorrhea

Study questions

To evaluate your understanding of this chapter, answer the following questions in the space provided; then compare your responses with the correct answers in Appendix B, pages 359 and 360.

1. What are the nursing interventions before and after an endoscopy?

2. What are the key goals for teaching a patient after pancreatic surgery?

3. What are the types of portal systemic shunts? _____

4. Which complication might result after a partial gastrectomy? _____

5. What is an abdominoperineal resection? _____

6. What dietary information should the nurse teach to the patient with a hiatal hernia? _____

7. Which foods should the patient with a gastric ulcer avoid? _____

8. What would the fecal occult blood test show if a patient has gastric cancer?

Study questions *(continued)*

9. How does ulcerative colitis differ from Crohn's disease? _____

_____

_____

10. Which foods should a patient with diverticulosis avoid? _____

_____

_____

11. What are the clinical manifestations of an intestinal obstruction? _____

_____

_____

12. Which nursing intervention is contraindicated in peritonitis? _____

_____

_____

13. What is the recommended diet for a patient with hemorrhoids? _____

_____

_____

14. Where does colorectal cancer commonly metastasize? _____

_____

_____

15. What is the recommended diet for a patient with cholecystitis? _____

_____

_____

16. What would blood chemistry tests reveal for a patient with hepatic cirrhosis?

_____

_____

17. How is Type A hepatitis transmitted? _____

_____

CHAPTER 5

Endocrine System

Learning objectives

Check off the items below once you've mastered them:

☐ Describe the psychosocial impact of endocrine disorders.

☐ Differentiate between modifiable and nonmodifiable risk factors in the development of an endocrine disorder.

☐ List three probable and three possible nursing diagnoses for a patient with an endocrine disorder.

☐ Identify the nursing interventions and responsibilities for a patient with any of the endocrine disorders.

☐ Write three goals for teaching a patient with any of the endocrine disorders.

I. Anatomy and physiology

A. Hypothalamus
  1. Controls temperature, respiration, and blood pressure
  2. Affects the emotional states of fear, anxiety, anger, rage, pleasure, and pain
  3. Produces hypothalamic-stimulating hormones, which affect the inhibition and release of pituitary hormones

B. Pituitary gland
  1. Considered the "master gland"
  2. Composed of anterior and posterior lobes
    a. Posterior lobe (neurohypophysis) secretes VASOPRESSIN (antidiuretic hormone: ADH) and oxytocin
    b. Anterior lobe (adenohypophysis) secretes follicle-stimulating hormone (FSH), luteinizing hormone (LH), prolactin, adrenocorticotropic hormone (ACTH), thyroid-stimulating hormone (TSH), and growth hormone (GH)
  3. Affects all hormonal activity; factors altering pituitary gland function affect all hormonal activity

C. Thyroid gland
  1. Accelerates cellular reactions, including basal metabolic rate (BMR) and growth
  2. Controlled by secretion of TSH
  3. Produces thyroxine (T_4), tri-iodothyronine (T_3), and thyrocalcitonin

D. Parathyroid glands
  1. Secrete parathyroid hormone (parathormone: PTH), which regulates calcium and phosphorus metabolism
  2. Require active form of vitamin D for PTH function

E. Adrenal glands
  1. Adrenal cortex secretes three major hormones
    a. Glucocorticoids (cortisol)
    b. MINERALOCORTICOIDS (aldosterone)
    c. Sex hormones (androgens, estrogens, and progesterone)
  2. Adrenal medulla secretes two hormones
    a. Norepinephrine
    b. Epinephrine

F. Pancreas
  1. Accessory gland of digestion
    a. Exocrine function: secretion of digestive enzymes
      (1) Amylase
      (2) Lipase
      (3) Trypsin

    b. Endocrine function: secretion of hormones from islets of
       Langerhans
       (1) Insulin
       (2) Glucagon
       (3) Somatostatin

2. Main pancreatic duct joins the common bile duct and empties into the
   duodenum at the ampulla of Vater

II. Physical assessment findings

A. Subjective data that commonly accompany endocrine disorders
  1. Changes in weight; hair quality and distribution; body proportions,
     muscle mass, and fat distribution
  2. Fatigue and weakness
  3. Change in mood or behavior
  4. Anorexia
  5. Constipation, diarrhea, urinary frequency
  6. Change in menses and libido
  7. History of infections
  8. Intolerance of heat or cold

B. Objective data for evaluating endocrine disorders
  1. Vital signs (VS)
  2. Skin color and temperature
  3. Change in level of consciousness
  4. Pattern and character of respirations
  5. Change in urinary patterns
  6. Change in thirst
  7. Abnormalities of nails
  8. Change in visual acuity

III. Diagnostic tests and procedures

A. Venous sampling
  1. Definition and purpose
    a. Procedure using a catheter
    b. Assessment of serial hormone levels after insertion of the catheter
  2. Nursing interventions and responsibilities
    a. Withhold food and fluids before the procedure
    b. Check the venipuncture site for bleeding after the procedure

B. Hematologic studies
  1. Definition and purpose
    a. Laboratory test of a blood sample
    b. Analysis for white blood cells (WBCs), red blood cells (RBCs),
      erythrocyte sedimentation rate (ESR), platelets, prothrombin time
      (PT), partial thromboplastin time (PTT), hemoglobin (Hgb), and
      hematocrit (Hct)

2. Nursing interventions and responsibilities
    a. Note current drug therapy that might alter test results
    b. Check the venipuncture site for bleeding after the procedure

C. Blood chemistry
    1. Definition and purpose
        a. Laboratory test of a blood sample
        b. Analysis for potassium, sodium, calcium, phosphorus, ketones, glucose, osmolality, chloride, blood urea nitrogen (BUN), creatinine, T_3, T_4, protein-bound iodine (PBI), cortisol
    2. Nursing interventions and responsibilities
        a. Withhold food and fluids, as directed, before the procedure
        b. Check for recent studies using radiopaque dyes that may alter test results
        c. Note pregnancy
        d. List current medications that contain iodine
        e. Check the venipuncture site for bleeding after the procedure

D. Fasting serum glucose and two-hour postprandial glucose test
    1. Definition and purpose
        a. Laboratory test of a blood sample
        b. Analysis to measure the body's use and disposal of glucose
    2. Nursing interventions and responsibilities
        a. Withhold food and fluids for 8 hours before fasting sample is drawn
        b. Withhold insulin until the test is completed
        c. Administer 100 grams of glucose orally and request the laboratory to draw blood 2 hours later
        d. Assess the patient for hypoglycemia or hyperglycemia

E. Glucose tolerance test (GTT)
    1. Definition and purpose
        a. Laboratory test of blood and urine
        b. Analysis to measure absorption of carbohydrates
    2. Nursing interventions and responsibilities
        a. List any medications that might interfere with the test
        b. Note pregnancy, trauma, or infectious disease
        c. Provide the patient with a high-carbohydrate diet 2 days before the test; then have the patient fast 12 hours before the test begins
        d. Instruct the patient to avoid smoking, caffeine, alcohol, and exercise for 8 hours before the procedure
        e. Withhold all medications after midnight
        f. Obtain fasting serum glucose and urine specimen
        g. Administer test load oral glucose and record time
        h. Request laboratory collection of serum glucose and urine specimens at 30, 60, 120, and 180 minutes
        i. Refrigerate samples

      j. Assess the patient for hyperglycemia or hypoglycemia

F. ACTH stimulation test
    1. Definition and purpose
        a. Laboratory test of a blood sample
        b. Analysis for cortisol
    2. Nursing interventions and responsibilities
        a. List any medications that might interfere with the test
        b. Monitor 24-hour I.V. infusion of ACTH after baseline serum sample is drawn
        c. Check the venipuncture site for bleeding

G. Dexamethasone suppression test
    1. Definition and purpose
        a. Laboratory test of urine samples
        b. Analysis of serum cortisol and urinary 17-hydroxycorticosteroids (17-OH-CS) after administration of dexamethasone
    2. Nursing interventions and responsibilities
        a. Administer dexamethasone and an antacid, as prescribed
        b. Obtain single urine and 24-hour urine samples, as directed
        c. List any medications that might interfere with the test

H. 24-hour urine test for 17-ketosteroids (17-KS) and 17-OH-CS
    1. Definition and purpose
        a. Laboratory test of urine samples
        b. Quantitative laboratory analysis of urine collected over 24 hours to determine hormone precursors
    2. Nursing interventions and responsibilities
        a. Withhold all medications for 48 hours before the test
        b. Instruct the patient to void and note the time (collection of urine starts with the next voiding)
        c. Place urine container on ice
        d. Measure each voided urine
        e. Instruct the patient to void at the end of the 24-hour period
        f. List any medications that might interfere with the test

I. Urine vanillylmandelic acid (VMA) test
    1. Definition and purpose
        a. Laboratory test of urine samples
        b. Quantitative analysis of urine collected over 24 hours to determine the end products of catecholamine metabolism (epinephrine and norepinephrine)
    2. Nursing interventions and responsibilities
        a. List any medications, previous tests, and medical conditions that might interfere with the test
        b. Restrict foods that contain vanilla, coffee, tea, citrus fruits, bananas, nuts, and chocolate for 3 days before 24-hour urine collection

     c. Instruct the patient to void and note the time (collection of urine starts with the next voiding)

     d. Place urine container on ice

     e. Measure each voided urine

     f. Instruct the patient to void at the end of the 24-hour period

J. BMR
  1. Definition and purpose
     a. Noninvasive test
     b. Indirect measurement of oxygen consumed by the body during a given time
  2. Nursing interventions and responsibilities
     a. List medications taken before the procedure
     b. Note environmental and emotional stressors

K. Visual acuity and field testing
  1. Definition and purpose
     a. Noninvasive test
     b. Measurement of central and peripheral vision
  2. Nursing interventions and responsibilities
     a. Ask the patient to wear or bring corrective lenses for the test
     b. Determine the patient's hearing and ability to follow directions

L. Computerized tomography (CT)
  1. Definition and purpose
     a. Noninvasive scan that may use I.V. injection of contrast dye
     b. Visualization of the sella turcica and abdomen
  2. Nursing interventions and responsibilities
     a. Explain the procedure
     b. Note the patient's allergies to iodine, seafood, and radiopaque dyes
     c. Allay the patient's anxiety
     d. Inform the patient about possible throat irritation and flushing of the face

M. Ultrasonography
  1. Definition and purpose
     a. Noninvasive procedure using echoes from sound waves
     b. Visualization of the thyroid, pelvis, and abdomen
  2. Nursing interventions and responsibilities
     a. Withhold food and fluids 8 to 12 hours before the test
     b. Determine the patient's ability to lie still
     c. Ask the patient not to smoke or chew gum for 8 to 12 hours before the test
     d. Administer an enema before the procedure, as directed
     e. Remove abdominal dressing before the procedure

N. Closed percutaneous thyroid biopsy
  1. Definition and purpose
     a. Procedure involving a percutaneous, sterile aspiration of a small amount of thyroid tissue
     b. Histologic evaluation
  2. Nursing interventions and responsibilities before the procedure
     a. Withhold food and fluids after midnight
     b. Obtain written, informed consent
  3. Nursing interventions and responsibilities after the procedure
     a. Maintain bed rest for 24 hours
     b. Monitor VS
     c. Check the biopsy site for bleeding
     d. Assess the patient for esophageal or tracheal puncture
O. Thyroid uptake (radioactive iodine uptake: RAIU)
  1. Definition and purpose
     a. Procedure using oral or I.V. radioactive iodine
     b. Measurement of the amount of radioactive iodine taken up by the thyroid gland in 24 hours
  2. Nursing interventions and responsibilities before the procedure
     a. Advise the patient not to eat iodine-rich foods, such as iodized salt or shellfish, for 24 hours before the test
     b. Discontinue all thyroid and cough medications 7 to 10 days before the test
     c. Schedule a thyroid scan before tests using iodine-based dyes
P. Thyroid scan
  1. Definition and purpose
     a. Procedure using an oral or I.V. radioactive isotope
     b. Visual imaging of radioactivity distribution in the thyroid gland
  2. Nursing interventions and responsibilities before the procedure
     a. Advise the patient not to eat iodine-rich foods, such as iodized salt or shellfish, for 24 hours before the test
     b. Discontinue all thyroid and cough medications 7 to 10 days before the test
     c. Schedule the scan before other tests using iodine-based dyes or radioactive iodine
Q. Arteriography
  1. Definition and purpose
     a. Procedure using an injection of a radiopaque dye through a catheter
     b. Fluoroscopic examination of the arterial blood supply to the parathyroid, adrenal, or pancreatic glands
  2. Nursing interventions and responsibilities before the procedure
     a. Obtain written, informed consent

   b. Note the patient's allergies to iodine, seafood, and radiopaque dyes
   c. Inform the patient about possible throat irritation and flushing of the face after the dye injection
   d. Withhold food and fluids after midnight
   3. Nursing interventions and responsibilities after the procedure
   a. Monitor VS
   b. Check the insertion site for bleeding

R. Sulkowitch's test
   1. Definition and purpose
   a. Laboratory test of urine
   b. Analysis to measure the amount of calcium being excreted
   2. Nursing interventions and responsibilities
   a. If hypercalcemia is indicated, collect a single urine sample before a meal
   b. If hypocalcemia is indicated, collect a single urine sample after a meal

IV. Psychosocial impact of endocrine disorders

A. Developmental impact
   1. Decreased self-esteem
   2. Changes in body image
   3. Embarrassment from the changes in body function and structure, such as changes in secondary sex characteristics and sexual functioning

B. Economic impact
   1. Disruption of employment
   2. Cost of vocational retraining
   3. Cost of medications
   4. Cost of special diet
   5. Cost of hospitalizations and follow-up care

C. Occupational and recreational impact
   1. Physical activity restrictions
   2. Adjustment to change in occupation

D. Social impact
   1. Social withdrawal and isolation
   2. Changes in eating patterns
   3. Changes in role performance
   4. Changes in sexual function

V. Risk factors for developing endocrine disorders

A. Modifiable risk factors
   1. Medication
   2. Stress

3. Diet
4. Obesity

B. Nonmodifiable risk factors
1. Family history of endocrine illness
2. History of trauma
3. Aging

VI. Nursing diagnostic categories for a patient with an endocrine disorder

A. Probable nursing diagnostic categories
1. Fluid volume excess
2. Fluid volume deficit
3. Altered nutrition: more than body requirements
4. Body image disturbance
5. Altered urinary elimination

B. Possible nursing diagnostic categories
1. Potential for injury
2. Social isolation
3. Knowledge deficit
4. Noncompliance
5. Sensory-perceptual alteration: visual
6. Sensory-perceptual alteration: tactile
7. Impaired skin integrity
8. Altered thought process

VII. Adrenalectomy

A. Definition — surgical of one or both adrenal glands

B. Preoperative nursing interventions and responsibilities
1. Complete patient and family preoperative teaching
   a. Determine the patient's understanding of the procedure
   b. Describe the operating room (OR), postanesthesia care unit (PACU), and preoperative and postoperative routines
   c. Demonstrate postoperative turning, coughing, and deep breathing (TCDB), splinting, leg exercises, and range-of-motion (ROM) exercises
   d. Explain the postoperative need for drainage tubes, surgical dressings, oxygen therapy, I.V. therapy, and pain control
2. Complete a preoperative checklist
3. Administer preoperative medications, as prescribed
4. Allay the patient's and family's anxiety about surgery
5. Document the patient's history and physical assessment data base
6. Administer steroids, as prescribed
7. Administer vasopressors, as prescribed

C. Postoperative nursing interventions and responsibilities
  1. Assess cardiac, respiratory, and neurologic status and fluid balance
     a. Monitor fluid intake and output and serum electrolyte levels
     b. Keep in mind that adrenalectomy disturbs mineralocorticoid and glucocorticoid secretion, resulting in altered fluid and electrolyte balance
  2. Assess pain and administer postoperative analgesics, as prescribed
  3. Assess for return of peristalsis; provide solid foods and liquids, as tolerated
  4. Administer I.V. fluids
  5. Allay the patient's anxiety
  6. Inspect the surgical dressing and change, as directed
  7. Reinforce TCDB and splinting of incision
  8. Keep the patient in semi-Fowler's position
  9. Provide incentive spirometry
  10. Maintain activity, as tolerated
  11. Monitor VS, urinary output (UO), intake and output (I/O), central venous pressure (CVP), laboratory studies, electrocardiogram (ECG), neurovital signs, daily weight, specific gravity, urine for glucose and ketones, and pulse oximetry
  12. Monitor and maintain position and patency of drainage tubes: nasogastric (NG), indwelling urinary (Foley), wound drainage
  13. Encourage the patient to express feelings about changes in body image and the need for lifelong medication replacement
  14. Administer antacids, as prescribed
  15. Maintain a quiet environment
  16. Administer hormone replacements, as prescribed
  17. Administer vasopressors, as prescribed

D. Possible surgical complications
  1. Shock
  2. Hypoglycemia
  3. Hemorrhage
  4. Peptic ulcers
  5. Adrenal crisis
  6. Pneumothorax
  7. Acute renal failure
  8. Infection

E. Postoperative teaching goals (instructions to the patient and family)
  1. Keep follow-up appointments
  2. Maintain a normal weight
  3. Know the action, side effects, and scheduling of medications
  4. Recognize the signs and symptoms of infection, hypovolemia, and hypoglycemia
  5. Avoid exposure to people with infections
  6. Alternate rest periods with activity

7. Complete incision care daily
8. Comply with lifelong hormone replacement
9. Identify ways to reduce stress
10. Wear a medical identification bracelet
11. Monitor blood pressure daily
12. Explore methods to reduce insomnia
13. Avoid extreme temperatures

VIII. Hypophysectomy

A. Definition – surgical removal of part or all of the pituitary gland

B. Preoperative nursing interventions and responsibilities
1. Complete patient and family preoperative teaching
    a Determine the patient's understanding of the procedure
    b. Describe the OR, PACU, and preoperative and postoperative routines
    c. Demonstrate postoperative TCDB, splinting, and leg and ROM exercises
    d. Explain the postoperative need for drainage tubes, surgical dressings, oxygen therapy, I.V. therapy, and pain control
2. Complete a preoperative checklist
3. Administer preoperative medications, as prescribed
4. Allay the patient's and family's anxiety about surgery
5. Document the patient's history and physical assessment data base
6. Administer steroids, as prescribed
7. Administer antibiotics, as prescribed

C. Postoperative nursing interventions and responsibilities
1. Assess cardiac, respiratory, and neurologic status and fluid balance
2. Assess pain and administer postoperative analgesics, as prescribed
3. Assess for return of peristalsis: provide solid foods and liquids, as tolerated
4. Administer I.V. fluids
5. Allay the patient's anxiety
6. Inspect the surgical dressing or nasal drip pad and change, as directed
7. Reinforce TCDB
8. Keep the patient in semi-Fowler's position
9. Provide incentive spirometry
10. Maintain activity: as tolerated
11. Monitor VS, UO, I/O, CVP, laboratory studies, neurovital signs, daily weight, specific gravity, urine glucose and ketones, and pulse oximetry
12. Monitor and maintain the position and patency of the Foley catheter
13. Precautions: seizure
14. Encourage the patient to express feelings about changes in body image and a fear of dying

15. Administer antibiotics, as prescribed
16. Administer hormone replacements, as prescribed
17. Observe the patient for signs of increased intracranial pressure (ICP)
18. Check for rhinorrhea
19. Provide mouth and eye care
20. Avoid brushing the patient's teeth
21. Administer stool softeners, as prescribed

D. Possible surgical complications
1. Diabetes insipidus
2. Increased ICP
3. Hemorrhage
4. Adrenal crisis
5. Thyroid storm
6. Meningitis
7. Diplopia

E. Postoperative teaching goals (instructions to the patient and family)
1. Keep follow-up appointments
2. Know the action, side effects, and scheduling of medications
3. Recognize the signs and symptoms of infection, seizure activity, and hormone deficiencies
4. Avoid coughing, blowing nose, lifting, straining at stool, and sneezing
5. Wear a medical identification bracelet
6. Comply with lifelong hormone replacement

IX. Parathyroid surgeries

A. Definition
1. Thyroidectomy: surgical removal of part or all of the thyroid gland
2. Parathyroidectomy: surgical removal of one or more parathyroid glands

B. Preoperative nursing interventions and responsibilities
1. Complete patient and family preoperative teaching
   a. Determine the patient's understanding of the procedure
   b. Describe the OR, PACU, and preoperative and postoperative routines
   c. Demonstrate postoperative TCDB, splinting, and leg and ROM exercises
   d. Explain the postoperative need for drainage tubes, surgical dressings, oxygen therapy, I.V. therapy, and pain control
2. Complete a preoperative checklist
3. Administer preoperative medications, as prescribed
4. Allay the patient's and family's anxiety about surgery
5. Document the patient's history and physical assessment data base
6. Administer iodine preparations and antithyroid medications, as prescribed

C. Surgical nursing interventions and responsibilities
   1. Assess respiratory status
   2. Assess pain and administer postoperative analgesics, as prescribed
   3. Assess for return of peristalsis: provide solid foods and liquids, as tolerated
   4. Administer I.V. fluids
   5. Allay the patient's anxiety
   6. Inspect the surgical dressing for bleeding, especially at the back of the neck, and change dressing, as directed
   7. Reinforce TCDB and splinting of incision
   8. Keep the patient in semi-Fowler's position, with neutral alignment and support to neck
   9. Provide incentive spirometry
   10. Maintain activity, as tolerated
   11. Provide humidified cold steam nebulizer
   12. Monitor VS, UO, I/O, CVP, laboratory studies, urine glucose and ketones, and pulse oximetry
   13. Monitor and maintain position and patency of wound drainage tubes
   14. Precautions: seizure
   15. Encourage the patient to express feelings about a fear of choking or loss of the voice
   16. Assess for tetany
   17. Assess for hoarseness and aphasia
   18. Assess for thyroid storm
   19. Discourage talking
   20. Have calcium gluconate and tracheostomy tray available
   21. Provide specific parathyroidectomy care
       a. Provide a high-calcium diet with vitamin D
       b. Administer calcium and vitamin D supplements, as prescribed

D. Possible surgical complications
   1. Hypocalcemia
   2. Laryngeal nerve damage
   3. Hypothyroidism
   4. Respiratory distress
   5. Hemorrhage
   6. Arrhythmias

E. Postoperative teaching goals (instructions to the patient and family)
   1. Keep follow-up appointments
   2. Know the action, side effects, and scheduling of medications
   3. Recognize the signs and symptoms of infection, seizure activity, and hypothyroidism
   4. Alternate periods of talking with voice rest
   5. Complete incision care daily
   6. Complete ROM exercises of the neck daily

X. Hyperthyroidism

A. Definition – increased synthesis of thyroid hormone from overactivity (Graves' disease) or change in thyroid gland (toxic nodular goiter)

B. Possible etiology
1. Autoimmune disease
2. Genetic
3. Psychological or physiologic stress
4. Thyroid adenomas
5. Pituitary tumors
6. Infection

C. Pathophysiology
1. Thyroid-stimulating antibodies (TSAb) have a slow, sustained, stimulating effect on thyroid metabolism
2. Accelerated metabolism causes increased synthesis of thyroid hormone

D. Possible clinical manifestations
1. Anxiety
2. Flushed, smoooth skin
3. Heat intolerance
4. Mood swings
5. Diaphoresis
6. Tachycardia
7. Palpitations
8. Dyspnea
9. Weakness
10. Increased hunger
11. Increased systolic blood pressure
12. Tachypnea
13. Fine hand tremors
14. Exophthalmos
15. Weight loss
16. Diarrhea
17. Hyperhydrosis
18. Bruit or thrill over thyroid

E. Possible diagnostic test findings
1. Thyroid scan: nodules
2. Blood chemistry: increased T_3, T_4, PBI, ^{131}Iodine; decreased TSH, cholesterol
3. ECG: atrial fibrillation
4. BMR: increased

F. Medical management
1. Diet: high-protein, high-carbohydrate, high-calorie; restrict stimulants, such as coffee and caffeine
2. I.V. therapy: heparin lock

   3. Activity: bed rest
   4. Monitoring: VS, I/O
   5. Laboratory studies: T_3, T_4
   6. Sedatives: phenobarbital (Luminal)
   7. Radiation therapy
   8. Thionamides: methimazole (Tapazole), propylthiouracil (Propyl-Thyracil)
   9. Iodine preparations: potassium iodide (SSKI), radioactive iodine
  10. Adrenergic blocking agents: propranolol (Inderal), reserpine (Serpasil), guanethidine sulfate (Ismelin)
  11. Vitamins: thiamine (vitamin B_1), ascorbic acid (vitamin C)
  12. Cardiac glycoside: digoxin (Lanoxin)
  13. Tranquilizers: diazepam (Valium), chlordiazepoxide (Librium)
  14. Glucocorticoids: cortisone acetate (Cortone), hydrocortisone sodium succinate (Solu-Cortef)
  15. I.V. glucose

G. Nursing interventions and responsibilities
   1. Maintain the patient's diet
   2. Avoid stimulants, such as drugs and foods that contain caffeine
   3. Administer I.V. fluids
   4. Assess fluid balance
   5. Monitor and record VS, UO, I/O, and laboratory studies
   6. Administer medications, as prescribed
   7. Weigh the patient daily
   8. Provide rest periods
   9. Provide a quiet, cool environment
  10. Provide eye and skin care
  11. Allay the patient's anxiety
  12. Encourage the patient to express feelings about changes in body image
  13. Provide postchemotherapeutic and postradiation nursing care
      a. Provide skin, mouth, and perineal care
      b. Encourage dietary intake
      c. Administer antiemetics and antidiarrheals, as prescribed
      d. Monitor for bleeding, infection, and electrolyte imbalance
      e. Provide rest periods

H. Teaching goals (instructions to the patient and family)
   1. Keep follow-up appointments
   2. Stop smoking
   3. Maintain a normal weight
   4. Know the action, side effects, and scheduling of medications
   5. Identify ways to reduce stress
   6. Recognize the signs and symptoms of thyroid storm
   7. Adhere to activity limitations
   8. Avoid exposure to people with infections
   9. Alternate rest periods with activity

10. Monitor self for infection
11. Follow dietary recommendations and restrictions
12. Maintain a quiet environment
13. State reasons for emotional changes

I. Possible medical complications
1. Thyroid storm (thyroid crisis): tachycardia, delirium, agitation, coma, death, hyperpyrexia, dehydration, arrhythmias, diarrhea
2. Cardiac arrhythmias
3. Diabetes mellitus

J. Possible surgical interventions: subtotal thyroidectomy when euthyroid state is established (see page 190)

XI. Hypothyroidism (myxedema)

A. Definition — underactive state of thyroid gland, resulting in absence or decreased secretion of thyroid hormone

B. Possible etiology
1. Autoimmune disease: Hashimoto's thyroiditis
2. Thyroidectomy
3. Overuse of antithyroid drugs
4. Malfunction of pituitary gland
5. Use of radioactive iodine

C. Pathophysiology
1. Thyroid gland fails to secrete a satisfactory quantity of thyroid hormone
2. Hyposecretion of thyroid hormone results in overall decrease in metabolism

D. Possible clinical manifestations
1. Fatigue
2. Weight gain
3. Dry, flaky skin
4. Edema
5. Cold intolerance
6. Coarse hair
7. Alopecia
8. Thick tongue, swollen lips
9. Mental sluggishness
10. Menstrual disorders
11. Constipation
12. Hypersensitivity to narcotics, barbiturates, and anesthetics
13. Anorexia
14. Decreased diaphoresis
15. Hypothermia

E. Possible diagnostic test findings
   1. Blood chemistry: decreased T_3, T_4, PBI, sodium; increased TSH, cholesterol
   2. BMR: decreased
   3. RAIU: decreased
   4. ECG: sinus bradycardia

F. Medical management
   1. Diet: high-fiber, high-protein, low-calorie with increased fluid intake
   2. Activity: as tolerated
   3. Monitoring: VS, UO, and I/O
   4. Laboratory studies: T_3, T_4, and sodium
   5. Stool softeners: docusate sodium (Colace)
   6. Thyroid hormone replacement: levothyroxine (Synthroid), liothyronine sodium (Cytomel), thyroglobulin (Proloid)

G. Nursing interventions and responsibilities
   1. Maintain the patient's diet
   2. Force fluids
   3. Assess fluid balance
   4. Monitor and record VS, UO, I/O, and laboratory studies
   5. Administer medications, as prescribed
   6. Encourage the patient to express feelings of depression
   7. Encourage physical activity and mental stimulation
   8. Provide a warm environment
   9. Avoid sedation: administer one-half to one-third the normal dose of sedatives or narcotics
   10. Check for constipation, infection, and edema
   11. Prevent skin breakdown
   12. Provide frequent rest periods

H. Teaching goals (instructions to the patient and family)
   1. Keep follow-up appointments
   2. Exercise regularly
   3. Maintain a normal weight
   4. Know the action, side effects, and scheduling of medications
   5. Recognize the signs and symptoms of myxedema coma
   6. Alternate rest periods with activity
   7. Monitor self for constipation
   8. Follow dietary recommendations and restrictions
   9. Use additional protection in cold weather
   10. Limit activity in cold weather
   11. Avoid using sedatives
   12. Complete skin care daily

I. Possible medical complications
   1. Coronary artery disease
   2. Congestive heart failure (CHF)

3. Acute organic psychosis
4. Angina
5. Myocardial infarction (MI)
6. Myxedema coma: hypoventilation, hypothermia, respiratory acidosis, syncope, bradycardia, hypotension, seizures, and cerebral hypoxia

J. Possible surgical interventions: none

XII. Thyroid cancer

A. Definition — malignant, primary tumor of the thyroid, which does not affect thyroid hormone secretion

B. Possible etiology
1. Chronic overstimulation of the pituitary gland
2. Chronic overstimulation of the thymus gland
3. Neck radiation

C. Pathophysiology
1. Unregulated cell growth and uncontrolled cell division result in the development of a neoplasm
2. Papillary carcinoma: well-differentiated columnar cells form a solitary nodule in the thyroid gland that spreads to the cervical lymph nodes
3. Follicular carcinoma: encapsulated, well-differentiated cells that invade blood vessels and lymphatics
4. Anaplastic carcinoma: either squamous, spindle, or small round cells
5. Medullary carcinoma: solid, differentiated tumor arising from calcitonin-producing C-cells

D. Possible clinical manifestations
1. Enlarged thyroid gland
2. Painless, firm, irregular, and enlarged thyroid nodule or mass
3. Palpable cervical lymph nodes
4. Dysphagia
5. Hoarseness
6. Dyspnea

E. Possible diagnostic test findings
1. RAIU: "cold" nodule
2. Thyroid biopsy: cytology positive for cancer cells
3. Thyroid function tests: normal
4. Blood chemistry: increased calcitonin, serotonin, and prostaglandins

F. Medical management
1. Diet: high-protein, high-carbohydrate, high-calorie with supplemental feedings
2. I.V. therapy: heparin lock
3. Activity: as tolerated
4. Monitoring: VS, I/O

   5. Laboratory studies: calcitonin, serotonin
   6. Radiation therapy
   7. Chemotherapy: chlorambucil (Leukeran), doxorubicin hydrochloride (Adriamycin), vincristine sulfate (Oncovin)
   8. Thyroid hormone replacement: levothyroxine (Synthroid), liothyronine sodium (Cytomel), thyroglobulin (Proloid)
   9. Pulse oximetry
  10. Antiemetic: Nabilone (Cesamet)

G. Nursing interventions and responsibilities
   1. Maintain the patient's diet
   2. Assess respiratory status
   3. Assess ability to swallow
   4. Monitor and record VS, I/O, and laboratory studies
   5. Administer medications, as prescribed
   6. Encourage the patient to express feelings about fear of dying
   7. Provide postchemotherapeutic and postradiation nursing care
      a. Provide skin, mouth, and perineal care
      b. Encourage dietary intake
      c. Administer antiemetics and antidiarrheals, as prescribed
      d. Monitor for bleeding, infection, and electrolyte imbalance
      e. Provide rest periods
   8. Provide information about the American Cancer Society

H. Teaching goals (instructions to the patient and family)
   1. Keep follow-up appointments
   2. Maintain a normal weight
   3. Know the action, side effects, and scheduling of medications
   4. Recognize the signs and symptoms of respiratory distress and difficulty swallowing
   5. Alternate rest periods with activity
   6. Follow dietary recommendations and restrictions
   7. Seek help from community agencies and resources

I. Possible medical complications
   1. Laryngotracheal obstruction
   2. Respiratory distress
   3. Esophageal obstruction

J. Possible surgical interventions
   1. Thyroidectomy (see page 190)
   2. Modified neck dissection

XIII. Simple goiter

A. Definition — enlarged thyroid gland

B. Possible etiology
   1. Decreased iodine intake

    2. Intake of goitrogenic foods: soybeans, peanuts, peaches, strawberries
    3. Use of goitrogenic drugs: iodine, lithium, propylthiouracil
    4. Genetic defects

C. Pathophysiology
    1. Low levels of thyroid hormone stimulate increased secretion of TSH by the pituitary gland
    2. TSH stimulation causes the thyroid to increase in size to compensate for the low levels of thyroid hormone

D. Possible clinical manifestations
    1. Dysphagia
    2. Enlarged thyroid gland
    3. Dyspnea

E. Possible diagnostic test findings
    1. Blood chemistry: normal or decreased T_4
    2. RAIU: normal or increased

F. Medical management
    1. Diet: avoid goitrogenic foods, use iodized salt
    2. Activity: as tolerated
    3. Monitoring: VS, I/O
    4. Laboratory studies: T_4
    5. Iodine preparations: potassium iodide (SSKI), radioactive iodine
    6. Thyroid hormone replacement: levothyroxine (Synthroid), liothyronine sodium (Cytomel), thyroglobulin (Proloid)
    7. Avoid goitrogenic drugs

G. Nursing interventions and responsibilities
    1. Maintain the patient's diet
    2. Assess respiratory status
    3. Monitor and record VS, I/O, and laboratory studies
    4. Administer medications, as prescribed
    5. Encourage the patient to express feelings about changes in body image
    6. Assess the patient's ability to swallow

H. Teaching goals (instructions to the patient and family)
    1. Keep follow-up appointments
    2. Know the action, side effects, and scheduling of medications
    3. Recognize the signs and symptoms of respiratory distress and difficulty swallowing
    4. Follow dietary recommendations and restrictions

I. Possible medical complications
    1. Respiratory distress
    2. Laryngotracheal obstruction

J. Possible surgical interventions: subtotal thyroidectomy (see page 190)

XIV. Hyperparathyroidism

A. Definition — overactivity of one or more parathyroid glands, resulting in increased PTH secretion

B. Possible etiology
   1. Chronic renal failure
   2. Bone disease
   3. Benign adenomas
   4. Hypertrophy of parathyroid gland
   5. Malignant tumors of parathyroid gland
   6. Vitamin D deficiency
   7. Malabsorption

C. Pathophysiology
   1. Excessive secretion of PTH leads to bone demineralization and hypocalcemia
   2. Hypercalcemia increases the risk of renal calculi

D. Possible clinical manifestations
   1. Renal colic
   2. Renal calculi
   3. Arrhythmias
   4. Constipation
   5. Bowel obstruction
   6. Anorexia
   7. Weight loss
   8. Nausea and vomiting
   9. Depression
   10. Mental dullness
   11. Fatigue
   12. Osteoporosis
   13. Muscle weakness
   14. Mood swings
   15. Deep bone pain
   16. Hematuria
   17. Paresthesia
   18. Thick nails
   19. Pathologic fractures

E. Possible diagnostic test findings
   1. ECG: shortened Q-T interval
   2. Urine chemistry: decreased phosphorus; increased calcium
   3. Blood chemistry: increased calcium, BUN, creatinine, chloride, alkaline phosphatase; decreased phosphorus
   4. X-ray: osteoporosis

F. Medical management
   1. Diet: low-calcium, high-fiber, high-phosphorus in small frequent feedings; increase fluid intake to 3,000 ml/day
   2. I.V. therapy: heparin lock
   3. Activity: as tolerated
   4. Monitoring: VS, UO, and I/O
   5. Laboratory studies: calcium, phosphorus, BUN, creatinine, potassium, and sodium
   6. Radiation therapy
   7. Treatments: strain urine, bed cradle
   8. Analgesic: oxycodone hydrochloride (Tylox)
   9. Diuretics: furosemide (Lasix), ethacrynic acid (Edecrin)
   10. Antacid: aluminum hydroxide gel (ALternaGEL)
   11. Estrogen: estrogen (Premarin)
   12. Antineoplastic: plicamycin (Mithracin)
   13. Phosphate salts: K-Phos, Neutra-Phos
   14. Dialysis using calcium-free dialysate
   15. I.V. saline

G. Nursing interventions and responsibilities
   1. Maintain the patient's diet
   2. Force fluids with acidifying solutions: cranberry juice
   3. Administer I.V. fluids
   4. Assess urinary status
   5. Monitor and record VS, UO, I/O, and laboratory studies
   6. Administer medications, as prescribed
   7. Encourage the patient to express feelings about chronic illness
   8. Encourage the patient to walk
   9. Prevent falls
   10. Strain urine
   11. Assess bone, flank pain
   12. Move the patient carefully to prevent pathologic fractures
   13. Limit strenuous activity
   14. Assess the patient for constipation
   15. Provide postchemotherapeutic and postradiation nursing care
       a. Provide skin, mouth, and perineal care
       b. Encourage dietary intake
       c. Administer antiemetics and antidiarrheals, as prescribed
       d. Monitor for bleeding, infection, and electrolyte imbalance
       e. Provide rest periods

H. Teaching goals (instructions to the patient and family)
   1. Keep follow-up appointments
   2. Exercise regularly
   3. Maintain a normal weight
   4. Know the action, side effects, and scheduling of medications
   5. Recognize the signs and symptoms of renal calculi

    6. Adhere to activity limitations
    7. Alternate rest periods with activity
    8. Follow dietary recommendations and restrictions
    9. Promote a safe environment
   10. Strain urine
   11. Prevent falls
   12. Prevent constipation

I. Possible medical complications
    1. Peptic ulcer
    2. Psychosis
    3. Arrhythmias
    4. Renal failure
    5. Pathologic fractures

J. Possible surgical interventions: parathyroidectomy (see page 190)

XV. Hypoparathyroidism

A. Definition — decrease in PTH secretion

B. Possible etiology
    1. Thyroidectomy
    2. Autoimmune disease
    3. Parathyroidectomy
    4. Radiation
    5. Use of radioactive iodine
    6. Parathyroid tumor

C. Pathophysiology
    1. Decreased PTH decreases stimulation to osteoclasts, resulting in decreased release of calcium and phosphorus from bone
    2. Decreased circulating PTH reduces GI absorption of calcium and increases absorption of phosphorus
    3. Decreased blood calcium causes a rise in serum phosphates and decreased phosphate excretion by the kidney

D. Possible clinical manifestations
    1. Lethargy
    2. Calcification of ocular lens
    3. Muscle and abdominal spasms
    4. Trousseau's sign: positive
    5. Chvostek's sign: positive
    6. Tingling in fingers
    7. Arrhythmias
    8. Seizures
    9. Visual disturbances: diplopia, photophobia, blurring
   10. Dyspnea
   11. Laryngeal stridor

   12. Personality changes
   13. Brittle nails
   14. Alopecia
   15. Deep tendon reflexes: increased

E. Possible diagnostic test findings
   1. Blood chemistry: decreased PTH, calcium; increased phosphorus
   2. Urine chemistry: decreased calcium
   3. X-ray: calcification of basal ganglia; increased bone density
   4. ECG: prolonged Q-T interval
   5. Sulkowitch's test: decreased

F. Medical management
   1. Diet: high-calcium, low-phosphorus, low-sodium with spinach restriction
   2. Activity: as tolerated
   3. I.V. therapy: heparin lock
   4. Monitoring: VS, UO, and I/O
   5. Laboratory studies: PTH, calcium, and phosphorus
   6. Precautions: seizure
   7. Antacids: aluminum hydroxide gel (ALternaGEL)
   8. Sedatives: phenobarbital (Luminal)
   9. Anticonvulsants: phenytoin (Dilantin), $MgSO_4$ (Epsom salt)
  10. Vitamins: ergocalciferol (vitamin D), dihydrotachysterol (Hytakerol)
  11. Oral calcium salts: calcium gluconate (Kalcinate), calcium carbonate (Os-Cal)
  12. Diuretic: chlorthalidone (Hygroton)
  13. Hormone replacement: parathyroid extract (PTH)
  14. I.V. calcium salts: calcium chloride or calcium gluconate

G. Nursing interventions and responsibilities
   1. Maintain the patient's diet
   2. Assess neurologic status
   3. Maintain seizure precautions
   4. Monitor and record VS, I/O, and laboratory studies
   5. Administer medications, as prescribed
   6. Allay the patient's anxiety
   7. Keep tracheostomy tray and I.V. calcium gluconate available
   8. Maintain a calm environment

H. Teaching goals (instructions to the patient and family)
   1. Keep follow-up appointments
   2. Know the action, side effects, and scheduling of medications
   3. Identify ways to reduce stress
   4. Recognize the signs and symptoms of seizure activity
   5. Follow dietary recommendations and restrictions
   6. Promote a safe environment
   7. Maintain a quiet environment

I. Possible medical complications
   1. CHF
   2. Mental retardation
   3. Blindness

J. Possible surgical interventions: none

XVI. Cushing's syndrome (hypercortisolism)

A. Definition
   1. Hyperactivity of the adrenal cortex that results in excessive secretion of glucocorticoids, particularly cortisol
   2. Possible increase in mineralocorticoids and sex hormones

B. Possible etiology
   1. Hyperplasia of the adrenal glands
   2. Hypothalamic stimulation of the pituitary gland
   3. Adenoma or carcinoma of the pituitary gland
   4. Exogenous secretion of ACTH by malignant neoplasms in the lungs or gallbladder
   5. Excessive or prolonged administration of glucocorticoids or ACTH
   6. Adenoma or carcinoma of the adrenal cortex

C. Pathophysiology
   1. Hypothalamic stimulation of the pituitary gland causes excessive secretion of ACTH
   2. Excessive secretion of ACTH causes increased plasma cortisol
   3. Secretion of hypothalamic corticotropin-regulatory hormone (CRH) is not diminished by elevated blood cortisol levels

D. Possible clinical manifestations
   1. Weight gain
   2. HIRSUTISM
   3. Amenorrhea
   4. Weakness and fatigue
   5. Pain in joints
   6. Ecchymosis
   7. Edema
   8. Hypertension
   9. Mood swings
   10. Fragile skin
   11. Purple striae on abdomen
   12. Poor wound healing
   13. Truncal obesity
   14. Buffalo hump
   15. Moon face
   16. Gynecomastia
   17. Enlarged clitoris

18. Decreased libido
19. Muscle wasting
20. Recurrent infections
21. Acne

E. Possible diagnostic test findings
1. Dexamethasone suppression test: no decrease in 17-OH-CS
2. X-ray: pituitary or adrenal tumor; osteoporosis
3. Angiography: pituitary or adrenal tumors
4. CT scan: pituitary or adrenal tumors
5. Urine chemistry: increased 17-OH-CS and 17-KS; decreased specific gravity; glycosuria
6. Blood chemistry: increased cortisol, aldosterone, sodium, ACTH; decreased potassium
7. Ultrasonography: pituitary or adrenal tumors
8. Hematology: increased WBCs, RBCs; decreased eosinophils
9. GTT: hyperglycemia

F. Medical management
1. Diet: low-sodium, low-carbohydrate, low-calorie, high-potassium, and high-protein
2. Activity: as tolerated
3. Monitoring: VS, I/O, UO, urine glucose and ketones, and specific gravity
4. Laboratory studies: sodium, potassium, cortisol, BUN, glucose, WBCs, and RBCs
5. Radiation therapy
6. Chemotherapy
7. Diuretics: furosemide (Lasix), ethacrynic acid (Edecrin)
8. Potassium supplements: potassium chloride (K-Lor), potassium gluconate (Kaon)
9. Adrenal suppressants: metyrapone (Metopirone), aminoglutethimide (Cytadren)
10. Antineoplastics: mitotane (Lysodren)

G. Nursing interventions and responsibilities
1. Maintain the patient's diet
2. Assess fluid balance
3. Monitor and record VS, UO, I/O, specific gravity, finger sticks, urine glucose and ketones, and laboratory studies
4. Assess edema
5. Check for infections of skin, respiratory, and urinary tracts
6. Protect the patient from falls and bruising
7. Protect from infection
8. Provide meticulous skin care
9. Limit water intake
10. Weigh the patient daily

11. Administer medications, as prescribed
12. Encourage the patient to express feelings about changes in body image and sexual function
13. Provide rest periods
14. Minimize environmental stress
15. Provide postchemotherapeutic and postradiation nursing care
    a. Provide skin, mouth, and perineal care
    b. Encourage dietary intake
    c. Administer antiemetics and antidiarrheals, as prescribed
    d. Monitor for bleeding, infection, and electrolyte imbalance
    e. Provide rest periods

H. Teaching goals (instructions to the patient and family)
    1. Keep follow-up appointments
    2. Maintain a normal weight
    3. Know the action, side effects, and scheduling of medications
    4. Identify ways to reduce stress
    5. Recognize the signs and symptoms of infection and fluid retention
    6. Adhere to activity limitations
    7. Avoid exposure to people with infections
    8. Alternate rest periods with activity
    9. Monitor self for infection
    10. Follow dietary recommendations and restrictions
    11. Promote a safe environment
    12. Maintain a quiet environment
    13. Wear a medical identification bracelet

I. Possible medical complications
    1. Adrenal insufficiency
    2. Infection
    3. Peptic ulcers
    4. Hypertension
    5. Fractures
    6. CHF
    7. Psychosis
    8. Arrhythmias
    9. Diabetes mellitus
    10. Arteriosclerosis
    11. Nephrosclerosis

J. Possible surgical interventions
    1. Adrenalectomy (see page 187)
    2. Hypophysectomy (see page 189)

XVII. Addison's disease

A. Definition — chronic hypoactivity of the adrenal cortex, resulting in insufficient secretion of glucocorticoids (cortisol) and mineralocorticoids (aldosterone)

B. Possible etiology
1. Idiopathic atrophy of adrenal glands
2. Surgical removal of adrenal glands
3. Autoimmune disease
4. Tuberculosis
5. Metastatic lesions from lung cancer
6. Pituitary hypofunction
7. Histoplasmosis
8. Trauma

C. Pathophysiology
1. Autoimmune theory: body produces adrenocorticol antibodies, resulting in adrenal hypofunction
2. Decreased aldosterone causes disturbances in sodium, water, and potassium metabolism
3. Decreased cortisol causes abnormal metabolism of fat, protein, and carbohydrate

D. Possible clinical manifestations
1. Hypoglycemia
2. Weakness and lethargy
3. Bronzed skin pigmentation of nipples, scars, and buccal mucosa
4. Dehydration
5. Anorexia
6. Thirst
7. Decreased pubic and axillary hair
8. Orthostatic hypotension
9. Diarrhea
10. Nausea
11. Weight loss
12. Depression

E. Possible diagnostic test findings
1. Blood chemistry: decreased Hct, Hgb, cortisol, glucose, sodium, chloride, aldosterone; increased BUN, potassium
2. Urine chemistry: decreased 17-KS and 17-OH-CS
3. BMR: decreased
4. Fasting blood sugar (FBS): hypoglycemia
5. ECG: prolonged P-R and Q-T intervals

F. Medical management
   1. Diet: high-carbohydrate, high-protein, high-sodium, low-potassium in small, frequent feedings before steroid therapy; high-potassium and low-sodium when on steroid therapy
   2. I.V. therapy: hydration, electrolyte replacement; heparin lock
   3. Activity: bed rest
   4. Monitoring: VS, UO, I/O, and specific gravity
   5. Laboratory studies: sodium, potassium, osmolality, cortisol, chloride, glucose, BUN, creatinine, Hgb, and Hct
   6. I.V. saline
   7. Vasopressor: phenylephrine hydrochloride (NeoSynephrine)
   8. Antacids: Magnesium and aluminum hydroxide (Maalox), aluminum hydroxide gel (Gelusil)
   9. Mineralocorticoids (aldosterone): fludrocortisone acetate (Florinef)
  10. Glucocorticoids: cortisone acetate (Cortone), hydrocortisone (Solu-Cortef)

G. Nursing interventions and responsibilities
   1. Maintain the patient's diet
   2. Adminster I.V. fluids
   3. Assess fluid balance
   4. Monitor and record VS, UO, I/O, specific gravity, and laboratory studies
   5. Weigh the patient daily
   6. Administer medications, as prescribed
   7. Keep the patient in bed
   8. Allay the patient's anxiety
   9. Assess edema
  10. Protect the patient from falls
  11. Encourage fluid intake
  12. Assist with activities of daily living (ADLs)
  13. Maintain a quiet environment
  14. Protect the patient from infection

H. Teaching goals (instructions to the patient and family)
   1. Keep follow-up appointments
   2. Avoid strenuous exercise, particularly in hot weather
   3. Maintain a normal weight
   4. Know the action, side effects, and scheduling of medications
   5. Identify ways to reduce stress
   6. Recognize the signs and symptoms of adrenal crisis
   7. Avoid exposure to people with infections
   8. Alternate rest periods with activity
   9. Monitor self for infection
  10. Follow dietary recommendations and restrictions
  11. Maintain a quiet environment
  12. Increase fluid intake in hot weather

13. Avoid using over-the-counter drugs
14. Wear a medical identification bracelet

I. Possible medical complications
   1. Addisonian crisis (adrenal crisis): marked hypotension, cyanosis, abdominal cramps, diarrhea, costovertebral tenderness, fever, confusion, coma
   2. Arrhythmias
   3. Hypovolemic shock
   4. Renal failure

J. Possible surgical interventions: none

XVIII. Pheochromocytoma

A. Definition – catecholamine-secreting neoplasm associated with hyperfunctioning adrenal medulla

B. Possible etiology
   1. Genetics
   2. Pregnancy
   3. Trauma

C. Pathophysiology
   1. Tumor in the adrenal medulla secretes large amounts of catecholamines (epinephrine and norepinephrine)
   2. Increased catecholamines cause hypertension, increased BMR, and hyperglycemia

D. Possible clinical manifestations
   1. Labile malignant hypertension
   2. Throbbing headaches
   3. Diaphoresis
   4. Palpitations
   5. Tachycardia
   6. Excessive anxiety
   7. Hyperactivity
   8. Dilated pupils
   9. Cold extremities
   10. Weakness
   11. Weight loss
   12. Dyspnea
   13. Vertigo
   14. Angina
   15. Nausea
   16. Vomiting
   17. Anorexia
   18. Visual disturbances
   19. Polyuria

20. Diarrhea
21. Tinnitus
22. Tremors

E. Possible diagnostic test findings
1. CT scan: adrenal tumor
2. Angiography: adrenal tumor
3. BMR: increased
4. VMA: increased
5. ECG: tachycardia
6. Blood chemistries: increased BUN, creatinine, glucose, and catecholamines
7. Urine chemistries: increased glucose and catecholamines

F. Medical management
1. Diet: high-calorie, high-vitamin and mineral with restricted use of stimulants, such as caffeine beverages
2. Activity: as tolerated
3. Monitoring: VS, UO, I/O, and urine glucose and ketones
4. Position: semi-Fowler's
5. Laboratory studies: BUN, creatinine, and glucose
6. Radiation therapy
7. Sedative: phenobarbital (Luminal)
8. Alpha adrenergic blockers: phentolamine (Regitine), phenoxybenzamine hydrochloride (Dibenzyline)
9. Beta adrenergic blocker: propranolol (Inderal)
10. Vasodilator: nitroprusside sodium (Nipride)
11. Tranquilizers: diazepam (Valium), chlordiazepoxide (Librium)
12. Catecholamine inhibitor: metyrosine (Demser)

G. Nursing interventions and responsibilities
1. Maintain the patient's diet
2. Assess cardiovascular status
3. Keep the patient in semi-Fowler's position
4. Monitor and record VS, UO, I/O, orthostatic blood pressure, specific gravity, urine glucose and ketones, neurovital signs, and laboratory studies
5. Weigh the patient daily
6. Administer medications, as prescribed
7. Encourage the patient to express feelings about fear of dying
8. Protect the patient from falls
9. Minimize environmental stress
10. Provide rest periods
11. Keep phentolamine (Regitine) available

H. Teaching goals (instructions to the patient and family)
1. Keep follow-up appointments
2. Stop smoking

3. Maintain a normal weight
4. Know the action, side effects, and scheduling of medications
5. Identify ways to reduce stress
6. Recognize the signs and symptoms of renal failure
7. Avoid exposure to people with infections
8. Alternate rest periods with activity
9. Monitor self for infection
10. Follow dietary recommendations and restrictions
11. Promote a safe environment
12. Maintain a quiet environment
13. Monitor blood pressure, urine glucose, and ketones daily

I. Possible medical complications
   1. Cardiac arrest
   2. Cerebral hemorrhage
   3. Blindness
   4. Renal failure
   5. MI
   6. CHF

J. Possible surgical interventions
   1. Adrenal medulla resection after administration of phentolamine (Regitine)
   2. Adrenalectomy (see page 187)

XIX. Hyperaldosteronism (primary aldosteronism, Conn's syndrome)

A. Definition—hypersecretion of aldosterone (mineralocorticoids) from adrenal cortex

B. Possible etiology
   1. Adenoma of adrenal cortex
   2. Adrenal hyperplasia
   3. Adrenal carcinoma

C. Pathophysiology: Aldosterone's primary effect on the renal tubules causes the kidneys to retain sodium and water and excrete potassium and hydrogen

D. Possible clinical manifestations
   1. Muscle weakness
   2. Polyuria
   3. POLYDIPSIA
   4. Metabolic alkalosis
   5. Hypertension
   6. Postural hypotension
   7. Headache
   8. Paresthesia

9. Pyelonephritis
10. Nocturia
11. Chvostek's sign: positive
12. Trousseau's sign: positive

E. Possible diagnostic test findings
   1. Blood chemistry: decreased potassium; increased sodium, carbon dioxide (CO_2)
   2. Arterial blood gases (ABGs): metabolic alkalosis
   3. Urine chemistry: increased aldosterone, protein, pH; decreased specific gravity

F. Medical management
   1. Diet: high-potassium, low-sodium
   2. Activity: as tolerated
   3. Monitoring: VS, U/O, and I/O
   4. Laboratory studies: potassium, sodium, calcium, and ABGs
   5. Potassium salts: potassium chloride (KCl), potassium gluconate (Kaon)
   6. Diuretics: spironolactone (Aldactone), acetazolamide (Diamox)
   7. Calcium salts: calcium gluconate (Kalcinate), calcium carbonate (Os-Cal)

G. Nursing interventions and responsibilities
   1. Maintain the patient's diet as tolerated
   2. Assess fluid balance
   3. Monitor and record VS, UO, I/O, orthostatic blood pressure, specific gravity, and laboratory studies
   4. Monitor laboratory results: ABGs, sodium, potassium, and calcium
   5. Administer medications, as prescribed
   6. Allay the patient's anxiety
   7. Weigh the patient daily
   8. Provide a quiet environment

H. Teaching goals (instructions to the patient and family)
   1. Keep follow-up appointments
   2. Maintain a normal weight
   3. Know the action, side effects, and scheduling of medications
   4. Recognize the signs and symptoms of fluid overload and muscle irritability
   5. Alternate rest periods with activity
   6. Follow dietary recommendations and restrictions
   7. Maintain a quiet environment

I. Possible medical complications
   1. Neuropathy
   2. Arrhythmias

J. Possible surgical interventions: adrenalectomy (see page 187)

XX. Diabetes mellitus

A. Definition
   1. Chronic disorder of carbohydrate metabolism with subsequent alteration of protein and fat metabolism
   2. Results from a disturbance in the production, action, and rate of utilization of insulin
   3. Five types of diabetes mellitus
      a. Type I (insulin-dependent diabetes mellitus [IDDM], or ketosis-prone): usually develops in childhood
      b. Type II (non-insulin-dependent diabetes mellitus [NIDDM], or ketosis-resistant): usually develops after age 30
      c. Gestational diabetes mellitus (GDM): occurs with pregnancy
      d. Secondary diabetes: induced by trauma, surgery, or medications; can be treated as Type I or Type II
      e. Maturity-onset diabetes (MODY): Type II that develops in teens and young adults under age 30

B. Possible etiology
   1. Failure of body to produce insulin
   2. Blockage of insulin supply
   3. Autoimmune disease
   4. Receptor defect in normally insulin-responsive cells
   5. Genetics
   6. Exposure to chemicals
   7. Hyperpituitarism
   8. Cushing's syndrome
   9. Hyperthyroidism
   10. Infection
   11. Surgery
   12. Stress
   13. Medications
   14. Pregnancy
   15. Trauma

C. Pathophysiology
   1. Type I (IDDM) results from an inability to produce endogenous insulin by the beta cells in the islets of Langerhans in the pancreas
   2. Type II (NIDDM) is a deficit in insulin release or an insulin-receptor defect in peripheral tissues
   3. Insulin deprivation of insulin-dependent cells leads to a marked decrease in the cellular rate of glucose uptake
   4. Glucogenesis increases because of decreased stimulation of glucose metabolism with resulting hyperglycemia and glycosuria
   5. Decreased insulin triggers release of free fatty acids that cannot be metabolized and are released as ketone bodies in blood urine

    6. Decreased insulin depresses protein synthesis, causing a release of amino acids that are converted by the liver into glucose and ketones

    7. The formation of urea results in overall nitrogen loss

D. Possible clinical manifestations
1. Weight loss
2. Anorexia
3. POLYPHAGIA
4. Acetone breath
5. Weakness
6. Fatigue
7. Dehydration
8. Pain
9. Paresthesia
10. Polyuria
11. Polydipsia
12. Kussmaul respirations
13. Multiple infections and boils
14. Flushed, warm, smooth, shiny skin
15. Atrophic muscles
16. Poor wound healing
17. Mottled extremities
18. Peripheral and visceral neuropathies
19. Retinopathy
20. Sexual dysfunction
21. Blurred vision

E. Possible diagnostic test findings
1. Blood chemistry: increased glucose, potassium, chloride, ketones, cholesterol, and triglycerides; decreased CO_2; pH less than 7.4
2. Urine chemistry: increased glucose, ketones
3. FBS: increased
4. GTT: hyperglycemia
5. Postprandial blood sugar: hyperglycemia
6. Glycosylated hemoglobin assay (GHb): increased

F. Medical management
1. Diet: individually prescribed diet based on ideal weight, metabolic activity, and personal activity levels
   a. Use the American Diabetes Association's exchange list for meal planning to design a diet that will distribute an individual's caloric needs, carbohydrate, fat, and protein intake (ratio 1:1:1) over 24 hours
   b. Avoid refined and simple sugars and saturated fats
   c. Limit cholesterol
   d. Include high fiber and high complex carbohydrates
2. Activity: as tolerated

3. Monitoring: VS, UO, and I/O
4. Laboratory studies: glucose, potassium, and pH
5. Hypoglycemics: short-acting (regular, Semilente); intermediate-acting (NPH, Lente); long-acting (PZI, Ultralente); tolbutamide (Orinase), chlorpropamide (Diabinese), acetohexamide (Dymelor), tolazamide (Tolinase), glyburide (DiaBeta, Micronase), glipizide (Glucotrol)
6. Vitamin and mineral supplements

G. Nursing interventions and responsibilities
1. Maintain the patient's diet
2. Force fluids
3. Assess acid-base and fluid balance
4. Monitor and record VS, UO, I/O, finger sticks for blood glucose, and laboratory studies
5. Administer medications, as prescribed
6. Encourage the patient to express feelings about diet, medication regimen, and body image changes
7. Encourage activity, as tolerated
8. Weigh the patient weekly
9. Provide meticulous skin and foot care
10. Monitor the patient for infection
11. Maintain a warm and quiet environment
12. Monitor wound healing
13. Observe for Somogyi phenomena
14. Provide information about the American Diabetes Association
15. Foster independence
16. Determine the patient's compliance to diet, exercise, and medication regimens

H. Teaching goals (instructions to the patient and family)
1. Keep follow-up appointments
2. Exercise regularly
3. Stop smoking
4. Maintain a normal weight
5. Know the action, side effects, and scheduling of medications
6. Identify ways to reduce stress
7. Recognize the signs and symptoms of hyperglycemia and hypoglycemia
8. Alternate rest periods with activity
9. Monitor self for infection, skin breakdown, changes in peripheral circulation, poor wound healing, and numbness in extremities
10. Follow dietary recommendations and restrictions
11. Maintain a quiet environment
12. Seek help from community agencies and resources
13. Know and use proper dietary substitutions if unable to take prescribed diet because of illness

14. Adjust diet and insulin for changes in work, exercise, trauma, infection, fever, and stress
15. Demonstrate administration of hypoglycemics
16. Demonstrate home blood glucose monitoring technique (HBGM)
17. Complete daily skin and foot care
18. Wear a medical identification bracelet
19. Carry an emergency supply of glucose
20. Seek counseling for sexual dysfunction and feelings about body image changes
21. Avoid use of over-the-counter medication
22. Avoid alcohol
23. Demonstrate use of the subcutaneous insulin infusion therapy (Insulin pump)
24. Adhere to the treatment regimen to prevent complications

I. Possible medical complications
1. Ketoacidosis (diabetic coma): abdominal pain; acetone breath; altered consciousness; hot, flushed skin; Kussmaul respirations; nausea; vomiting; hypotension; oliguria; tachycardia
2. Insulin reaction (hypoglycemia): hunger, weakness, hand tremors, pallor, tachycardia, diaphoresis, irritability, confusion, diplopia, slurred speech, headaches
3. Infections
4. Peripheral neuropathies
5. Glaucoma
6. Impotence
7. Coronary artery disease
8. Gangrene
9. Cerebrovascular accident (CVA)
10. Chronic renal failure
11. Nonketotic hyperosmolar coma syndrome (HNKS): severe dehydration, severe hypotension, fever, stupor, and seizures
12. Hypovolemia
13. Diabetic retinopathy
14. Peripheral vascular disease

J. Possible surgical interventions: none

XXI. Diabetes insipidus

A. Definition—deficiency of ADH (vasopressin) that is secreted by the posterior lobe of the pituitary gland (neurohypophysis)

B. Possible etiology
1. Trauma to posterior lobe of pituitary gland
2. Tumor of posterior lobe of pituitary gland
3. Brain surgery
4. Head injury

    5. Idiopathic
    6. Meningitis

C. Pathophysiology
    1. Decreased ADH reduces the ability of distal and collecting renal tubules to concentrate urine
    2. Copious, dilute urine and intense thirst result

D. Possible clinical manifestations
    1. Polyuria (greater than 5 liters/day)
    2. Polydipsia (4 to 40 liters/day)
    3. Fatigue
    4. Dehydration
    5. Weight loss
    6. Muscle weakness and pain
    7. Headache
    8. Tachycardia

E. Possible diagnostic test findings
    1. Urine chemistry: specific gravity less than 1.004, osmolality 50 to 200 mOsm/kg
    2. Blood chemistry: decreased ADH by radioimmunoassay
    3. Water deprivation test: inability to concentrate urine

F. Medical management
    1. Diet: regular with restriction of foods that exert a diuretic effect
    2. I.V. therapy: hydration, electrolyte replacement; heparin lock
    3. Activity: bed rest
    4. Monitoring: VS, UO, CVP, and I/O
    5. Laboratory studies: potassium, sodium, BUN, creatinine, specific gravity, and osmolality
    6. Treatments: Foley catheter
    7. ADH stimulant: carbamazepine (Tegretol)
    8. ADH replacement: lypressin (Diapid nasal spray), vasopressin (Pitressin)
    9. Radiation

G. Nursing interventions and responsibilities
    1. Maintain the patient's diet
    2. Force fluids
    3. Administer I.V. fluids
    4. Assess fluid balance
    5. Maintain patency of Foley catheter
    6. Monitor and record VS, UO, CVP, I/O, specific gravity, and laboratory studies
    7. Administer medications, as prescribed
    8. Allay the patient's anxiety
    9. Weigh the patient daily

10. Provide postchemotherapeutic and postradiation nursing care
    a. Provide skin, mouth, and perineal care
    b. Encourage dietary intake
    c. Administer antiemetics and antidiarrheals, as prescribed
    d. Monitor for bleeding, infection, and electrolyte imbalance
    e. Provide rest periods

H. Teaching goals (instructions to the patient and family)
    1. Keep follow-up appointments
    2. Maintain a normal weight
    3. Know the action, side effects, and scheduling of medications
    4. Recognize the signs and symptoms of dehydration
    5. Follow dietary recommendations and restrictions
    6. Wear a medical identification bracelet
    7. Increase fluid intake in hot weather

I. Possible medical complications
    1. Dehydration
    2. Arrhythmias
    3. Hypovolemic shock

J. Possible surgical interventions: none

XXII. Hyperpituitarism (acromegaly)

A. Definition—hypersecretion of growth hormone by the anterior pituitary gland (adenohypophysis)

B. Possible etiology
    1. Prolactin-secreting benign adenomas
    2. Growth-hormone secreting tumors
    3. Cushing's syndrome caused by pituitary dysfunction
    4. LH-, FSH-, or TSH-secreting adenomas
    5. Adrenalectomy
    6. Pregnancy

C. Pathophysiology
    1. Excessive secretion of growth hormone occurs after epiphyseal closing
    2. Excessive secretion of growth hormone causes overdevelopment of cartilage, bone, soft tissue; thickens skin; and enlarges sweat glands, sebaceous glands, and gonads
    3. Growth-hormone-induced hypermetabolism causes hormone alterations

D. Possible clinical manifestations
    1. Coarse facial features
    2. Enlarged tongue
    3. Protruding jaw
    4. Spiderlike fingers
    5. Wide hands and feet

6. Weakness
7. Impotence
8. Infertility
9. Thick skin and nails
10. Diplopia
11. Cranial nerve palsies
12. Joint deformities
13. Pain in joints
14. Deepening of voice
15. Diaphoresis
16. Hirsutism
17. Headache

E. Possible diagnostic test findings
   1. Insulin tolerance test: hyperglycemia
   2. CT scan: enlarged pituitary
   3. Visual fields: hemianopia, diplopia
   4. X-rays: thickened long bones and skull
   5. Blood chemistry: increased phosphorus, prolactin, glucose, somatotropin; decreased FSH
   6. Urine chemistry: increased calcium, glucose

F. Medical management
   1. Activity: as tolerated
   2. Monitoring: VS, UO, and I/O
   3. Laboratory studies: glucose, potassium, and calcium
   4. Radiation therapy
   5. Dopaminergics: levodopa (Larodopa), bromocriptine mesylate (Parlodel)
   6. Hormones: somatotropin (Humatrope), ethinyl estradiol (Estinyl), testosterone (Delatestryl), levothyroxine sodium (Synthroid), liothyronine (Cytomel), diethylstilbesterol
   7. Glucocorticoids: cortisone acetate (Cortone), hydrocortisone (Cortef), hydrocortisone sodium succinate (Solu-Cortef)
   8. Ergot alkaloid: methysergide maleate (Sansert)
   9. Mineralocorticoid: fludrocortisone acetate (Florinef)
   10. Cryosurgery
   11. Thermocoagulation
   12. Ultrasound therapy

G. Nursing interventions and responsibilities
   1. Assess fluid balance
   2. Monitor and record VS, UO, I/O, urine glucose and ketones, finger sticks, and laboratory studies
   3. Administer medications, as prescribed
   4. Encourage the patient to express feelings about changes in body image and sexual dysfunction

5. Maintain activity, as tolerated
6. Provide skin care
7. Position and support painful joints
8. Protect the patient from falls
9. Monitor for infection
10. Provide postchemotherapeutic and postradiation nursing care
    a. Provide skin, mouth, and perineal care
    b. Encourage dietary intake
    c. Administer antiemetics and antidiarrheals, as prescribed
    d. Monitor for bleeding, infection, and electrolyte imbalance
    e. Provide rest periods

H. Teaching goals (instructions to the patient and family)
   1. Keep follow-up appointments
   2. Know the action, side effects, and scheduling of medications
   3. Identify ways to reduce stress
   4. Avoid exposure to people with infections
   5. Alternate rest periods with activity
   6. Monitor self for infection
   7. Promote a safe environment
   8. Maintain a quiet environment
   9. Wear a medical identification bracelet
   10. Carry emergency adrenal hormone replacement drugs

I. Possible medical complications
   1. Blindness
   2. Visual disturbances
   3. Diabetes mellitus
   4. Cushing's syndrome
   5. Hyperthyroidism
   6. Hypertension
   7. CHF
   8. Angina
   9. Cardiomyopathy
   10. Hyperparathyroidism
   11. Renal calculi
   12. Cardiac arrest

J. Possible surgical interventions: hypophysectomy (see page 189)

XXIII. Hypopituitarism (Simmonds' disease)

A. Definition—hypofunction of anterior pituitary gland (adenohypophysis), resulting in insufficient or absent quantities of anterior pituitary gland hormones or target organ hormones

B. Possible etiology
   1. Adenomas or carcinomas of pituitary gland

2. Postpartum hemorrhage
3. Head trauma
4. Necrosis of pituitary gland (Sheehan's syndrome)
5. Radiation of head
6. Hypophysectomy
7. Insufficient hypothalamic releasing factors

C. Pathophysiology
1. Decreased pituitary function results in decreased amounts of GH, TSH, and ACTH
2. With progressive loss of pituitary function, levels of FSH and LH also decrease

D. Possible clinical manifestations
1. Lethargy
2. Decreased strength
3. Decreased tolerance for cold temperatures
4. Hypothermia
5. Hypotension
6. Emaciation
7. Decreased axillary and pubic hair
8. Atrophy of gonads and thyroid
9. Impotence
10. Weight loss
11. Pallor
12. Decreased libido
13. Amenorrhea
14. Dry skin
15. Decreased perspiration
16. Recurrent infections
17. Headaches

E. Possible diagnostic test findings
1. Blood chemistry: decreased cortisol, growth hormone, ACTH, TSH, LH, FSH, glucose, and gonadotropins
2. RAIU: decreased
3. FBS: decreased glucose
4. GTT: decreased glucose
5. Hematology: decreased Hgb, and Hct
6. CT scan: adenohypophyseal tumor
7. Visual fields: hemianopia and loss of color vision
8. Angiography: adenohypophyseal tumor
9. Urine chemistry: decreased gonadotropins, 17-OH-CS, and 17-KS
10. Skull X-ray: adenohypophyseal tumor

F. Medical management
1. Diet: high-protein
2. Activity: as tolerated

3. Monitoring: VS, UO, I/O, and laboratory studies
4. Radiation therapy
5. Dopaminergics: levodopa (Larodopa), bromocriptine mesylate (Parlodel)
6. Hormones: somatotropin (Humatrope), ethinyl estradiol (Estinyl), testosterone (Delatestryl), levothyroxine sodium (Synthroid), liothyronine (Cytomel)
7. Glucocorticoids: cortisone acetate (Cortone), hydrocortisone (Cortef), hydrocortisone sodium succinate (Solu-Cortef)

G. Nursing interventions and responsibilities
1. Maintain the patient's diet
2. Assess fluid balance
3. Monitor and record VS, UO, I/O, urine glucose and ketones, and laboratory studies
4. Administer medications, as prescribed
5. Encourage the patient to express feelings about changes in body image and sexual dysfunction
6. Maintain activity, as tolerated
7. Prevent falls
8. Monitor for infection
9. Maintain a warm environment
10. Provide skin care
11. Allay the patient's anxiety
12. Reinforce the need to eat
13. Provide postchemotherapeutic and postradiation nursing care
    a. Provide skin, mouth, and perineal care
    b. Encourage dietary intake
    c. Administer antiemetics and antidiarrheals, as prescribed
    d. Monitor for bleeding, infection, and electrolyte imbalance
    e. Provide rest periods

H. Teaching goals (instructions to the patient and family)
1. Keep follow-up appointments
2. Maintain a normal weight
3. Know the action, side effects, and scheduling of medications
4. Recognize the signs and symptoms of dehydration
5. Avoid exposure to people with infections
6. Monitor self for infection
7. Follow dietary recommendations and restrictions
8. Promote a safe environment
9. Maintain a quiet environment
10. Alternate rest periods with activity
11. Wear a medical identification bracelet

12. Identify ways to reduce stressful stimuli

I. Possible medical complications
   1. Death
   2. Hypothyroidism
   3. Adrenal insufficiency

J. Possible surgical interventions
   1. Hypophysectomy (see page 189)
   2. Resection of pituitary gland

Points to remember

Factors altering the function of the pituitary gland—the master gland—affect all hormonal activity.

Changes in secondary sex characteristics and sexual function that accompany diseases of the endocrine system may embarrass some patients.

Disturbances in mineralocorticoid and glucocorticoid secretion alter fluid and electrolyte balance.

A patient with hyperthyroidism is susceptible to complications, including thyroid storm, arrhythmias, and diabetes mellitus.

Cushing's syndrome is associated with excessive ACTH secretion.

Diabetes insipidus involves a deficiency of ADH.

Glossary

The following terms are defined in Appendix A, page 354.

hirsutism

mineralocorticoid

polydipsia

polyphagia

vasopressin

Study questions

To evaluate your understanding of this chapter, answer the following questions in the space provided; then compare your responses with the correct answers in Appendix B, pages 360 and 361.

1. Which foods should a patient avoid before a urine VMA test? _____

_____

_____

2. In which ways can an endocrine disorder affect a patient developmentally?

_____

_____

3. What should the patient learn about hormone replacement after an adrenalectomy? _____

_____

4. Which complications might follow a hypophysectomy? _____

_____

_____

5. What type of diet and dietary supplements would be prescribed for the patient after a parathyroidectomy? _____

_____

6. What are the signs and symptoms of thyroid storm? _____

_____

_____

7. What are the clinical manifestations of hypothyroidism? _____

_____

_____

8. What would blood chemistry tests reveal about a patient with thyroid cancer?

_____

_____

Study questions *(continued)*

9. Which medications might a physician prescribe for a patient with a simple goiter? _____

_____

10. Which conditions in hyperparathyroidism are caused by increased PTH secretion? _____

_____

11. What is a key nursing intervention for a patient with hypoparathyroidism?

_____

_____

12. Which diagnostic tests would indicate that a patient has Cushing's syndrome?

_____

_____

13. Which results of the urine chemistry test indicate Addison's disease?

_____

_____

14. What are the pathophysiologic events in pheochromocytoma? _____

_____

_____

15. Which acid-base imbalance is associated with hyperaldosteronism?

_____

_____

16. What are two key clinical manifestations of diabetes insipidus? _____

_____

_____

17. What is acromegaly? _____

_____

CHAPTER 6

Renal and Urologic System

Learning objectives

Check off the items below once you've mastered them:

☐ Describe the psychosocial impact of renal and urologic disorders.

☐ Differentiate between modifiable and nonmodifiable risk factors in the development of a renal or urologic disorder.

☐ List three probable and three possible nursing diagnoses for a patient with a renal or urologic disorder.

☐ Identify the nursing interventions and responsibilities for a patient with a renal or urologic disorder.

☐ Write three goals for teaching a patient with a renal or urologic disorder.

I. Anatomy and physiology

A. Kidneys
1. Two bean-shaped organs
2. Four components: cortex, medulla, renal pelvis, and nephron
   a. Cortex
      (1) Makes up the outer layer of the kidney
      (2) Contains the glomeruli, proximal tubules of the nephron, and distal tubules of the nephron
   b. Medulla
      (1) Makes up the inner layer of the kidney
      (2) Contains the loops of Henle and the collecting tubules
   c. Renal pelvis: collects urine from the calices
   d. Nephron
      (1) Makes up the functional unit of the kidney
      (2) Contains the Bowman's capsule and the glomerulus
      (3) Contains the renal tubule, which consists of proximal convoluted, loop of Henle, distal convoluted, and collecting segments

B. Ureter
1. This tubule extends from the renal pelvis to the bladder floor
2. Ureter transports urine from the kidney to the bladder
3. Ureterovesical sphincter prevents reflux of urine from the bladder into the ureter

C. Bladder
1. Muscular, distendable sac that stores urine
2. Total capacity of approximately 1 liter

D. Urethra
1. This tubule extends from the bladder to the urinary meatus
2. Urethra transports urine from the bladder to the urinary meatus

E. Urine formation
1. Blood from the renal artery is filtrated across the glomerular capillary membrane in the Bowman's capsule
2. Filtration requires adequate intravascular volume and adequate cardiac output
3. Composition of formed filtrate is similar to blood plasma without proteins
4. Formed filtrate moves through the tubules of the nephron, which reabsorb and secrete electrolytes, water, glucose, amino acids, ammonia, and bicarbonate
5. Antidiuretic hormone (ADH) and aldosterone control the reabsorption of water and electrolytes

F. Blood pressure control
1. Regulation of fluid volume by the kidney affects blood pressure

2. Renin-angiotensin system is activated by decreased blood pressure
3. Renal disease can alter the renin-angiotensin system

G. Prostate gland
 1. This fibrous capsule is connected to and surrounds the male urethra
 2. Prostate gland contains ducts that secrete the alkaline portion of seminal fluid and that open into the prostatic portion of the urethra

II. Physical assessment findings

A. Subjective data commonly accompanying renal disorders
 1. Changes in pattern of urination: frequency, nocturia, hesitancy, urgency, dribbling, incontinence, and retention
 2. Changes in appearance of urine: dilute, concentrated, HEMATURIA, and PYURIA
 3. Dysuria
 4. Pain
 5. Chills and fever

B. Objective data to evaluate in renal disorders
 1. Urine output: POLYURIA, OLIGURIA, and ANURIA
 2. Specific gravity
 3. Hematuria
 4. Urine pH
 5. Periorbital and peripheral edema
 6. Bladder distention
 7. Skin coloring
 8. Comparison of total intake and output (I/O)
 9. Muscle tremors
 10. Pattern and character of respirations
 11. Size of prostate gland
 12. Temperature
 13. Weight

III. Diagnostic tests and procedures

A. Urinalysis
 1. Definition and purpose
   a. Laboratory test of urine
   b. Microscopic examination for color, appearance, pH, specific gravity, protein, glucose, ketones, red blood cells (RBCs), white blood cells (WBCs), and casts
 2. Nursing interventions and responsibilites
   a. Wash perineal area
   b. Obtain first morning urine specimen

B. Urine culture and sensitivity
 1. Definition and purpose

  a. Laboratory test of urine
  b. Microscopic examination for bacteria
 2. Nursing interventions and responsibilities
  a. Clean perineal area and urinary meatus with bacteriostatic solution
  b. Collect midstream sample in sterile container

C. 24-hour urine collection
 1. Definition and purpose
  a. Laboratory test of urine
  b. Quantitative analysis of samples collected over 24 hours to determine kidney function
 2. Nursing interventions and responsibilities
  a. Instruct the patient to void and note time (collection starts with the next voiding)
  b. Place urine container on ice
  c. Measure each voided urine
  d. Instruct the patient to void at the end of the 24-hour period
  e. Note medications that might alter tests results

D. Blood chemistry
 1. Definition and purpose
  a. Laboratory test of blood sample
  b. Analysis for potassium, sodium, calcium, phosphorus, glucose, bicarbonate, blood urea nitrogen (BUN), creatinine, protein, albumin, and osmolality
 2. Nursing interventions and responsibilities
  a. Withhold food and fluids before the procedure, as directed
  b. Check the site for bleeding after the procedure

E. Kidneys, ureters, bladder (KUB) X-ray
 1. Definition and purpose
  a. Noninvasive examination of the renal system
  b. Radiographic picture of the kidneys, ureters, and bladder
 2. Nursing interventions and responsibilities
  a. Schedule the x-ray before other examinations requiring contrast medium
  b. Ensure that the patient removes metallic belts

F. I.V. pyelogram (IVP)
 1. Definition and purpose
  a. Procedure using an injection of a radiopaque dye
  b. Fluoroscopic examination of kidneys, ureters, and bladder
 2. Nursing interventions and responsibilities before the procedure
  a. Note the patient's allergies to iodine, seafood, and radiopaque dyes
  b. Withhold food and fluids after midnight
  c. Administer laxatives, as prescribed

       d. Inform the patient about possible throat irritation and flushing of the face
    3. Nursing interventions and responsibilities after the procedure
       a. Instruct the patient to drink at least 1 liter of fluids
       b. Check the venipuncture site for bleeding

G. Cystoscopy
    1. Definition and purpose
       a. Procedure using a cystoscope
       b. Direct visualization of the bladder
    2. Nursing interventions and responsibilities before the procedure
       a. Withhold food and fluids
       b. Allay the patient's anxiety
       c. Obtain written, informed consent
       d. Administer enemas and medications, as prescribed
    3. Nursing interventions and responsibilities after the procedure
       a. Administer analgesics and sitz baths, as prescribed
       b. Monitor I/O and vital signs (VS)
       c. Check the patient's urine for clots
       d. Force fluids

H. Renal angiography
    1. Definition and purpose
       a. Procedure using an injection of a radiopaque dye through a catheter
       b. Radiographic examination of the renal arterial supply
    2. Nursing interventions and responsibilities before the procedure
       a. Allay the patient's anxiety
       b. Inform the patient about a possible burning feeling after dye is injected
       c. Obtain written, informed consent
       d. Withhold food and fluids after midnight
       e. Instruct the patient to void immediately before procedure
       f. Administer enemas, as prescribed
    3. Nursing interventions and responsibilities after the procedure
       a. Assess VS and peripheral pulses
       b. Inspect the catheter insertion site for bleeding
       c. Force fluids

I. Renal scan
    1. Definition and purpose
       a. Procedure using an I.V. injection of a radioisotope
       b. Visual imaging of blood flow distribution to the kidneys
    2. Nursing interventions and responsibilities before the procedure
       a. Assist with administering radioisotope as necessary
       b. Check the patient's history for allergies
    3. Nursing interventions and responsibilities after the procedure

       a. Assess the patient for signs of delayed allergic reaction, such as itching and hives

       b. Wear gloves when caring for incontinent patients and double-bag linens

J. Renal biopsy
1. Definition and purpose
   a. Percutaneous procedure to remove a small amount of renal tissue
   b. Histologic evaluation
2. Nursing interventions and responsibilities before the procedure
   a. Assess baseline clotting studies and VS
   b. Withhold food and fluids after midnight
   c. Obtain written, informed consent
3. Nursing interventions and responsibilities after the procedure
   a. Monitor and record VS, hemoglobin (Hgb) and hematocrit (Hct)
   b. Check biopsy site for bleeding

K. Cystourethrogram
1. Definition and purpose
   a. Procedure calling for the insertion of a catheter and the introduction of dye
   b. Visualization of the bladder and ureters
2. Nursing interventions and responsibilities
   a. Allay the patient's anxiety
   b. Advise the patient about voiding requirements during the procedure
   c. Monitor voiding after the procedure

L. Cystometrogram (CMG)
1. Definition and purpose
   a. Procedure to test the urinary bladder
   b. Graphic recording of the pressures exerted at varying phases of filling of the bladder
2. Nursing interventions and responsibilities before the procedure
   a. Allay the patient's anxiety
   b. Advise the patient about voiding requirements during the procedure
   c. Monitor voiding after the procedure

M. Hematologic studies
1. Definition and purpose
   a. Laboratory test of blood sample
   b. Analysis of blood sample for WBCs, RBCs, erythrocyte sedimentation rate (ESR), platelets, prothrombin time (PT), partial thromboplastin time (PTT), Hgb, and Hct
2. Nursing interventions and responsibilities
   a. Explain the purpose of the procedure
   b. Check the venipuncture site for bleeding

IV. Psychosocial impact of renal and urologic disorders

A. Developmental impact
   1. Body image changes
   2. Feeling of lack of control over body functions
   3. Fear of rejection
   4. Embarrassment from changes in body function and structure
   5. Decreased self-esteem

B. Economic impact
   1. Cost of renal dialysis and organ transplant
   2. Cost of hospitalizations and follow-up care
   3. Cost of medications
   4. Cost of special diet
   5. Disruption of employment

C. Occupational and recreational impact
   1. Restrictions in physical activity
   2. Changes in leisure activity

D. Social impact
   1. Changes in eating patterns
   2. Social isolation
   3. Changes in elimination patterns and modes
   4. Changes in sexual function

V. Risk factors for developing renal and urologic disorders

A. Modifiable risk factors
   1. Diet: high-sodium, high-calcium
   2. Exposure to chemical and environmental pollutants
   3. Smoking
   4. Contact sports
   5. Culturally based reluctance to discuss hygiene and health habits

B. Nonmodifiable risk factors
   1. History of renal dysfunction
   2. History of hypertension
   3. Aging
   4. Family history of renal disease

VI. Nursing diagnostic categories for a patient with a renal or urologic disorder

A. Probable nursing diagnostic categories
   1. Fluid volume deficit (regulatory failure)
   2. Fluid volume excess
   3. Altered urinary elimination
   4. Pain

5. Sexual dysfunction
6. Body image disturbance
7. Self-esteem disturbance

B. Possible nursing diagnostic categories
   1. Impaired skin integrity
   2. Noncompliance
   3. Activity intolerance
   4. Anticipatory grieving
   5. Impaired gas exchange

VII. Kidney transplantation

A. Definition – implantation of a kidney to a person who requires dialysis during the last stage of renal disease

B. Preoperative nursing interventions and responsibilities
   1. Complete patient and family preoperative teaching
      a. Determine the patient's understanding of the procedure
      b. Describe the operating room (OR), postanesthesia unit (PACU), and preoperative and postoperative routines
      c. Demonstrate postoperative turning, coughing, and deep breathing (TCDB), splinting, leg exercises, and range-of-motion (ROM) exercises
      d. Explain the postoperative need for drainage tubes, surgical dressings, oxygen therapy, I.V. therapy, and pain control
   2. Complete a preoperative checklist
   3. Administer preoperative medications, as prescribed
   4. Allay the patient's and family's anxiety about surgery
   5. Document the patient's history and physical assessment data base
   6. Verify histocompatability tests
   7. Administer immunosuppressive drugs, as prescribed, for 2 days before the transplantation
   8. Maintain protective isolation
   9. Administer transfusion therapy, as prescribed
   10. Administer I.V. therapy, as prescribed
   11. Monitor urinary output (UO)
   12. Verify that hemodialysis was completed 24 hours before transplant

C. Postoperative nursing interventions and responsibilities
   1. Assess cardiac and respiratory status and fluid balance
   2. Assess pain and administer postoperative analgesics, as prescribed
   3. Assess for return of peristalsis; give solid foods and liquids, as tolerated
   4. Administer I.V. fluids and transfusion therapy, as prescribed
   5. Allay the patient's anxiety
   6. Inspect the surgical dressing and change, as directed
   7. Reinforce TCDB and splinting of incision

8. Keep the patient in semi-Fowler's position
9. Provide incentive spirometry, intermittent positive pressure breathing (IPPB)
10. Maintain activity: as tolerated, increase walking
11. Monitor and record VS, UO, I/O, central venous pressure (CVP), laboratory studies, urine for blood, electrocardiogram (ECG), specific gravity, daily weight, pulse oximetry, and creatinine levels
12. Monitor and maintain position and patency of drainage tubes: indwelling urinary catheter (Foley), nasogastric (NG), wound drainage
13. Isolation precautions: protective
14. Encourage the patient to express feelings about chronicity of illness, fear of dying, guilt
15. Administer antifungals, as prescribed
16. Administer immunosuppressive agents with synthetic prostaglandins, as prescribed
17. Administer corticosteroids, as prescribed
18. Assess for organ rejection
19. Monitor for infection
20. Provide mouth and skin care
21. Administer antibiotics, as prescribed
22. Administer antilymphocytic globulin (ALG) and antithymocytic globulin (ATG or RATG)), as prescribed
23. Prepare for hemodialysis
24. Avoid prolonged periods of sitting
25. Promote live donor and recipient relationship
26. Monitor for depression
27. Monitor for edema of the scrotum, labia, or thigh ipsilateral to the graft
28. Assess the allograft site for pain and edema

D. Possible surgical complications
1. Renal graft rejection
2. Gastrointestinal hemorrhage
3. Acute renal failure
4. Bladder and ureter fistulas
5. Candidiasis of mouth
6. Hypertension
7. Cerebrovascular accident (CVA)
8. Gastric ulcer
9. Liver failure
10. Depression
11. Psychosis
12. Congestive heart failure
13. Hypovolemia

E. Postoperative teaching goals (instructions to the patient and family)
1. Keep follow-up appointments

   2. Stop smoking
   3. Maintain a normal weight
   4. Know the action, side effects, and scheduling of medications
   5. Recognize the signs and symptoms of infection and rejection
   6. Avoid contact sports
   7. Complete incision care daily
   8. Adhere to a low-sodium and low-protein diet
   9. Avoid exposure to people with infections
  10. Monitor stool for occult blood
  11. Monitor self for infection

VIII. Kidney surgery

A. Definition
   1. Nephrectomy: surgical removal of the entire kidney
   2. Lithotomy: surgical removal of renal calculi

B. Preoperative nursing interventions and responsibilities
   1. Complete patient and family preoperative teaching
     a. Determine the patient's understanding of the procedure
     b. Describe the OR, PACU, and preoperative and postoperative routines
     c. Demonstrate postoperative TCDB, splinting, and leg and ROM exercises
     d. Explain the postoperative need for drainage tubes, surgical dressings, oxygen therapy, I.V. therapy, and pain control
   2. Complete a preoperative checklist
   3. Administer preoperative medications, as prescribed
   4. Allay the patient's and family's anxiety about surgery
   5. Document the patient's history and physical assessment data base
   6. Administer antibiotics, as prescribed

C. Postoperative nursing interventions and responsibilities
   1. Assess cardiac, respiratory, and neurologic status and fluid balance
   2. Assess pain and administer analgesics, as prescribed
   3. Assess for return of peristalsis; give solid foods, as tolerated, with increased fluids
   4. Administer I.V. fluids, transfusion therapy, and IVH, as prescribed
   5. Allay the patient's anxiety
   6. Inspect the surgical dressing and change as directed
   7. Reinforce TCDB and splinting of incision
   8. Keep the patient in semi-Fowler's position
   9. Provide incentive spirometry
  10. Maintain activity: as tolerated, active and passive ROM exercises, increase walking
  11. Monitor and record VS, UO, I/O, CVP, laboratory studies, urine for blood, daily weight, specific gravity, and pulse oximetry

12. Monitor and maintain position and patency of drainage tubes: NG, Foley, wound drainage, nephrostomy, suprapubic, ureteral
13. Encourage the patient to express feelings about changes in body image and a fear of dying
14. Administer antibiotics, as prescribed
15. Administer stool softeners, as prescribed
16. Do not irrigate or manipulate the nephrostomy tube
17. Apply antiembolism stockings

D. Possible surgical complications
   1. Hemorrhage
   2. Atelectasis
   3. Pneumothorax
   4. Pneumonia
   5. Paralytic ileus

E. Postoperative teaching goals (instructions to the patient and family)
   1. Keep follow-up appointments
   2. Know the action, side effects, and scheduling of medications
   3. Recognize the signs and symptoms of infection and renal failure
   4. Complete incision care daily
   5. Avoid using over-the-counter medications
   6. Increase fluid intake and drink lots of cranberry juice
   7. Avoid lifting, straining, horseback riding, and contact sports
   8. Void frequently

IX. Prostate surgery

A. Definition
   1. Transurethral resection of prostate (TURP): insertion of a resectoscope into the urethra to excise prostatic tissue
   2. Suprapubic prostatectomy: low abdominal incision into the bladder to the anterior aspect of the prostate to remove large tumors of the prostate
   3. Retropubic prostatectomy: low midline incision below the bladder into prostatic capsule to remove a mass in the pelvic area
   4. Perineal prostatectomy: incision through the perineum to remove the prostate and surrounding tissue

B. Preoperative nursing interventions and responsibilities
   1. Complete patient and family preoperative teaching
      a. Determine the patient's understanding of the procedure
      b. Describe the OR, PACU, and preoperative and postoperative routines
      c. Demonstrate postoperative TCDB, splinting, and leg and ROM exercises
      d. Explain the postoperative need for drainage tubes, surgical dressings, oxygen therapy, I.V. therapy, and pain control
   2. Complete a preoperative checklist

3. Administer preoperative medications, as prescribed
4. Allay the patient's and family's anxiety about surgery
5. Document the patient's history and physical assessment data base
6. Administer antibiotics, as prescribed

C. Postoperative nursing interventions and responsibilities
1. Assess cardiac and respiratory status and fluid balance
2. Assess pain and administer postoperative analgesics, as prescribed
3. Assess for return of peristalsis; provide a high-protein, high-fiber, acid-ash diet, as tolerated, with increased fluids
4. Administer I.V. fluids
5. Allay the patient's anxiety
6. Inspect the surgical dressing and change, as directed
7. Reinforce TCDB and splinting of incision
8. Keep the patient in semi-Fowler's position
9. Provide incentive spirometry
10. Maintain activity: as tolerated, progressive ambulation
11. Monitor and record VS, UO, I/O, laboratory studies, urine for blood, stool counts, and pulse oximetry
12. Monitor and maintain position and patency of drainage tubes: NG, Foley, wound drainage, suprapubic
13. Encourage the patient to express feelings about changes in body image and fear of sexual dysfunction
14. Administer stool softeners, as prescribed
15. Maintain closed continuous bladder irrigation
16. Administer antibiotics, as prescribed
17. Provide treatments: sitz baths
18. Administer anticholinergics, as prescribed
19. Administer antispasmodics, as prescribed
20. Avoid rectal temperatures and enemas
21. Administer urinary antiseptics, as prescribed
22. Monitor urinary patterns after removal of catheters

D. Possible surgical complications
1. Hemorrhage
2. Shock
3. Infection
4. Epididymitis
5. Impotence

E. Postoperative teaching goals (instructions to the patient and family)
1. Keep follow-up appointments
2. Stop smoking
3. Know the action, side effects, and scheduling of medications
4. Recognize the signs and symptoms of infection, bleeding, and urinary tract obstruction
5. Complete incision care daily

6. Avoid using over-the-counter medications
7. Avoid Valsalva's maneuver, lifting, exercising vigorously, or prolonged sitting in the car
8. Increase fluid intake
9. Complete perineal strengthening exercises daily
10. Avoid alcohol and caffeine

X. Urinary diversion

A. Definition
1. Ureterosigmoidostomy: ureters are excised from the bladder and implanted into the sigmoid colon; urine flows through the colon and is excreted through the rectum
2. Nephrostomy: percutaneous insertion of catheter into kidney
3. Ileal conduit: ureters are implanted into a segment of the ileum that has been resected from the intestinal tract with the formation of an abdominal stoma
4. Cutaneous ureterostomy: ureters are excised from the bladder and brought through the abdominal wall to create a stoma

B. Preoperative nursing interventions and responsibilities
1. Complete patient and family preoperative teaching
   a. Determine the patient's understanding of the procedure
   b. Describe the OR, PACU, and preoperative and postoperative routines
   c. Demonstrate postoperative TCDB, splinting, and leg and ROM exercises
   d. Explain the postoperative need for drainage tubes, surgical dressings, oxygen therapy, I.V. therapy, and pain control
2. Complete a preoperative checklist
3. Administer preoperative medications, as prescribed
4. Allay the patient's and family's anxiety about surgery
5. Document the patient's history and physical assessment data base
6. Administer bowel preparation, as prescribed

C. Postoperative nursing interventions and responsibilities
1. Assess renal status and fluid balance
2. Assess pain and administer postoperative analgesics, as prescribed
3. Assess for return of peristalsis; provide acid-ash diet, as tolerated, with increased fluids; avoid giving milk and dairy products
4. Administer I.V. fluids
5. Allay the patient's anxiety
6. Inspect the surgical dressing and change, as directed
7. Reinforce TCDB and splinting of incision
8. Keep the patient in semi-Fowler's position
9. Provide incentive spirometry
10. Maintain activity: as tolerated, increased walking

11. Monitor and record VS, UO, I/O, laboratory studies, daily weight, specific gravity, and pulse oximetry
12. Monitor and maintain position and patency of drainage tubes: NG, Foley, wound drainage
13. Encourage the patient to express feelings about changes in body image, embarrassment, and sexual dysfunction
14. Administer antibiotics, as prescribed
15. Administer antispasmodics, as prescribed
16. Apply and change ostomy bags
17. Provide skin care, particularly around the stoma
18. Apply antiembolism stockings

D. Possible surgical complications
   1. Chronic renal failure
   2. Infection
   3. Urinary and rectal fistulas
   4. Hemorrhage
   5. Peritonitis
   6. Ureteral obstruction
   7. Stomal stenosis
   8. Bowel obstruction
   9. Renal calculi

E. Postoperative teaching goals (instructions to the patient and family)
   1. Keep follow-up appointments
   2. Know the action, side effects, and scheduling of medications
   3. Recognize the signs and symptoms of infection and stomal stenosis
   4. Complete stoma and skin care daily
   5. Use ostomy bags and leg bags
   6. Increase fluid intake
   7. Follow dietary recommendations and restrictions
   8. Avoid enemas and laxatives
   9. Empty urinary diversion appliances frequently

XI. Cystitis

A. Definition—inflammation of the urinary bladder related to a superficial infection that does not extend to the bladder mucosa

B. Possible etiology
   1. Stagnation of urine in the bladder
   2. Obstruction of the urethra
   3. Sexual intercourse
   4. Incorrect aseptic technique during catheterization
   5. Incorrect perineal care
   6. Kidney infection
   7. Radiation
   8. Diabetes mellitus

9. Pregnancy

C. Pathophysiology
 1. Bacterial infection from a secondary source spreads to the bladder, causing an inflammatory response
 2. Cell destruction from trauma to the bladder wall, particularly the trigone area, initiates an acute inflammatory reaction

D. Possible clinical manifestations
 1. Frequency of urination
 2. Urgency of urination
 3. Burning or pain on urination
 4. Lower abdominal discomfort
 5. Dark, odoriferous urine
 6. Flank tenderness or suprapubic pain
 7. Nocturia
 8. Low-grade fever
 9. Urge to bear down on urination
 10. Dysuria
 11. Dribbling

E. Possible diagnostic test findings
 1. Urine culture and sensitivity: positive identification of organisms *(E. coli, P. vulgaris, S. faecalis)*
 2. Urine chemistry: hematuria, pyuria; increased protein, leukocytes, specific gravity
 3. Cystoscopy: obstruction or deformity

F. Medical management
 1. Diet: acid-ash diet with increased intake of fluids and vitamin C
 2. Activity: as tolerated
 3. Monitoring: VS, UO, and I/O
 4. Laboratory studies: specific gravity, urine culture and sensitivity
 5. Treatments: sitz baths
 6. Antibiotics: trimethoprim and sulfamethoxazole (Bactrim), cephalexin (Keflex)
 7. Analgesics: oxycodone hydrochloride (Tylox)
 8. Urinary antiseptics: phenazopyridine (Pyridium)
 9. Antipyretics: acetaminophen (Tylenol)

G. Nursing interventions and responsibilities
 1. Maintain the patient's diet
 2. Force fluids (cranberry or orange juice) to 3,000 ml/day
 3. Assess renal status
 4. Monitor and record VS, UO, I/O, and laboratory studies
 5. Administer medications, as prescribed
 6. Allay the patient's anxiety
 7. Maintain treatments: sitz baths, perineal care

    8. Encourage voiding every 2 to 3 hours

H. Teaching goals (instructions to the patient and family)
1. Keep follow-up appointments
2. Stop smoking
3. Know the action, side effects, and scheduling of medications
4. Recognize the signs and symptoms of recurrent infection
5. Avoid coffee, tea, alcohol, and cola
6. Increase fluid intake to 3,000 ml/day using orange juice and cranberry juice
7. Void every 2 to 3 hours and after intercourse
8. Perform perineal care correctly
9. Avoid bubble baths, vaginal deodorants, and tub baths

I. Possible medical complications
1. Chronic cystitis
2. Urethritis
3. Pyelonephritis

J. Possible surgical interventions: none

XII. Glomerulonephritis

A. Definition—inflammation of the capillary loops in the glomeruli of the kidney

B. Possible etiology
1. Injected serum proteins
2. Systemic lupus erythematosus
3. Group A beta-hemolytic streptococcal infection

C. Pathophysiology
1. Antigen-antibody complexes are filtered and trapped within the glomeruli, causing inflammation
2. Inflammation occludes the glomeruli, causing decreased glomerular filtration and retention of protein wastes and electrolytes

D. Possible clinical manifestations
1. Bradycardia
2. Pharyngitis and tonsillitis
3. Peripheral and periorbital edema
4. Lethargy and malaise
5. Anorexia
6. Elevated temperature
7. Hypertension
8. Tea-colored urine
9. Flank pain
10. Dyspnea
11. Visual disturbances

12. Dizziness
13. Oliguria
14. Seizures
15. Weight loss
16. Dehydration

E. Possible diagnostic test findings
1. Urine chemistry: increased RBCs, WBCs, protein, casts, specific gravity
2. Blood chemistry: increased BUN, creatinine; decreased protein, creatine clearance, C-reactive protein, albumin
3. Hematology: decreased Hgb, Hct; increased ESR
4. Renal biopsy: inflammation of the glomerular capillaries

F. Medical management
1. Diet: high-carbohydrate, high-vitamin, with restricted intake of sodium, protein, potassium, and fluids
2. I.V. therapy: heparin lock
3. Activity: bed rest
4. Monitoring: VS, UO, I/O, and ECG
5. Laboratory studies: BUN, creatinine, specific gravity, sodium, potassium, glucose, Hgb, and Hct
6. Antibiotics: penicillin V potassium (Pen-Vee K), ampicillin (Omnipen)
7. Antihypertensives: diazoxide (Hyperstat), hydralazine hydrochloride (Apresoline)
8. Cardioglycoside: digoxin (Lanoxin)
9. Immunosuppressants: cyclophosphamide (Cytoxan), azathioprine (Imuran)
10. Antacids: magnesium and aluminum hydroxide (Maalox), aluminum hydroxide gel (ALternaGEL)
11. Corticosteroid: prednisone (Deltasone)
12. Diuretics: chlorthalidone (Hygroton), furosemide (Lasix)
13. Peritoneal dialysis and hemodialysis
14. Anticoagulants: warfarin sodium (Coumadin), heparin sodium (Lipo-Hepin)
15. Precautions: seizure

G. Nursing interventions and responsibilities
1. Maintain the patient's diet
2. Restrict fluids
3. Reinforce TCDB
4. Assess renal, respiratory, cardiovascular, and neurologic status and fluid balance
5. Monitor and record VS, UO, I/O, ECG, laboratory studies, urine glucose and ketones, hematuria, weight, and specific gravity
6. Administer medications, as prescribed
7. Encourage the patient to express feelings about changes in body image

8. Maintain seizure precautions
9. Protect the patient from falls
10. Monitor for bleeding and infection
11. Provide skin and mouth care

H. Teaching goals (instructions to the patient and family)
1. Keep follow-up appointments
2. Stop smoking
3. Maintain a normal weight
4. Know the action, side effects, and scheduling of medications
5. Recognize the signs and symptoms of renal failure
6. Avoid exposure to people with infections
7. Alternate rest periods with activity
8. Monitor self for infection
9. Follow dietary recommendations and restrictions

I. Possible medical complications
1. Metabolic acidosis
2. Chronic renal failure
3. Hypertensive encephalopathy
4. Congestive heart failure (CHF)
5. Nephrotic syndrome
6. Pulmonary edema

J. Possible surgical interventions: none

XIII. Pyelonephritis

A. Definition — inflammation of renal pelvis

B. Possible etiology
1. Enteric bacteria
2. Ureterovesical reflux
3. Urinary tract obstruction
4. Pregnancy
5. Trauma
6. Urinary tract infection
7. Incorrect aseptic technique
8. Diabetes mellitus
9. Staphylococcal or streptococcal infections

C. Pathophysiology
1. Bacterial infection from a secondary source spreads to the renal pelvis, causing an inflammatory response
2. Cell destruction from trauma to the renal pelvis initiates an inflammatory reaction

D. Possible clinical manifestations
1. Elevated temperature

    2. Chills
    3. Nausea and vomiting
    4. Flank pain
    5. Chronic fatigue
    6. Bladder irritability
    7. Hypertension
    8. Dysuria
    9. Burning on urination
  10. Frequency of urination
  11. Urgency of urination
  12. Headache
  13. Anorexia
  14. Weight loss
  15. Odoriferous, concentrated urine

E. Possible diagnostic test findings
    1. IVP: atrophy, blockage, or deformity of kidney
    2. Urine culture and sensitivity: bacteria
    3. Urine chemistry: pyuria, hematuria; leukocytes, WBCs, and casts; specific gravity greater than 1.025; albuminuria
    4. Hematology: increased WBCs
    5. 24-hour urine collection: decreased creatinine clearance

F. Medical management
    1. Diet: soft, high-calorie, low-protein
    2. I.V. therapy: heparin lock
    3. Activity: as tolerated
    4. Monitoring: VS, UO, I/O, urine pH, and specific gravity
    5. Laboratory studies: WBCs, urine protein, and urine culture and sensitivity
    6. Treatments: warm, moist compresses to flank
    7. Fluid intake: 3,000 ml/day
    8. Analgesic: meperidine hydrochloride (Demerol)
    9. Antibiotics: cefazolin (Ancef), cefoxitin (Mefoxin), trimethoprim and sufamethoxazole (Bactrim)
  10. Urinary antiseptic: phenazopyridine (Pyridium)
  11. Antiemetic: prochlorperazine (Compazine)
  12. Alkalinizers: potassium acetate, sodium bicarbonate
  13. Sedative: phenobarbital (Luminal)
  14. Peritoneal dialysis and hemodialysis

G. Nursing interventions and responsibilities
    1. Maintain the patient's diet
    2. Force fluids to 3,000 ml/day
    3. Assess renal status and fluid balance
    4. Monitor and record VS, UO, I/O, laboratory studies, daily weight, specific gravity, and urine for blood, protein, and pH

5. Administer medications, as prescribed
6. Allay the patient's anxiety
7. Continue giving hot, moist compresses; warm baths
8. Prevent chilling
9. Provide rest periods
10. Provide skin, mouth, and perineal care
11. Encourage frequent voiding

H. Teaching goals (instructions to the patient and family)
1. Keep follow-up appointments
2. Know the action, side effects, and scheduling of medications
3. Recognize the signs and symptoms of urinary tract infection
4. Alternate rest periods with activity
5. Follow dietary recommendations and restrictions
6. Void frequently

I. Possible medical complications
1. Chronic renal failure
2. Hypertension
3. Septicemia

J. Possible surgical interventions: none

XIV. Urolithiasis

A. Definition—stones in kidney, ureters, or bladder

B. Possible etiology
1. Diet high in calcium, vitamin D, milk, protein, oxalate, alkali
2. Gout
3. Hyperparathyroidism
4. Urinary tract infection
5. Urinary stasis
6. Dehydration
7. Idiopathic
8. Immobility
9. Genetics
10. Hypercalcemia
11. Urinary tract obstruction
12. Leukemia
13. Polycythemia vera
14. Chemotherapy

C. Pathophysiology
1. Crystalline substances that normally are dissolved and excreted in the urine form precipitates
2. Stones are composed of calcium phosphate, oxalate, or uric acid

D. Possible clinical manifestations
  1. Flank pain
  2. Costovertebral tenderness
  3. Cool, moist skin
  4. RENAL COLIC
  5. Frequency of urination
  6. Urgency of urination
  7. Diaphoresis
  8. Chills and fever
  9. Pallor
  10. Nausea and vomiting
  11. Syncope
  12. Dysuria

E. Possible diagnostic test findings
  1. KUB: stones
  2. IVP: stones
  3. Urine chemistry: pyuria, proteinuria, hematuria, presence of WBCs, increased specific gravity
  4. Cystoscopy: visualization of stones
  5. 24-hour urine collection: increased uric acid, oxalate, calcium, phosphorus, creatinine
  6. Blood chemistry: increased calcium, phosphorus, creatinine, BUN, uric acid, protein, alkaline phosphatase

F. Medical management
  1. Diet
     a. For calcium stones—acid-ash with limited intake of calcium and milk products
     b. For oxalate stones—alkaline-ash with limited intake of foods high in oxalate (cola, tea)
     c. For uric acid stones—alkaline-ash with limited intake of foods high in purine
  2. I.V. therapy: heparin lock
  3. Activity: as tolerated
  4. Monitoring: VS, UO, I/O, and urine pH
  5. Laboratory studies: creatinine, BUN, phosphorus, calcium, and protein
  6. Treatments: strain urine, moist heat to flank, hot baths
  7. Force fluids to 3,000 ml/day
  8. Antigout agent: sulfinpyrazone (Anturane)
  9. Analgesic: meperidine hydrochloride (Demerol)
  10. Antibiotics: cefazolin (Ancef), cefoxitin (Mefoxin)
  11. Antiemetic: prochlorperazine (Compazine)
  12. Acidifiers: ammonium chloride, methenamine mandelate (Mandelamine)
  13. Alkalinizers: potassium acetate, sodium bicarbonate
  14. Chemolysis

15. Electrohydraulic lithotripsy
16. Ultrasonic lithotripsy
17. Laser impulse
18. Extra corporeal shock wave lithotripsy
19. Percutaneous nephrostolithotomy (PCNL)
20. Prevention of cystinuria: tiopronin (Thiola)

G. Nursing interventions and responsibilities
   1. Maintain the patient's diet
   2. Force fluids to 3,000 ml/day
   3. Assess renal status
   4. Monitor and record VS, UO, I/O, daily weight, specific gravity, laboratory studies, and urine pH
   5. Administer medications, as prescribed
   6. Allay the patient's anxiety
   7. Continue straining urine and giving warm baths and warm soaks to flank
   8. Assess pain

H. Teaching goals (instructions to the patient and family)
   1. Keep follow-up appointments
   2. Exercise regularly
   3. Know the action, side effects, and scheduling of medications
   4. Recognize the signs and symptoms of urinary tract infection
   5. Alternate rest periods with activity
   6. Monitor self for infection
   7. Follow dietary recommendations and restrictions
   8. Increase fluid intake—especially during hot weather, illness, and exercise
   9. Void when urge is felt
   10. Test urine pH
   11. Increase fluids at night and void frequently

I. Possible medical complications
   1. Chronic urinary tract infection
   2. Renal obstruction
   3. Ureterovesical reflux
   4. Hydronephrosis
   5. Pyelonephritis

J. Possible surgical interventions: lithotomy (see page 235)

XV. Acute renal failure

A. Definition—sudden inability of the kidneys to regulate fluid and electrolyte balance and remove toxic products from the body

B. Possible etiology
   1. CHF

2. Cardiogenic shock
3. Hemorrhage
4. Burns
5. Septicemia
6. Hypotension
7. Acute tubular necrosis
8. Acute vasoconstriction
9. Endocarditis
10. Malignant hypertension
11. Diabetes mellitus
12. Dehydration
13. Tumor
14. Blood transfusion reaction
15. Cardiopulmonary bypass
16. Nephrotoxins: antibiotics, X-ray dyes, pesticides, anesthetics
17. Renal calculi
18. Benign prostatic hypertrophy
19. Acute glomerulonephritis
20. Trauma
21. Congenital deformity
22. Anaphylaxis
23. Collagen diseases

C. Pathophysiology
 1. Decreased perfusion of the kidney results in decreased blood flow and glomerular filtrate, ischemia, and oliguria
 2. Damaged nephrons are unable to absorb and secrete water, electrolytes, glucose, amino acids, ammonia, and bicarbonate
 3. Disorder may progress from anuric or oliguric phase through diuretic phase to convalescence phase to recovery of function
 4. Disorder may develop into chronic renal failure

D. Possible clinical manifestions
 1. Urine output less than 400 ml/day for 1 to 2 weeks followed by diuresis (3 to 5 liters/day) for 2 to 3 weeks
 2. Lethargy
 3. Drowsiness
 4. Stupor
 5. Coma
 6. Irritability
 7. Headache
 8. Costovertebral pain
 9. Circumoral numbness
10. Tingling extremities
11. Anorexia
12. Restlessness
13. Weight gain

14. Nausea and vomiting
15. Pallor
16. Epistaxis
17. Ecchymosis
18. Diarrhea or constipation
19. Stomatitis
20. Thick, tenacious sputum

E. Possible diagnostic test findings
   1. Blood chemistry: increased potassium, phosphorus, magnesium, BUN, creatinine, and uric acid; decreased calcium, carbon dioxide (CO_2), and sodium
   2. Hematology: decreased Hgb, Hct, erythrocytes; increased PT and PTT
   3. Urine chemistry: albuminuria, proteinuria, increased sodium; casts, RBCs, and WBCs; specific gravity greater than 1.025, then fixed at less than 1.010
   4. IVP: decreased renal perfusion and function
   5. Phenolsulfonphthalein (PSP): decreased
   6. Arterial blood gases (ABGs): metabolic acidosis

F. Medical management
   1. Diet: low-protein, increased-carbohydrate, moderate-fat, and moderate-calorie with potassium, sodium and phosphorus intake regulated according to serum levels
   2. I.V. therapy: electrolyte replacement, heparin lock
   3. Position: semi-Fowler's
   4. Activity: bed rest, active and passive ROM and isometric exercises
   5. Monitoring: VS, UO, I/O, ECG, and CVP
   6. Laboratory studies: BUN, creatinine, phosphorus, calcium, potassium, sodium, Hgb, Hct, and specific gravity
   7. Nutritional support: total parental nutrition (TPN)
   8. Treatments: Foley catheter, incentive spirometry, cooling blanket
   9. Fluids: restrict intake to amount needed to replace fluid loss
   10. Transfusion therapy: packed RBCs
   11. Antibiotics: cefazolin (Ancef), cefoxitin (Mefoxin)
   12. Analgesic: oxycodone hydrochloride (Tylox)
   13. Diuretics: furosemide (Lasix), mannitol (Osmitrol)
   14. Antacid: aluminum hydroxide gel (ALternaGEL)
   15. Antiemetic: prochlorperazine (Compazine)
   16. Cation exchange resins: sodium polystyrene sulfonate (Kayexalate)
   17. Chelating agent: dimercaprol (BAL)
   18. Beta adrenergic: dopamine hydrochloride (Intropin)
   19. Anticonvulsant: phenytoin (Dilantin)
   20. Peritoneal dialysis and hemodialysis
   21. Antipyretic: acetaminophen (Tylenol)
   22. Precautions: seizure
   23. Alkalinizing agent: sodium bicarbonate

24. Continuous arteriovenous hemofiltration (CAVH)

G. Nursing interventions and responsibilities
1. Maintain the patient's diet
2. Restrict fluids
3. Administer I.V. fluids
4. Assess fluid balance, respiratory, cardiovascular, and neurologic status
5. Keep the patient in semi-Fowler's position
6. Monitor and record VS, UO, I/O, CVP, daily weight, specific gravity, laboratory studies, stool for occult blood, and urine glucose and ketones
7. Administer TPN
8. Administer medications, as prescribed
9. Encourage the patient to express feelings about changes in body image
10. Monitor for arrhythmias
11. Provide cooling blanket
12. Monitor the patient for infection
13. Maintain a quiet environment
14. Maintain seizure precautions
15. Monitor the patient for bleeding
16. Protect the patient from falls
17. Encourage TCDB
18. Allay the patient's anxiety
19. Observe for uremic frost
20. Provide skin and mouth care using plain water
21. Monitor neurovital signs

H. Teaching goals (instructions to the patient and family)
1. Keep follow-up appointments
2. Avoid using over-the-counter medications
3. Stop smoking
4. Maintain a normal weight
5. Know the action, side effects, and scheduling of medications
6. Recognize the signs and symptoms of renal failure, urinary tract infection, respiratory infection
7. Avoid exposure to people with infections
8. Alternate rest periods with activity
9. Monitor self for infection
10. Follow dietary recommendations and restrictions
11. Maintain a quiet environemnt

I. Possible medical complications
1. Chronic renal failure
2. Decubiti
3. Contractures
4. Atelectasis
5. Gastrointestinal hemorrhage

6. Convulsions
7. Arrhythmias
8. Cardiac arrest
9. Pericarditis
10. Potassium intoxication
11. Pulmonary edema
12. Pulmonary infection
13. CHF
14. Hypertension
15. Anemia
16. Metabolic acidosis
17. Peripheral neuropathy
18. Hypocalcemia

J. Possible surgical interventions: none

XVI. Chronic renal failure

A. Definition—progressive, irreversible destruction of kidneys, resulting in loss of renal function

B. Possible etiology
1. Recurrent urinary tract infection
2. Exacerbations of nephritis
3. Urinary tract obstructions
4. Diabetes mellitus
5. Hypertension
6. Congenital abnormalities
7. Systemic lupus erythematosus
8. Nephrotoxins
9. Dehydration

C. Pathophysiology
1. Scarred nephrons are unable to absorb and secrete water, glucose, amino acids, ammonia, bicarbonate, and electrolytes
2. First stage: renal reserve is diminished, but metabolic wastes do not accumulate although renal damage exists
3. Second stage: renal insufficiency occurs and metabolic wastes begin to accumulate; kidneys are less able to correct metabolic imbalances
4. Third stage: uremia occurs with decreased urine output; increased accumulation of metabolic wastes; and disturbed fluid, electrolyte, and acid-base balances

D. Possible clinical manifestations
1. Muscle twitching
2. Paresthesia
3. Bone pain
4. Pruritus

    5. Decreased urinary output
    6. Stomatitis
    7. Lethargy
    8. Seizures
    9. Brittle nails and hair
  10. Kussmaul respirations
  11. Uremic frost
  12. Ecchymosis

E. Possible diagnostic test findings
    1. Urine chemistry: proteinuria, increased WBCs, sodium; decreased and fixed specific gravity
    2. Blood chemistry: increased BUN, creatinine, phosphorus, lipids; decreased calcium, CO_2, albumin
    3. ABGs: metabolic acidosis
    4. Hematology: decreased Hgb, Hct, platelets
    5. Glucose tolerance test: decreased

F. Medical management
    1. Diet: low-protein, low-sodium, low-potassium, low-phosphorus, with high-calorie and high-carbohydrate
    2. Dietary restrictions: limit fluids
    3. I.V. therapy: heparin lock
    4. Activity: as tolerated
    5. Monitoring: VS, UO, and I/O
    6. Laboratory studies: BUN, creatinine, potassium, sodium, Hgb, Hct, glucose, albumin, and platelets
    7. Treatments: tepid baths
    8. Transfusion therapy: platelets
    9. Antibiotics: cefazolin (Ancef), cefoxitin (Mefoxin)
  10. Analgesic: oxycodone hydrochloride (Tylox)
  11. Diuretic: furosemide (Lasix)
  12. Antacids: aluminum hydroxide gel (ALternaGEL), magnesium and aluminum hydroxide (Maalox)
  13. Antiemetic: prochlorperazine (Compazine)
  14. Cation exchange resin: sodium polystyrene sulfonate (Kayexalate)
  15. Chelating agent: dimercaprol (BAL)
  16. Beta adrenergic: dopamine hydrochloride (Intropin)
  17. Anticonvulsant: phenytoin (Dilantin)
  18. Peritoneal dialysis and hemodialysis
  19. Antipyretic: acetaminophen (Tylenol)
  20. Precautions: seizure
  21. Alkalinizing agent: sodium bicarbonate
  22. Cardioglycoside: digoxin (Lanoxin)
  23. Stool softener: docusate sodium (Colace)
  24. Antiarrhythmic: procainamide (Pronestyl)

25. Antianemics: ferrous sulfate (Feosol), iron dextran (Imferon), epoietin alfa (recombinant human erythropoietin; Epogen)
26. Vitamins: pyridoxine hydrochloride (vitamin B_6), ascorbic acid (vitamin C)
27. Calcium supplements: calcium carbonate (Os-Cal)

G. Nursing interventions and responsibilities
1. Maintain the patient's diet
2. Restrict fluids
3. Assess renal, respiratory, and cardiovascular status and fluid balance
4. Monitor and record VS, UO, I/O, ECG, specific gravity, daily weight, laboratory studies, neurovital signs, neurovascular checks, urine for glucose and ketones, and urine, stool, and emesis for occult blood
5. Administer medications, as prescribed
6. Encourage the patient to express feelings about chronicity of illness
7. Provide treatments: tepid baths
8. Maintain a cool and quiet environment
9. Provide skin and mouth care using plain water
10. Maintain seizure precautions
11. Monitor for ecchymosis
12. Monitor for infection
13. Avoid giving the patient intramuscular injections
14. Protect the patient from falls

H. Teaching goals (instructions to the patient and family)
1. Keep follow-up appointments
2. Stop smoking
3. Maintain a normal weight
4. Know the action, side effects, and scheduling of medications
5. Recognize the signs and symptoms of infection
6. Avoid exposure to people with infection
7. Alternate rest periods with activity
8. Monitor self for infection
9. Follow dietary recommendations and restrictions
10. Promote a safe environment
11. Maintain a quiet environment
12. Complete skin and mouth care daily

I. Possible medical complications
1. Arrhythmias
2. Gastrointestinal bleeding
3. CHF
4. Pericardial effusion
5. Hyperphosphatemia
6. Pleural effusion
7. Dehydration
8. Hyperparathyroidism

     9. Renal osteodystrophy
   10. Uremia

J. Possible surgical interventions: kidney transplantation (see page 233)

XVII. Bladder cancer

A. Definition — malignant tumor that ulcerates mucosal lining of the bladder

B. Possible etiology
    1. Exposure to industrial chemicals
    2. Cigarette smoking
    3. Chronic bladder irritation
    4. Radiation
    5. Excessive intake of coffee, phenacetin, sodium, saccharin, sodium cyclamate
    6. Drug induced: cyclophosphamide (Cytoxan)

C. Pathophysiology
    1. Unregulated cell growth and uncontrolled cell division in bladder's transitional epithelium around trigone result in the development of a neoplasm
    2. Tumor metastasizes to ureters, prostate gland, vagina, rectum, and periaortic lymph nodes

D. Possible clinical manifestations
    1. Painless hematuria
    2. Dysuria
    3. Frequency of urination
    4. Anuria
    5. Urgency of urination
    6. Chills
    7. Flank or pelvic pain
    8. Elevated temperature
    9. Peripheral edema

E. Possible diagnostic test findings
    1. Cystoscopy: mass
    2. IVP: mass or obstruction
    3. KUB: mass or obstruction
    4. Cytologic exam: cytology positive for malignant cells
    5. Urine chemistry: hematuria
    6. Hematology: decreased RBCs, Hgb, Hct

F. Medical management
    1. I.V. therapy: heparin lock
    2. Activity: as tolerated
    3. Monitoring: VS, UO, and I/O
    4. Laboratory studies: Hgb and Hct

5. Radiation therapy
6. Chemotherapy
7. Treatments: Foley catheter
8. Transfusion therapy: packed RBCs
9. Sedative: phenobarbital (Luminal)
10. Antispasmotic: phenazopyridine (Pyridium)
11. Antineoplastics: 5-fluorouracil (Adrucil), methotrexate (Rheumatrex), bleomycin (Blenoxane), thiotepa (Thiotepa), doxorubicin hydrochloride (Adriamycin)
12. Antiemetic: nabilone (Cesamet)

G. Nursing interventions and responsibilities
1. Maintain the patient's diet
2. Force fluids
3. Administer I.V. fluids
4. Assess renal status
5. Monitor and record VS, UO, I/O, and laboratory studies
6. Administer medications, as prescribed
7. Encourage the patient to express feelings about a fear of dying
8. Provide postchemotherapeutic and postradiation nursing care
   a. Provide skin, mouth, and perineal care
   b. Encourage dietary intake
   c. Administer antiemetics and antidiarrheals, as prescribed
   d. Monitor the patient for bleeding, infection, and electrolyte imbalance
   e. Provide rest periods
9. Provide information about the American Cancer Society

H. Teaching goals (instructions to the patient and family)
1. Keep follow-up appointments
2. Stop smoking
3. Maintain a normal weight
4. Know the action, side effects, and scheduling of medications
5. Recognize the signs and symptoms of urinary tract infection and renal failure
6. Avoid exposure to people with infections
7. Alternate rest periods with activity
8. Monitor self for infection
9. Follow dietary recommendations and restrictions
10. Seek help from community agencies and resources

I. Possible medical complications
1. Ureteral obstruction
2. Vesicorectal and vesicovaginal fistulas

J. Possible surgical interventions
1. Ureterosigmoidostomy (see page 238)
2. Ileal conduit (see page 238)

3. Cutaneous ureterostomy (see page 238)
4. Cystectomy

XVIII. Benign prostatic hypertrophy (BPH)

A. Definition—hyperplasia of the lateral and subcervical lobes of the prostate gland that results in enlargement of the structure

B. Possible etiology
   1. Unknown
   2. Hormonal

C. Pathophysiology
   1. Enlarged prostate gland compresses urethra, resulting in urinary obstruction and retention
   2. Obstruction causes hydroureter and hydronephrosis

D. Possible clinical manifestations
   1. Nocturia
   2. Urgency, frequency, and burning on urination
   3. Decreased force and amount of stream
   4. Hesitancy
   5. Dysuria
   6. Urinary retention
   7. Urinary tract infection
   8. Dribbling

E. Possible diagnostic test findings
   1. Rectal examination: enlarged prostate gland by palpation
   2. Urine chemistry: bacteria, hematuria, alkaline pH, increased specific gravity
   3. Blood chemistry: increased BUN, creatinine
   4. PSP: decreased
   5. IVP: urethral obstruction, hydronephrosis
   6. Cystoscopy: enlarged prostate gland, obstructed urine flow, urinary stasis
   7. CMG: abnormal pressure recordings
   8. Urinary flow rate determination: volume small, flow pattern prolonged, peak flow low

F. Medical management
   1. Diet: force fluids
   2. Position: semi-Fowler's
   3. Activity: as tolerated
   4. Monitoring: VS, UO, and I/O
   5. Laboratory studies: BUN, and creatinine
   6. Treatments: Foley catheter, hot baths
   7. Antibiotics: trimethoprim and sulfamethoxazole (Bactrim), cephalexin (Keflex)

8. Analgesic: oxycodone hydrochloride (Tylox)
9. Urinary antiseptic: phenazopyridine (Pyridium)
10. Antianxiety: diazepam (Valium)
11. Alpha-blocker: phenoxybenzamine (Dibenzyline)
12. Alpha-adrenergic antagonists: prazosin (Minipress), terazosin (Hytrin)

G. Nursing interventions and responsibilities
1. Force fluids
2. Assess fluid balance
3. Keep the patient in semi-Fowler's position
4. Monitor and record: VS, UO, I/O, and laboratory studies
5. Administer medications, as prescribed
6. Encourage the patient to express feelings about changes in body image and fear of sexual dysfunction
7. Maintain position and patency of Foley catheter to straight drainage
8. Maintain activity, as tolerated
9. Provide hot baths
10. Provide privacy while urinating
11. Monitor for urinary tract infection

H. Teaching goals (instructions to the patient and family)
1. Keep follow-up appointments
2. Stop smoking
3. Maintain a normal weight
4. Know the action, side effects, and scheduling of medications
5. Recognize the signs and symptoms of urinary retention and infection

I. Possible medical complications
1. Chronic renal failure
2. Hydronephrosis
3. Hydroureter
4. Renal calculi
5. Cystitis

J. Possible surgical interventions
1. Suprapubic cystotomy with insertion of suprapubic catheter
2. TURP (see page 236)
3. Prostatectomy (see page 236)
4. Transurethral dilation of prostate gland (TUDP)

Points to remember

Renal disease can alter the renin-angiotensin system, which controls blood pressure.

Specific gravity of urine, the patient's daily weight, and accurate fluid output measurements are important, objective assessments for renal function.

A midstream urine sample should be collected for a urine culture and sensitivity test.

After a kidney transplantation, the nurse should assess the allograft site for pain and edema.

A patient with urolithiasis (calcium calculi) should follow an acid-ash diet with limited intake of calcium and milk products.

The nurse should observe the patient with acute renal failure for uremic frost.

Glossary

The following terms are defined in Appendix A, page 354.

anuria   polyuria

hematuria   pyuria

oliguria   renal colic

Study questions

To evaluate your understanding of this chapter, answer the following questions in the space provided; then compare your responses with the correct answers in Appendix B, pages 361 and 362.

1. Which isolation precautions would be used for a patient after kidney transplantation? _____

2. Which nursing intervention is contraindicated in a patient with a nephrostomy tube? _____

3. What are the four types of urinary diversions? _____

4. What would urine and blood chemistry tests reveal about a patient with glomerulonephritis? _____

5. What type of diet would the physician prescribe for a patient with pyelonephritis? _____

6. Which foods can cause urolithiasis? _____

7. What type of diet would the physician prescribe for a patient with acute renal failure? _____

8. Which diagnostic tests might be prescribed for a patient with a diagnosis of bladder cancer? _____

9. What are the key clinical manifestations of BPH? _____

CHAPTER 7

Respiratory System

Learning objectives

Check off the following items once you've mastered them:

- [ ] Describe the psychosocial impact of respiratory disorders.

- [ ] Differentiate between modifiable and nonmodifiable risk factors in the development of a respiratory disorder.

- [ ] List three probable and three possible nursing diagnoses for a patient with a respiratory disorder.

- [ ] Identify the nursing interventions and responsibilities for a patient with a respiratory disorder.

- [ ] Write three goals for teaching a patient with a respiratory disorder.

I. Anatomy and physiology

A. Nares
  1. Filters out particles
  2. Humidifies inspired air
  3. Contains olfactory receptor sites

B. Paranasal sinuses
  1. Air-filled, cilia-lined cavities
  2. Function: to trap particles

C. Pharynx
  1. Serves as a passageway to digestive and respiratory tracts
  2. Maintains air pressure in the middle ear
  3. Contains mucosal lining that humidifies and warms inspired air and traps particles

D. Larynx
  1. Known as the "voice box"
  2. Connects the upper and lower airways
  3. Contains vocal cords that produce sounds and initiate the cough reflex

E. Trachea
  1. Consists of smooth muscle
  2. Contains C-shaped cartilagenous rings
  3. Connects the larynx to the bronchi

F. Bronchi and bronchioles
  1. Bronchi and bronchioles are formed by branching of the trachea
  2. Right main bronchus is slightly larger and more vertical than the left
  3. Bronchioles branch into terminal bronchioles, which end in alveoli

G. Alveoli
  1. Clustered microscopic sacs enveloped by capillaries
  2. Gases exchange in the alveoli
  3. Coating of surfactant reduces surface tension to keep alveoli from collapsing
  4. Diffusion of gases occurs across the alveolar-capillary membrane

H. Lungs
  1. Composed of three lobes on the right side and two lobes on the left side
  2. Covered by pleura
  3. Regulate air exchange by concentration gradient

I. Pleura
  1. Visceral pleura covers the lungs
  2. Parietal pleura lines the thoracic cavity
  3. Pleural fluid lubricates the pleura to reduce friction during respiration

II. Physical assessment findings

A. Subjective data that often accompany respiratory disorders
   1. Difficulty breathing
   2. Chest pain
   3. Voice change
   4. Dysphagia
   5. Fatigue
   6. Weight change
   7. Cough

B. Objective data to evaluate in respiratory disorders
   1. DYSPNEA
   2. Sputum
   3. Clubbing of fingers
   4. Adventitious sounds: CRACKLES, RHONCHI, wheezing, and pleural friction rub
   5. Fremitus
   6. Crepitus
   7. Pattern and character of respirations
   8. Thoracic anatomy
   9. Change in mentation
   10. Skin color and temperature

III. Diagnostic tests and procedures

A. Bronchoscopy
   1. Definition and purpose
      a. Procedure using a bronchoscope
      b. Direct visualization of the trachea and bronchial tree
   2. Nursing interventions and responsibilities before the procedure
      a. Withhold food and fluids
      b. Allay the patient's anxiety
   3. Nursing interventions and responsibilities after the procedure
      a. Check cough and gag reflex
      b. Assess sputum
      c. Assess respiratory status
      d. Withhold food and fluids until gag reflex returns
      e. Check vasovagal response

B. Chest X-ray
   1. Definition and purpose
      a. Noninvasive examination
      b. Radiographic picture of lung tissue
   2. Nursing interventions and responsibilities
      a. Determine the patient's ability to inhale and hold breath
      b. Ensure that the patient removes jewelry

C. Pulmonary angiography
  1. Definition and purpose
      a. Procedure using an injection of a radiopaque dye through a catheter
      b. Radiographic examination of the pulmonary circulation
  2. Nursing interventions and responsibilities before the procedure
      a. Note the patient's allergies to iodine, seafood, and radiopaque dyes
      b. Instruct the patient about possible flushing of the face or burning in the throat after dye is injected
  3. Nursing interventions and responsibilities after the procedure
      a. Assess peripheral neurovascular status
      b. Check the insertion site for bleeding

D. Sputum studies
  1. Definition and purpose
      a. Laboratory test
      b. Microscopic evaluation of sputum that includes culture and sensitivity, gram stain, and acid-fast bacillus
  2. Nursing interventions and responsibilities: obtain early-morning sterile specimen from suctioning or expectoration

E. Thoracentesis
  1. Definition and purpose
      a. Procedure using needle aspiration of intrapleural fluid under local anesthesia
      b. Specimen examination or removal of pleural fluid
  2. Nursing interventions and responsibilities during the procedure
      a. Reassure the patient
      b. Place the patient in the proper position (either sitting on the edge of the bed or lying partially on the side, partially on the back)
  3. Nursing interventions and responsibilities after the procedure
      a. Assess the patient's respiratory status
      b. Position the patient on the affected side, as ordered, for at least 1 hour to seal the puncture site
      c. Monitor vital signs frequently
      d. Check the puncture site for fluid leakage

F. Pulmonary function tests (PFTs)
  1. Definition and purpose
      a. Noninvasive test
      b. Measurement of lung volumes, ventilation, and diffusing capacity
  2. Nursing interventions and responsibilities
      a. Document bronchodilators or narcotics used before testing
      b. Allay the patient's anxiety during testing

G. Arterial blood gases (ABGs)
  1. Definition and purpose
      a. Laboratory test

b. Assessment of arterial blood for tissue oxygenation, ventilation, and acid-base status
   2. Nursing interventions and responsibilities before the procedure
   a. Note temperature
   b. Document oxygen and assisted mechanical ventilation used
   3. Nursing interventions and responsibilities after the procedure
   a. Apply pressure to the site for 5 minutes
   b. Apply a pressure dressing

H. Lung scan
   1. Definition and purpose
   a. Procedure using visual inhalation or I.V. injection of radioisotopes
   b. Imaging of distribution and blood flow in the lungs
   2. Nursing interventions and responsibilities
   a. Allay the patient's anxiety
   b. Determine the patient's ability to lie still during procedure
   c. Check the catheter insertion site for bleeding after the procedure

I. Mantoux intradermal skin test
   1. Definition and purpose
   a. Procedure involving the administration of tuberculin
   b. Detection of tuberculosis antibodies
   2. Nursing interventions and responsibilities
   a. Document current dermatitis or rashes
   b. Document history of positive results in past skin testing
   c. Circle and record test site
   d. Note date for follow-up reading

J. Laryngoscopy
   1. Definition and purpose
   a. Procedure using a laryngoscope
   b. Direct visualization of the larynx
   2. Nursing interventions and responsibilities before the procedure
   a. Withhold food or fluids for 6 to 8 hours before the test
   b. Explain that the patient will receive a sedative to promote relaxation
   c. Make sure a consent form has been signed
   3. Nursing interventions and responsibilities after the procedure
   a. Assess respiratory status
   b. Allay the patient's anxiety

K. Lung biopsy
   1. Definition and purpose
   a. Procedure involving the percutaneous removal of a small amount of lung tissue
   b. Histologic evaluation
   2. Nursing interventions and responsibilities before the procedure
   a. Withhold food and fluids

        b. Obtain written, informed consent
    3. Nursing interventions and responsibilities after the procedure
        a. Observe the patient for signs of pneumothorax and air embolism
        b. Check the patient for HEMOPTYSIS and hemorrhage
        c. Monitor and record vital signs (VS)
        d. Check the insertion site for bleeding

L. Hematologic studies
    1. Definition and purpose
        a. Laboratory test of a blood sample
        b. Analysis for red blood cells (RBCs), white blood cells (WBCs), prothrombin time (PT), partial thromboplastin time (PTT), erythrocyte sedimentation rate (ESR), platelets, hemoglobin (Hgb), and hematocrit (Hct)
    2. Nursing interventions and responsibilities
        a. Note current drug therapy before the procedure
        b. Check the site for bleeding after the procedure

M. Blood chemistry
    1. Definition and purpose
        a. Laboratory test of a blood sample
        b. Analysis for potassium, sodium, calcium, phosphorus, glucose, bicarbonate, blood urea nitrogen (BUN), creatinine, protein, albumin, and osmolality
    2. Nursing interventions and responsibilities
        a. Withhold food and fluids before the procedure, as directed
        b. Check the site for bleeding after the procedure

IV. Psychosocial impact of respiratory disorders

A. Developmental impact
    1. Decreased self-esteem
    2. Fear of dying

B. Economic impact
    1. Disruption or loss of employment
    2. Cost of hospitalizations and home health care

C. Occupational and recreational impact
    1. Restrictions in work activity
    2. Changes in leisure activities

D. Social impact
    1. Changes in sexual function
    2. Social isolation
    3. Changes in role performance

V. Possible risk factors

A. Modifiable risk factors
1. Crowded living conditions
2. Inadequate knowledge of risk factors
3. Exposure to chemical and environmental pollutants
4. Cigarette or pipe smoking
5. Use of chewing tobacco
6. Alcohol abuse

B. Nonmodifiable risk factors
1. Aging
2. History of allergies
3. Previous respiratory illness
4. Family history of respiratory illness
5. Family history of allergies

VI. Nursing diagnostic categories for a patient with a respiratory disorder

A. Probable nursing diagnostic categories
1. Impaired physical mobility
2. Altered cerebral tissue perfusion
3. Altered peripheral tissue perfusion
4. Altered cardiopulmonary tissue perfusion
5. Disturbed sleep

B. Possible nursing diagnostic categories
1. Ineffective breathing patterns
2. Impaired gas exchange
3. Ineffective airway clearance
4. Anxiety
5. Fear
6. Activity intolerance
7. Impaired verbal communication
8. Noncompliance
9. Aspiration
10. Altered nutrition: less than body requirements

VII. Laryngectomy

A. Definitions
1. Partial laryngectomy: surgical excision of a lesion on one vocal cord
2. Total laryngectomy: surgical removal of the larynx, hyoid bone, and tracheal rings with closure of the pharynx and formation of a permanent tracheostomy

B. Preoperative nursing interventions and responsibilities
1. Complete patient and family preoperative teaching

      a. Determine the patient's understanding of the procedure
      b. Describe the operating room (OR), postanesthesia care unit (PACU), and preoperative and postoperative routines
      c. Demonstrate postoperative turning, coughing, and deep breathing (TCDB), splinting, leg exercises, and range-of-motion (ROM) exercises
      d. Explain the postoperative need for drainage tubes, surgical dressings, oxygen therapy, I.V. therapy, and pain control
  2. Complete a preoperative checklist
  3. Administer preoperative medications, as prescribed
  4. Allay the patient's and family's anxiety about surgery
  5. Document the patient's history and physical assessment data base
  6. Establish methods of communication: writing, call bell
  7. Encourage the patient to express feelings about changes in body image and loss of voice

C. Postoperative nursing interventions and responsibilities
  1. Assess respiratory status
  2. Assess pain and administer postoperative analgesics, as prescribed
  3. Assess for return of peristalsis; provide solid foods and liquids, as tolerated
      a. Increase calories
      b. Increase protein
  4. Administer I.V. fluids and nasogastric (NG) tube feedings
  5. Allay the patient's anxiety
  6. Inspect the surgical dressing and change, as directed
  7. Reinforce TCDB
  8. Keep the patient in semi-Fowler's position
  9. Provide tracheal suction
 10. Increase activity, as tolerated
 11. Administer oxygen via high humidity tracheostomy mask
 12. Monitor and record VS, urinary output (UO), intake and output (I/O), laboratory studies, and pulse oximetry
 13. Monitor and maintain position and patency of drainage tubes: wound drainage
 14. Assess the color, amount, and consistency of sputum
 15. Encourage the patient to express feelings about changes in body image and loss of voice
 16. Provide oral hygiene
 17. Reinforce method of communication established preoperatively
 18. Reinforce speech therapy
 19. Assess gag and cough reflex and ability to swallow
 20. Provide stoma and laryngectomy care
 21. Reinforce increased intake of fluids
 22. Observe for hemorrhage and edema in the neck
 23. Arrange for referrals to community agencies

D. Possible surgical complications
   1. Hemorrhage
   2. Atelectasis
   3. Pneumonia
   4. Aspiration

E. Postoperative teaching goals (instructions to the patient and family)
   1. Keep follow-up appointments
   2. Communicate using esophageal speech or artificial larynx
   3. Know the action, side effects, and scheduling of medications
   4. Recognize the signs and symptoms of infection
   5. Avoid swimming, showering, and using aerosal sprays
   6. Complete stoma and laryngectomy care daily
   7. Suction laryngectomy using clean technique
   8. Protect the neck from injury
   9. Demonstrate ways to prevent debris from entering the stoma
   10. Seek help from community agencies and resources

VIII. Radical neck dissection

A. Definition—surgical excision of the sternocleidomastoid and omohyoid muscles, muscles of the floor of the mouth, submaxillary gland, internal jugular vein, external carotid artery, and cervical chain of lymph nodes in addition to laryngectomy

B. Preoperative nursing interventions and responsibilities
   1. Complete patient and family preoperative teaching
      a. Determine the patient's understanding of the procedure
      b. Describe the OR, PACU, and preoperative and postoperative routines
      c. Demonstrate postoperative TCDB, splinting, and leg and ROM exercises
      d. Explain the postoperative need for drainage tubes, surgical dressings, oxygen therapy, I.V. therapy, and pain control
   2. Complete a preoperative checklist
   3. Administer preoperative medications, as prescribed
   4. Allay the patient's and family's anxiety about surgery
   5. Document the patient's history and physical assessment data base
   6. Establish methods of communication: writing, call bell

C. Postoperative nursing interventions and responsibilities
   1. Assess cardiac, respiratory, and neurologic status
   2. Assess pain and administer postoperative analgesics, as prescribed
   3. Assess for the return of peristalsis; provide solid foods and liquids, as tolerated
   4. Administer I.V. fluids, NG tube feedings, and transfusion therapy, as prescribed
   5. Allay the patient's anxiety
   6. Inspect the surgical dressing and change, as directed

7. Reinforce TCDB
8. Keep the patient in high-Fowler's position
9. Provide tracheal suction
10. Maintain activity: as tolerated, active and passive ROM and isometric exercises
11. Administer oxygen via high humidity tracheostomy mask
12. Monitor and record VS, UO, I/O, laboratory studies, and pulse oximetry
13. Monitor and maintain position and patency of drainage tubes: NG, indwelling urinary catheter (Foley), and wound drainage
14. Assess gag and cough reflex and ability to swallow
15. Encourage the patient to express feelings about changes in body image and loss of voice
16. Provide stoma and laryngectomy care; arrange for referrals to community agencies for follow-up care
17. Reinforce increased intake of fluids
18. Observe the patient for hemorrhage and edema in the neck
19. Provide suture line care
20. Reinforce method of communication established preoperatively
21. Reinforce speech therapy

D. Possible surgical complications
1. Tracheostomy stenosis
2. Aspiration
3. Pneumonia
4. Hemorrhage

E. Postoperative teaching goals (instructions to the patient and family)
1. Keep follow-up appointments
2. Communicate using esophageal speech or artificial larynx
3. Know the action, side effects, and scheduling of medications
4. Recognize the signs and symptoms of infection and tracheostomy stenosis
5. Avoid swimming, showering, and using aerosol sprays
6. Protect neck from injury
7. Seek help from community agencies and resources
8. Suction laryngectomy using clean technique
9. Complete incision, stoma, and laryngectomy care daily
10. Demonstrate ways to prevent debris from entering the stoma
11. Complete ROM exercises for arms, shoulders, and neck daily
12. Use artificial larynx

IX. Pulmonary resections

A. Definition
1. Lobectomy: surgical removal of one lobe of the lung
2. Wedge resection: surgical removal of a wedge-shaped section of a lobe

3. Pneumonectomy: surgical removal of a lung

B. Preoperative nursing interventions and responsibilities
1. Complete patient and family preoperative teaching
   a. Determine the patient's understanding of the procedure
   b. Describe the OR, PACU, and preoperative and postoperative routines
   c. Demonstrate postoperative TCDB, splinting, and leg and ROM exercises
   d. Explain the postoperative need for drainage tubes, chest tubes, surgical dressings, oxygen therapy, I.V. therapy, and pain control
2. Complete a preoperative checklist
3. Administer preoperative medications, as prescribed
4. Allay the patient's and family's anxiety about surgery
5. Document the patient's history and physical assessment data base

C. Postoperative nursing interventions and responsibilities
1. Assess cardiac and respiratory status
2. Assess pain and administer postoperative analgesics, as prescribed
3. Assess for return of peristalsis; provide solid foods and liquids, as tolerated
4. Administer I.V. fluids
5. Allay the patient's anxiety
6. Inspect the surgical dressing and change, as directed
7. Reinforce TCDB and splinting of incision
8. Maintain the patient's position: for pneumonectomy patient, on the back or the side of the surgery; for lobectomy or wedge resection patient, on the back or the side opposite the surgery
9. Provide incentive spirometry, suction, chest physiotherapy (CPT), postural drainage
10. Maintain activity: as tolerated, active and passive ROM and isometric exercises
11. Administer oxygen and maintain endotracheal tube to ventilator
12. Monitor and record VS, UO, I/O, laboratory studies, electrocardiogram (ECG), hemodynamic variables, and pulse oximetry
13. Monitor and maintain position and patency of drainage tubes: NG, Foley, chest tube
14. Assess chest tube insertion site for subcutaneous air and drainage
15. Encourage the patient to express feelings about a fear of dying
16. Administer antibiotics, as prescribed

D. Possible surgical complications
1. Hemorrhage
2. Pneumonia

E. Postoperative teaching goals (instructions to the patient and family)
1. Keep follow-up appointments
2. Exercise regularly
3. Stop smoking

4. Maintain a normal weight
5. Know the action, side effects, and scheduling of medications
6. Recognize the signs and symptoms of infection and respiratory distress
7. Complete incision care daily
8. Maintain active ROM exercises to operative shoulder

X. Embolectomy

A. Definition – removal of an embolus from an artery using a balloon-tipped catheter

B. Preoperative nursing interventions and responsibilities
1. Complete patient and family preoperative teaching
   a. Determine the patient's understanding of the procedure
   b. Describe the OR, PACU, and preoperative and postoperative routines
   c. Demonstrate postoperative TCDB, splinting, and leg and ROM exercises
   d. Explain the postoperative need for drainage tubes, surgical dressings, oxygen therapy, I.V. therapy, and pain control
2. Complete a preoperative checklist
3. Administer preoperative medications, as prescribed
4. Allay the patient's and family's anxiety about surgery
5. Document the patient's history and physical assessment data base
6. Obtain a baseline vascular assessment
7. Administer anticoagulants, as prescribed
8. Administer antispasmodics, as prescribed
9. Administer thrombolytics, as prescribed
10. Provide a bed cradle
11. Avoid bumping the bed
12. Maintain extremity in slightly dependent position

C. Postoperative nursing interventions and responsibilities
1. Assess cardiac, respiratory, and neurologic status
2. Assess pain and administer postoperative analgesics, as prescribed
3. Assess for return of peristalsis; provide solid foods and liquids, as tolerated
4. Administer I.V. fluids
5. Allay the patient's anxiety
6. Inspect the surgical dressing and change, as directed
7. Reinforce TCDB
8. Keep the patient in semi-Fowler's position
9. Provide incentive spirometry
10. Maintain activity: as tolerated, active and passive ROM and isometric exercises
11. Administer oxygen

12. Monitor and record VS, UO, I/O, laboratory studies, neurovascular checks, and pulse oximetry
13. Administer anticoagulants, as prescribed
14. Provide bed cradle
15. Check site for bleeding
16. Maintain pressure dressing

D. Possible surgical complications
   1. Hemorrhage
   2. Embolism
   3. Thrombosis

E. Postoperative teaching goals (instructions to the patient and family)
   1. Keep follow-up appointments
   2. Exercise regularly
   3. Stop smoking
   4. Maintain a normal weight
   5. Know the action, side effects, and scheduling of medications
   6. Recognize the signs and symptoms of infection and bleeding
   7. Avoid prolonged sitting
   8. State cautions of long-term anticoagulant therapy
   9. Complete incision care daily

XI. Vena caval filter and plication of inferior vena cava

A. Definition
   1. Vena caval filter: surgical insertion of an intracaval filter (umbrella) to partially occlude the inferior vena cava and prevent pulmonary emboli
   2. Plication: surgical suturing and placement of Teflon clips to partially occlude the inferior vena cava and prevent pulmonary emboli

B. Preoperative nursing interventions and responsibilities
   1. Complete patient and family preoperative teaching
      a. Determine the patient's understanding of the procedure
      b. Describe the OR, PACU, and preoperative and postoperative routines
      c. Demonstrate postoperative TCDB, splinting, and leg and ROM exercises
      d. Explain the postoperative need for drainage tubes, surgical dressings, oxygen therapy, I.V. therapy, and pain control
   2. Complete a preoperative checklist
   3. Administer preoperative medications, as prescribed
   4. Allay the patient's and family's anxiety about surgery
   5. Document the patient's history and physical assessment data base

C. Postoperative nursing interventions and responsibilities
   1. Assess cardiac and respiratory status
   2. Assess pain and administer postoperative analgesics, as prescribed

3. Assess for return of peristalsis; provide solid foods and liquids, as tolerated
4. Administer I.V. fluids
5. Allay the patient's anxiety
6. Inspect the surgical dressing and change, as directed
7. Reinforce TCDB
8. Keep the patient in semi-Fowler's position, with the foot of the bed elevated
9. Provide incentive spirometry
10. Maintain activity: as tolerated, active and passive ROM, and isometric exercises
11. Administer oxygen
12. Monitor and record VS, UO, I/O, laboratory studies, neurovascular checks, and pulse oximetry
13. Check the insertion site for bleeding and hematoma
14. Assess peripheral edema
15. Apply antiembolism stockings
16. Avoid hip flexion

D. Possible surgical complications
   1. Embolism
   2. Infection

E. Postoperative teaching goals (instructions to the patient and family)
   1. Keep follow-up appointments
   2. Stop smoking
   3. Maintain a normal weight
   4. Know the action, side effects, and scheduling of medications
   5. Recognize the signs and symptoms of infection and edema
   6. Avoid prolonged sitting or crossing legs when sitting
   7. Complete incision care daily
   8. Walk daily
   9. Elevate legs when sitting
   10. Wear antiembolism stockings
   11. Adhere to long-term anticoagulant therapy

XII. Pneumonia

A. Definition—bacterial, viral, or fungal infection that causes inflammation of the alveolar spaces

B. Possible etiology
   1. Organisms: *E. coli, H. influenzae, S. aureus*
   2. Aspiration of food
   3. Aspiration of fluid
   4. Chemical irritants

C. Pathophysiology
   1. Microorganisms enter the alveolar spaces by droplet inhalation
   2. Inflammation occurs and alveolar fluid increases
   3. Ventilation decreases as secretions thicken

D. Possible clinical manifestations
   1. Cough
   2. Malaise
   3. Chills
   4. Shortness of breath
   5. Dyspnea
   6. Elevated temperature
   7. Crackles
   8. Rhonchi
   9. Pleural friction rub
   10. Pleuritic pain
   11. Sputum production
       a. Rusty, green, or bloody (pneumococcal pneumonia)
       b. Yellow-green (bronchopneumonia)

E. Possible diagnostic test findings
   1. Sputum studies: identification of organism
   2. Chest X-ray: pulmonary infiltrates
   3. Hematology: increased WBCs, ESR
   4. ABGs: hypoxemia, respiratory alkalosis

F. Medical management
   1. Diet: high-calorie, high-protein
   2. Dietary recommendation: force fluids
   3. I.V. therapy: hydration, heparin lock
   4. Oxygen therapy
   5. Intubation and mechanical ventilation
   6. Position: semi-Fowler's
   7. Activity: bed rest, active and passive ROM and isometric exercises
   8. Monitoring: VS, UO, and I/O
   9. Laboratory studies: WBCs, sputum culture, blood culture, and throat culture
   10. Nutritional support: total parental nutrition (TPN)
   11. Treatments: Foley catheter, CPT, postural drainage, and incentive spirometry
   12. Antibiotics: pencillin G potassium (Pentids), ampicillin (Omnipen)
   13. Antipyretics: aspirin, acetaminophen (Tylenol)
   14. Bronchodilators: metaproterenol sulfate (Alupent), isoetharine (Bronkosol)
   15. Specialized bed: rotation (Rotorest)
   16. Pulse oximetry

G. Nursing interventions and responsibilities
   1. Maintain the patient's diet
   2. Force fluids to 3 to 4 liters/day
   3. Administer I.V. fluids
   4. Administer oxygen
   5. Provide suction, TCDB
   6. Assess respiratory status
   7. Keep the patient in semi-Fowler's position
   8. Monitor and record VS, UO, I/O, laboratory studies, and pulse oximetry
   9. Administer medications, as prescribed
   10. Encourage the patient to express feelings about fear of suffocation
   11. Monitor and record color, consistency, and amount of sputum
   12. Allay the patient's anxiety
   13. Prevent spread of infection
   14. Provide oral hygiene
   15. Provide information about the American Lung Association

H. Teaching goals (instructions to the patient and family)
   1. Keep follow-up appointments
   2. Stop smoking
   3. Know the action, side effects, and scheduling of medications
   4. Recognize the signs and symptoms of respiratory infections
   5. Avoid exposure to people with infections
   6. Alternate rest periods with activity
   7. Monitor self for infection
   8. Follow dietary recommendations and restrictions
   9. Increase fluid intake to 3,000 ml/day

I. Possible medical complications
   1. Congestive heart failure (CHF)
   2. Pulmonary edema
   3. Respiratory failure

J. Possible surgical interventions: none

XIII. Chronic obstructive pulmonary disease (COPD)

A. Definition
   1. COPD is group of diseases that result in persistent obstruction of bronchial air flow
   2. Diseases include emphysema, asthma, bronchiectasis, and bronchitis
   3. In emphysema the stimulus to breathe is low PO_2 instead of increased PCO_2

B. Possible etiology
   1. Congential weakness
   2. Respiratory irritants: smoke, polluted air, chemical irritants

3. Respiratory tract infections
4. Genetic predisposition

C. Pathophysiology
  1. Bronchiectasis: infection destroys the bronchial mucosa, which is replaced by fibrous scar tissue; loss of resilience and dilation of airways causes pooling of secretions, obstruction of air flow, and decreased perfusion
  2. Asthma: irritants to bronchial tree cause bronchoconstriction, resulting in narrowed inflamed airways, dyspnea, and mucus production
  3. Bronchitis: excessive bronchial mucus production causes chronic or recurrent productive cough
  4. Emphysema: destruction of elastin alters alveolar walls and narrows airways, resulting in enlargement of air spaces distal to terminal bronchioles, trapped air, and coalesced alveoli

D. Possible clinical manifestations
  1. Cough
  2. Dyspnea
  3. Sputum production
  4. Weight loss
  5. Barrel chest (emphysema)
  6. Hemoptysis
  7. Exertional dyspnea
  8. Clubbing of fingers
  9. Malaise
  10. Wheezes
  11. Crackles
  12. Anemia
  13. Anxiety
  14. Diaphoresis
  15. Use of accessory muscles
  16. Orthopnea

E. Possible diagnostic test findings
  1. Chest X-ray: congestion, hyperinflation
  2. ABGs: respiratory acidosis, hypoxemia
  3. Sputum studies: positive identification of organism
  4. PFTs: increased residual volume, increased functional residual capacity, decreased vital capacity

F. Medical management
  1. Diet: high in protein, carbohydrates, vitamin C, calories, and nitrogen
  2. Dietary recommendation: force fluids to 3,000 ml/day
  3. I.V. therapy: heparin lock
  4. Oxygen therapy: 2 to 3 liters/minute
  5. Intubation and mechanical ventilation

   6. Position: high-Fowler's
   7. Activity: as tolerated
   8. Monitoring: VS, UO, and I/O
   9. Laboratory studies: ABGs, WBCs, and sputum studies
   10. Treatments: CPT, postural drainage, intermittent positive pressure breathing (IPPB), and incentive spirometry
   11. Antibiotics: ampicillin (Omnipen), tetracycline (Achromycin), cefixime (Suprax)
   12. Antacid: aluminum hydroxide gel (ALternaGEL)
   13. Bronchodilators: terbutaline (Brethine), aminophylline (Aminophyllin), isoproterenol (Isuprel)
   14. Steroids: hydrocortisone (Solu-Cortef), methylprednisolone sodium succinate (Solu-Medrol)
   15. Expectorant: guaifenesin (Robitussin)
   16. Beta-adrenergic drug: epinephrine hydrochloride (Adrenalin)
   17. Respiratory inhalant: cromolyn sodium (Intal)

G. Nursing interventions and responsibilities
   1. Maintain the patient's diet
   2. Administer small, frequent feedings
   3. Force fluids
   4. Administer low-flow oxygen
   5. Provide CPT, IPPB, TCDB, postural drainage, incentive spirometry, and suction
   6. Assess respiratory status
   7. Reinforce pursed-lip breathing
   8. Keep the patient in high-Fowler's position
   9. Monitor and record VS, UO, I/O, and laboratory studies
   10. Administer medications, as prescribed
   11. Encourage the patient to express feelings about fear of suffocation
   12. Activity, as tolerated
   13. Monitor and record the color, amount, and consistency of sputum
   14. Allay the patient's anxiety
   15. Weigh the patient daily
   16. Provide information about the American Lung Association

H. Teaching goals (instructions to the patient and family)
   1. Keep follow-up appointments
   2. Exercise regularly
   3. Stop smoking
   4. Maintain a normal weight
   5. Know the action, side effects, and scheduling of medications
   6. Identify ways to reduce stress
   7. Recognize the signs and symptoms of respiratory infection and hypoxia
   8. Adhere to activity limitations
   9. Avoid exposure to people with infections

10. Alternate rest periods with activity
11. Monitor self for infection
12. Follow dietary recommendations and restrictions
13. Maintain a quiet environment
14. Seek help from community agencies and resources
15. Demonstrate pursed-lip and diaphragmatic breathing
16. Avoid exposure to chemical irritants and pollutants
17. Demonstrate deep-breathing and coughing exercises
18. Avoid eating gas-producing foods, spicy foods, and extremely hot or cold foods

I. Possible medical complications
1. From emphysema
    a. Pulmonary hypertension
    b. Right-sided congestive heart failure
    c. Spontaneous pneumothorax
2. Carbon dioxide narcosis
3. Acute respiratory failure
4. Pneumonia

J. Possible surgical interventions: none

XIV. Adult respiratory distress syndrome (ARDS, shock lung)

A. Definition – clinical syndrome of respiratory insufficiency

B. Possible etiology
1. Viral pneumonia
2. Fat emboli
3. Sepsis
4. Decreased surfactant production
5. Fluid overload
6. Shock
7. Trauma
8. Neurologic injuries
9. Oxygen toxicity

C. Pathophysiology
1. Damaged capillary membranes cause interstitial edema and intra-alveolar hemorrhage
2. Decreased gas exchange results
3. Cellular damage causes decreased surfactant production, resulting in hypoxemia

D. Possible clinical manifestations
1. Dyspnea
2. TACHYPNEA
3. Cyanosis
4. Cough

    5. Crackles
    6. Rhonchi
    7. Anxiety
    8. Restlessness
    9. Decreased breath sounds

E. Possible diagnostic test findings
    1. ABGs: respiratory acidosis, hypoxemia that does not respond to increased percentage of oxygen
    2. Chest X-ray: interstitial edema
    3. Sputum studies: organism
    4. Blood cultures: organism

F. Medical management
    1. Diet: restrict fluid intake
    2. I.V. therapy: heparin lock
    3. Oxygen therapy
    4. Intubation and mechanical ventilation using positive end expiratory pressure (PEEP)
    5. Position: high-Fowler's
    6. Activity: bed rest; active ROM and isometric exercises
    7. Monitoring: VS, UO, I/O, central venous pressure (CVP), ECG, and hemodynamic variables
    8. Laboratory studies: ABGs, sputum studies, blood cultures, Hgb, and Hct
    9. Nutritional support: TPN
   10. Treatments: Foley catheter, CPT, postural drainage, and suction
   11. Transfusion therapy: platelets, packed RBCs
   12. Antibiotics: amoxicillin (Amoxil), ampicillin (Omnipen)
   13. Analgesic: morphine sulfate (Roxanol)
   14. Diuretics: furosemide (Lasix), ethacrynic acid (Edecrin)
   15. Anticoagulant: heparin (Lipo-Hepin)
   16. Steroids: hydrocortisone (Solu-Cortef), methylprednisolone sodium succinate (Solu-Medrol)
   17. Antacid: aluminum hydroxide gel (ALternaGEL)
   18. Neuromucular blocking agents: pancuronium bromide (Pavulon), vecuronium bromide (Norcuron)
   19. Mucosal barrier fortifier: sucralfate (Carafate)
   20. Pulse oximetry

G. Nursing interventions and responsibilities
    1. Maintain fluid restrictions
    2. Administer I.V. fluids
    3. Monitor mechanical ventilation
    4. Provide suction, TCDB, and postural drainage
    5. Assess respiratory status
    6. Keep the patient in high-Fowler's position

7. Monitor and record VS, UO, CVP, hemodynamic variables, I/O, specific gravity, laboratory studies, and pulse oximetry
8. Administer TPN
9. Administer medications, as prescribed
10. Encourage the patient to express feelings about fear of suffocation
11. Organize nursing care to allow rest periods
12. Weigh the patient daily
13. Allay the patient's anxiety
14. Maintain bed rest

H. Teaching goals (instructions to the patient and family)
1. Keep follow-up appointments
2. Stop smoking
3. Know the action, side effects, and scheduling of medications
4. Recognize the signs and symptoms of respiratory distress
5. Adhere to activity limitations
6. Avoid exposure to people with respiratory infections
7. Alternate rest periods with activity
8. Monitor self for infection
9. Demonstrate deep breathing and coughing exercises
10. Avoid exposure to chemical irritants and pollutants

I. Possible medical complications
1. Pulmonary edema
2. Atelectasis

J. Possible surgical interventions: none

XV. Tuberculosis, pulmonary (TB)

A. Definition—airborne, infectious, communicable disease that can occur acutely or chronically

B. Possible etiology: *Mycobacterium tuberculosis*

C. Pathophysiology
1. Alveoli become the focus of infection from inhaled droplets containing bacteria
2. Tubercle bacilli multiply, spread through the lymphatics, and drain into the systemic circulation
3. In the lung tissue, macrophages surround the bacilli and form tubercles
4. Tubercles go through the process of caseation, liquefaction, and cavitation

D. Possible clinical manifestations
1. Fatigue
2. Malaise
3. Irritability

4. Night sweats
5. Tachycardia
6. Weight loss
7. Anorexia
8. Cough
9. Yellow and mucoid sputum
10. Dyspnea
11. Hemoptysis
12. Crackles
13. Elevated temperature

E. Possible diagnostic test findings
   1. Chest X-ray: active or calcified lesions
   2. Sputum cultures: positive acid-fast bacillus; positive *M. tuberculosis*
   3. Hematology: increased WBCs, ESR
   4. Mantoux skin test: positive

F. Medical management
   1. Diet: high-carbohydrate, high-protein, high-vitamin B_6 and C, high calorie
   2. I.V. therapy: heparin lock
   3. Activity: bed rest, active ROM and isometric exercises
   4. Monitoring: VS, UO, and I/O
   5. Laboratory studies: ABGs and sputum studies
   6. Treatments: CPT, postural drainage, and incentive spirometry
   7. Precautions: respiratory
   8. Antibiotic: streptomycin
   9. Antituberculosis: isoniazid (INH), ethambutol (Myambutol), rifampin (Rifadin), pyrazinamide (PMS Pyrazinamide)

G. Nursing interventions and responsibilities
   1. Maintain the patient's diet
   2. Provide small frequent meals
   3. Provide suction, TCDB, CPT, and postural drainage
   4. Assess respiratory status
   5. Monitor and record VS, UO, I/O, and laboratory studies
   6. Administer medications, as prescribed
   7. Allay the patient's anxiety
   8. Maintain respiratory precautions
   9. Force fluids
   10. Maintain bed rest
   11. Instruct the patient to cover nose and mouth when sneezing
   12. Provide frequent oral hygiene
   13. Provide ultraviolet light or well-ventilated room
   14. Provide information about the American Lung Association

H. Teaching goals (instructions to the patient and family)
   1. Keep follow-up appointments

2. Stop smoking
3. Maintain a normal weight
4. Know the action, side effects, and scheduling of medications
5. Identify ways to reduce stress
6. Recognize the signs and symptoms of respiratory infection
7. Adhere to activity limitations
8. Avoid exposure to people with infections
9. Alternate rest periods with activity
10. Monitor self for infection
11. Follow dietary recommendations and restrictions
12. Seek help from community agencies and resources
13. Demonstrate methods to prevent spread of droplets of sputum
14. Provide adequate air ventilation in rooms

I. Possible medical complications
1. Atelectasis
2. Spontaneous pneumothorax

J. Possible surgical intervention: lobectomy (see page 269)

XVI. Pneumothorax

A. Definition
1. Loss of negative intrapleural pressure results in collapse of the lung
2. Types include spontaneous, open, tension

B. Possible etiology
1. Blunt chest trauma
2. Rupture of a bleb
3. CVP line insertion
4. Thoracentesis
5. Penetrating chest injuries

C. Pathophysiology
1. The loss of negative intrapleural pressure causes the collapse of the lung
2. Surface area for gas exchange is reduced, resulting in hypoxia and hypercarbia
3. Spontaneous pneumothorax occurs with the rupture of a bleb
4. Open pneumothorax occurs when an opening through the chest wall allows the entrance of positive atmospheric pressure into the pleural space
5. Tension pneumothorax occurs when there is a buildup of positive pressure in the pleural space

D. Possible clinical manifestations
1. Sharp pain that increases with exertion
2. Diminished or absent breath sounds unilaterally
3. Dyspnea

4. Tracheal shift
5. Anxiety
6. Diaphoresis
7. Tachycardia
8. Tachypnea
9. Decreased chest expansion unilaterally
10. Subcutaneous emphysema
11. Pallor
12. Cough

E. Possible diagnostic test findings
1. Chest X-ray: pneumothorax
2. ABGs: respiratory acidosis, hypoxemia
3. Ventilation-perfusion scintigraphy: decreased
4. Ventilation-perfusion (V/Q) defects: V/Q mismatches

F. Medical management
1. Oxygen therapy
2. Position: high-Fowler's
3. Activity: out of bed to chair, active ROM exercises to affected arm
4. Monitoring: VS and I/O
5. Laboratory studies: ABGs
6. Treatments: incentive spirometry
7. Insertion: chest tube to water-seal drainage
8. Thoracentesis
9. Analgesic: oxycodone hydrochloride (Tylox)

G. Nursing interventions and responsibilities
1. Administer oxygen
2. Provide TCDB and incentive spirometry
3. Assess respiratory status
4. Maintain chest tube to water-seal drainage
5. Keep the patient in high-Fowler's position
6. Monitor and record VS, chest tube drainage, air leak or subcutaneous emphysema, and laboratory studies
7. Administer medications, as prescribed
8. Allay the patient's anxiety
9. Assess the patient's pain

H. Teaching goals (instructions to the patient and family)
1. Keep follow-up appointments
2. Stop smoking
3. Know the action, side effects, and scheduling of medications
4. Recognize the signs and symptoms of pneumothorax and respiratory infection
5. Avoid heavy lifting

I. Possible medical complications
   1. Mediastinal shift
   2. Respiratory insufficiency
   3. Infection

J. Possible surgical interventions: none

XVII. Pulmonary embolism

A. Definition
   1. Undissolved substance in the pulmonary vasculature that obstructs blood flow
   2. Three types
      a. Fat
      b. Air
      c. Thrombus

B. Possible etiology
   1. Flat, long bone fractures
   2. Thrombophlebitis
   3. Venous stasis
   4. Hypercoagulability
   5. Abdominal surgery
   6. Malignant tumors
   7. Prolonged bedrest
   8. Obesity

C. Pathophysiology
   1. Air, fat, or the tail of a thrombus that breaks off travels from the venous circulation to the right side of the heart and pulmonary artery
   2. Blood flow is obstructed by the embolism, resulting in pulmonary hypertension and possible infarction

D. Possible clinical manifestations
   1. Dyspnea
   2. Tachycardia
   3. Elevated temperature
   4. Cough
   5. Hemoptysis
   6. Chest pain
   7. Tachypnea
   8. Anxiety
   9. Crackles
   10. Hypotension
   11. Arrhythmias

E. Possible diagnostic test findings
   1. Chest X-ray: dilated pulmonary arteries
   2. ABGs: respiratory alkalosis, hypoxemia

   3. Lung scan: decreased pulmonary circulation, blood flow obstruction
   4. Angiography: location of embolism, filling defect of pulmonary artery
   5. Blood chemistry: increased lactic dehydrogenase (LDH)
   6. ECG: tachycardia, nonspecific ST changes
F. Medical management
   1. I.V. therapy: hydration, heparin lock
   2. Oxygen therapy
   3. Intubation and mechanical ventilation
   4. Position: high-Fowler's
   5. Activity: bed rest; active and passive ROM and isometric exercises
   6. Monitoring: VS, UO, CVP, ECG, I/O, and neurovascular checks
   7. Laboratory studies: ABGs, PT, and PTT
   8. Treatments: Foley catheter, incentive spirometry
   9. Analgesic: meperidine hydrochloride (Demerol)
  10. Diuretics: furosemide (Lasix), ethacrynic acid (Edecin)
  11. Anticoagulants: heparin (Lipo-Hepin), warfarin sodium (Coumadin)
  12. Fibrinolytics: streptokinase, urokinase
  13. Pulse oximetry

G. Nursing interventions and responsibilities
   1. Administer I.V. fluids
   2. Administer oxygen
   3. Provide suction and TCDB
   4. Assess respiratory status
   5. Keep the patient in high-Fowler's position
   6. Monitor and record VS, UO, CVP, I/O, urine for blood, laboratory studies, and pulse oximetry
   7. Administer medications, as prescribed
   8. Allay the patient's anxiety
   9. Monitor and record color, consistency, and amount of sputum
  10. Assess for positive Homans' sign

H. Teaching goals (instructions to the patient and family)
   1. Keep follow-up appointments
   2. Exercise regularly
   3. Stop smoking
   4. Maintain a normal weight
   5. Know the action, side effects, and scheduling of medications
   6. Identify ways to reduce stress
   7. Recognize the signs and symptoms of respiratory distress
   8. Avoid several activities
      a. Prolonged sitting and standing
      b. Wearing constrictive clothing
      c. Crossing legs when seated
      d. Using oral contraceptives

I. Possible medical complications: pulmonary infarction

J. Possible surgical interventions
    1. Vein ligation
    2. Plication of inferior vena cava (see page 272)
    3. Embolectomy (see page 271)

XVIII. Lung cancer

A. Definition—malignant tumor of the lung that may be primary or metastatic

B. Possible etiology
    1. Cigarette smoking
    2. Exposure to environmental pollutants
    3. Exposure to occupational pollutants

C. Pathophysiology
    1. Unregulated cell growth and uncontrolled cell division result in the development of a neoplasm
    2. Four histologic types include epidermoid (squamous), adenocarcinoma, large cell anaplastic, small cell anaplastic
    3. Lungs are a common target site for metastasis from other organs

D. Possible clinical manifestations
    1. Cough
    2. Dyspnea
    3. Hemoptysis
    4. Chest pain
    5. Chills
    6. Fever
    7. Weight loss
    8. Weakness
    9. Anorexia
    10. Wheezing
    11. Fatigue

E. Possible diagnostic test findings
    1. Chest X-ray: lesion or mass
    2. Bronchoscopy: positive biopsy
    3. Angiography: involvement of pulmonary artery or pulmonary veins
    4. Sputum studies: positive cytology for cancer cells
    5. Lung scan: mass

F. Medical management
    1. Diet: high-protein, high-calorie
    2. I.V. therapy: heparin lock
    3. Oxygen therapy
    4. Intubation and mechanical ventilation
    5. Position: semi-Fowler's
    6. Actvity: as tolerated, active and passive ROM exercises

7. Monitoring: VS, UO, and I/O
8. Laboratory studies: ABGs
9. Nutritional support: TPN
10. Radiation therapy
11. Antineoplastics: cyclophosphamide (Cytoxan), doxorubicin hydrochloride (Adriamycin)
12. Treatment: incentive spirometry
13. Isotope implant
14. Laser photocoagulation
15. Diuretics: furosemide (Lasix), ethacrynic acid (Edecrin)
16. Chemotherapy: BCG vaccine (not FDA-approved for this use)
17. Analgesics: meperidine hydrochloride (Demerol), morphine sulfate (Roxanol)
18. Antiemetic: nabilone (Cesamet)
19. Pulse oximetry

G. Nursing interventions and responsibilities
1. Maintain the patient's diet
2. Encourage fluids
3. Administer I.V. fluids
4. Administer oxygen
5. Provide suction, and TCDB
6. Assess respiratory status
7. Keep the patient in semi-Fowler's position
8. Monitor and record VS, UO, I/O, laboratory studies, and pulse oximetry
9. Administer TPN
10. Administer medications, as prescribed
11. Encourage the patient to express feelings about changes in body image and a fear of dying
12. Assess the patient's pain and administer analgesics as prescribed
13. Provide postchemotherapeutic and postradiation nursing care
    a. Provide skin, mouth, and perineal care
    b. Encourage dietary intake
    c. Administer antiemetics and antidiarrheals, as prescribed
    d. Monitor for bleeding, infection, and electrolyte imbalance
    e. Provide rest periods
14. Provide information about the American Cancer Society

H. Teaching goals (instructions to the patient and family)
1. Keep follow-up appointments
2. Exercise regularly
3. Stop smoking
4. Maintain a normal weight
5. Know the action, side effects, and scheduling of medications
6. Demonstrate deep breathing and coughing exercises
7. Alternate rest periods with activity

  8. Follow dietary recommendations and restrictions

I. Possible medical complications
  1. Respiratory insufficiency
  2. Pneumonia

J. Possible surgical interventions
  1. Lung resection (see page 269)
  2. Lobectomy (see page 269)
  3. Wedge resection (see page 269)
  4. Pneumonectomy (see page 270)

XIX. Laryngeal cancer

A. Definition—benign or malignant tumor of the larynx

B. Possible etiology
  1. Cigarette smoking
  2. Alcohol abuse
  3. Exposure to environmental pollutants
  4. Exposure to radiation
  5. Voice strain

C. Pathophysiology
  1. Unregulated cell growth and uncontrolled cell division result in the development of a neoplasm through the growth of abnormal cells
  2. Most laryngeal cancers are squamous cell carcinomas
  3. Intrinsic cancer is cancer within the larynx
  4. Extrinsic cancer is cancer outside the larynx

D. Possible clinical manifestations
  1. Throat pain
  2. Burning sensation
  3. Palpable lump in neck
  4. Dysphagia
  5. Dyspnea
  6. Cough
  7. Hemoptysis
  8. Progressive hoarseness
  9. Sore throat
  10. Weakness
  11. Weight loss
  12. Foul breath

E. Possible diagnostic test findings
  1. Laryngoscopy: lesions, ulcerations, positive biopsy
  2. Biopsy: cytology positive for cancer cells
  3. Computed tomography (CT): laryngeal tumor
  4. Magnetic resonance imaging (MRI): laryngeal tumor

F. Medical management
   1. Diet: high-calorie, high-vitamin, high-protein
   2. I.V. therapy: heparin lock
   3. Oxygen therapy
   4. Position: semi-Fowler's
   5. Activity: as tolerated
   6. Monitoring: VS, UO, and I/O
   7. Laboratory studies: Hgb, Hct, and ABGs
   8. Nutritional support: TPN, NG tube feedings, and gastrostomy feedings
   9. Radiation therapy
  10. Chemotherapy
  11. Treatment: incentive spirometry
  12. Analgesic: oxycodone hydrochloride (Tylox)
  13. Antineoplastics: methotrexate sodium (Mexate), vincristine sulfate (Oncovin), bleomycin sulfate (Blenoxane), cisplatin (Platinol)
  14. Antiemetic: nabilone (Cesamet)

G. Nursing interventions and responsibilities
   1. Maintain high-calorie, high-vitamin, high-protein diet
   2. Administer I.V. fluids
   3. Administer oxygen
   4. Provide incentive spirometry, TCDB
   5. Assess respiratory status
   6. Maintain activity, as tolerated
   7. Keep the patient in semi-Fowler's position
   8. Monitor and record VS, UO, I/O, and laboratory studies
   9. Administer TPN, NG tube feedings, and gastrostomy feedings
  10. Administer medications, as prescribed
  11. Encourage the patient to express feelings about potential loss of voice and changes in body image
  12. Monitor and record the color, amount, and consistency of sputum
  13. Provide postchemotherapeutic and postradiation nursing care
    a. Provide skin, mouth, and perineal care
    b. Encourage dietary intake
    c. Administer antiemetics and antidiarrheals, as prescribed
    d. Monitor for bleeding, infection, and electrolyte imbalance
    e. Provide rest periods
  14. Provide information about the Lost Chord Club, New Voice Club, and International Association of Laryngectomies

H. Teaching goals (instructions to the patient and family)
   1. Keep follow-up appointments
   2. Stop smoking
   3. Maintain a normal weight
   4. Know the action, side effects, and scheduling of medications
   5. Recognize the signs and symptoms of respiratory distress

6. Limit using voice
7. Avoid exposure to people with infections
8. Alternate rest periods with activity
9. Monitor self for infection
10. Follow dietary recommendations and restrictions
11. Seek help from community agencies and resources

I. Possible medical complications
   1. Laryngeal obstruction
   2. Respiratory distress

J. Possible surgical interventions
   1. Partial laryngectomy (see page 266)
   2. Total laryngectomy (see page 266)
   3. Radical neck dissection (see page 268)

Points to remember

Objective assessment findings in respiratory disorders include dyspnea, adventitious sounds, sputum, clubbing of fingers, fremitus, crepitus, and a change in patterns and character of respirations.

After a bronchoscopy, food and fluids should be withheld until the patient's gag reflex returns.

After any surgery on the respiratory tract, TCDB should be encouraged frequently.

The stimulus for breathing in emphysema is low PO_2.

The patient with ARDS, pneumothorax, or pulmonary embolism should be placed in high-Fowler's position.

Respiratory precautions should be used for the patient with TB.

Lung cancer has been linked to cigarette smoking and environmental and occupational pollutants.

Glossary

The following terms are defined in Appendix A, page 354.

crackles

dyspnea

hemoptysis

rhonchi

tachypnea

Study questions

To evaluate your understanding of this chapter, answer the following questions in the space provided; then compare your responses with the correct answers in Appendix B, pages 362 and 363.

1. Which nursing interventions are appropriate after a bronchoscopy?

_____

_____

2. What is removed in a total laryngectomy? _____

_____

_____

3. What is a key postoperative assessment for a patient with a radical neck dissection? _____

_____

4. How should a patient be positioned after a pneumonectomy? _____

_____

_____

5. Which surgical complications may follow an embolectomy? _____

_____

_____

6. What is the purpose of a vena caval filter? _____

_____

_____

7. What are the clinical manifestations for a patient with pneumonia?

_____

_____

8. What are the four diseases associcated with COPD? _____

_____

_____

Study questions *(continued)*

9. In a patient with ARDS, what would the ABG analysis reveal? ⎯⎯⎯⎯⎯⎯

10. How is TB spread? ⎯⎯⎯⎯⎯⎯⎯⎯⎯⎯⎯⎯⎯⎯⎯⎯⎯

11. What is the key clinical manifestation of pneumothorax? ⎯⎯⎯⎯⎯⎯

12. What should a patient with pulmonary embolism avoid? ⎯⎯⎯⎯⎯⎯

13. What are the four histologic types of lung cancer? ⎯⎯⎯⎯⎯⎯

14. Which antineoplastic agents might be used to treat laryngeal cancer?

CHAPTER 8

Integumentary System

Learning objectives

Check off the following items once you've mastered them:

☐ Describe the psychosocial impact of integumentary system disorders.

☐ Differentiate between modifiable and nonmodifiable risk factors in the development of an integumentary system disorder.

☐ List three probable and three possible nursing diagnoses for a patient with an integumentary system disorder.

☐ Identify the nursing interventions and responsibilities for a patient with an integumentary system disorder.

☐ Write goals for teaching a patient with an integumentary system disorder.

I. Anatomy and physiology

A. Skin: first line of defense against microorganisms; composed of three layers
  1. Epidermis
     a. Outer avascular layer composed of dense squamous cells that constantly shed
     b. Keratinocytes and melanocytes in this layer
  2. Dermis:
     a. Origin of hair, nails, sebaceous glands, eccrine sweat glands, apocrine sweat glands
     b. Collagen layer that supports the epidermis and contains nerves and blood vessels
  3. Subcutaneous tissue (hypodermis)
     a. Third layer of skin is composed of loose connective tissue filled with fatty cells
     b. It provides heat, insulation, shock absorption, and a reserve of calories

B. Hair
  1. It protects and covers the body, except for the palms, lips, soles of the feet, nipples, and external genitalia
  2. Hormones stimulate differential growth

C. Nails
  1. Composed of dead cells filled with keratin
  2. Protect the tips of the fingers and toes

D. Glandular appendages
  1. Three types are sebaceous, eccrine, and apocrine
  2. Sebaceous glands (oil), which lubricate hair and epidermis, are stimulated by sex hormones
  3. Eccrine sweat glands regulate body temperature through water secretion
  4. Apocrine sweat glands — located in the axilla, nipple, anal, and pubic areas — secrete odorless fluid; decomposition of this fluid by bacteria causes odor

II. Physical assessment findings

A. Subjective data that often accompany integumentary disorders
  1. Change in skin color, texture, and temperature
  2. Perspiration or dryness
  3. Itching
  4. Brittle, thick, or soft nails
  5. Fever
  6. Hair loss
  7. Rash

B. Objective data to evaluate in integumentary disorders
   1. Pattern of pigmentation and hair distribution
   2. Skin texture, turgor, color, and temperature
   3. Peripheral edema
   4. TROPHIC changes: skin, hair, and nails
   5. Skin lesions: type, shape, and character
   6. PRURITUS
   7. NEVI and scars
   8. Elevated body temperature
   9. Erythema
   10. Petechiae and ecchymosis

III. Diagnostic tests and procedures

A. Blood chemistry
   1. Definition and purpose
      a. Laboratory test of a blood sample
      b. Analysis for potassium, sodium, calcium, phosphorus, ketones, glucose, osmolality, chloride, blood urea nitrogen (BUN), and creatinine
   2. Nursing interventions and responsibilities
      a. Withhold food and fluids before the procedure, as directed
      b. Check the site for bleeding after the procedure

B. Hematologic studies
   1. Definition and purpose
      a. Laboratory test of a blood sample
      b. Analysis for red blood cells (RBCs), white blood cells (WBCs), erythrocyte sedimentation rate (ESR), platelets, prothrombin time (PT), partial thromboplastin time (PTT), hemoglobin (Hgb), hematocrit (Hct)
   2. Nursing interventions and responsibilities: check the site for bleeding

C. Skin biopsy (punch biopsy)
   1. Definition and purpose
      a. Procedure using a circular punch instrument to remove a small amount of skin tissue
      b. Histologic evaluation
   2. Nursing interventions and responsibilities: check the site for bleeding and infection

D. Skin testing
   1. Definition and purpose
      a. Procedure using a patch, scratch, or intradermal technique
      b. Administration of an allergen to the skin's surface or into the dermis
   2. Nursing interventions and responsibilities
      a. Keep the area dry

      b. Record the site, date, and time of test
      c. Inspect the site for erythema, papules, VESICLES, edema, and induration
      d. Record the date and time for follow-up site reading

E. Skin scrapings
  1. Definition and purpose
      a. Procedure calling for cells scraped by a scalpel and covered with potassium hydroxide
      b. Microscopic examination of scales, nails, and hair
  2. Nursing interventions and responsibilities: check scraping site for bleeding and infection

F. Skin studies
  1. Definition and purpose
      a. Laboratory test
      b. Microscopic examination of skin, including gram stain, culture and sensitivity, cytology, and immunofluorescence (IF)
  2. Nursing interventions and responsibilities
      a. Follow laboratory procedure guidelines
      b. Note current antibiotic therapy

G. Wood's light
  1. Definition and purpose
      a. Procedure using ultraviolet (UV) light
      b. Direct examination of skin
  2. Nursing interventions and responsibilities
      a. Explain procedure
      b. Allay the patient's anxiety

IV. Psychosocial impact of integumentary disorders

A. Developmental impact
  1. Changes in body image
  2. Fear of rejection
  3. Changes in role performance
  4. Decreased self-esteem

B. Economic impact
  1. Cost of cosmetics
  2. Disruption or loss of employment
  3. Cost of hospitalizations and follow-up care
  4. Cost of medications

C. Occupational and recreational impact
  1. Restrictions in physical activity
  2. Changes in leisure activity

D. Social impact
  1. Social isolation (from embarrassment about changes in skin appearance)
  2. Sexual dysfunction

V. Possible risk factors for integumentary disorders

A. Modifiable risk factors
  1. Infection
  2. Occupation
  3. Exposure to chemical and environmental pollutants
  4. Exposure to radiation
  5. Exposure to sun
  6. Personal hygiene habits
  7. Climate
  8. Use of cosmetics and soaps
  9. Stress
  10. Nutritional deficiencies
  11. Medications
  12. Crowded living conditions

B. Nonmodifiable risk factors
  1. Aging
  2. History of endocrine, vascular, or immune disorders
  3. Family history of skin disease or allergies
  4. History of allergies
  5. Exposure to communicable disease
  6. Pregnancy
  7. Menopause

VI. Nursing diagnostic categories for a patient with an integumentary disorder

A. Probable nursing diagnostic categories
  1. Impaired skin integrity
  2. Body image disturbance
  3. Self-esteem disturbance
  4. Pain
  5. Sensory-perceptual alteration: tactile

B. Possible nursing diagnostic categories
  1. Ineffective breathing patterns
  2. Ineffective individual coping
  3. Fluid volume deficit
  4. Potential for infection
  5. Anxiety
  6. Social isolation

VII. Skin graft

A. Definition
  1. Replacement of damaged skin with healthy skin to protect underlying structures or to reconstruct areas for cosmetic or functional purposes
  2. Split-thickness graft: graft of half of the epidermis, which is removed by a dermatome
  3. Full-thickness graft: graft of the entire epidermis
  4. Pinch graft: graft of a small piece of skin, obtained by elevating the skin with a needle and removing it with scissors

B. Preoperative nursing interventions and responsibilities
  1. Complete patient and family preoperative teaching
     a. Determine the patient's understanding of the procedure
     b. Describe the operating room (OR), postanesthesia care unit (PACU), and preoperative and postoperative routines
     c. Demonstrate postoperative turning, coughing, and deep breathing (TCDB), splinting, leg exercises, and range-of-motion (ROM) exercises
     d. Explain the postoperative need for drainage tubes, surgical dressings, oxygen therapy, I.V. therapy, and pain control
  2. Complete a preoperative checklist
  3. Administer preoperative medications, as prescribed
  4. Allay the patient's and family's anxiety about surgery
  5. Document the patient's history and physical assesssment data base
  6. Prepare the donor and graft sites

C. Postoperative nursing interventions and responsibilities
  1. Assess pain and administer postoperative analgesics, as prescribed
  2. Assess for return of peristalsis; provide solid foods and liquids, as tolerated
  3. Administer I.V. fluids
  4. Allay the patient's anxiety
  5. Provide hydrotherapy, as directed
  6. Reinforce TCDB
  7. Provide incentive spirometry
  8. Maintain activity: as tolerated, active and passive ROM and isometric exercises
  9. Avoid weight bearing on the extremity with the graft site
  10. Monitor and record vital signs (VS), urinary output (UO), intake and output (I/O), and neurovascular checks distal to the recipient site
  11. Elevate and immobilize the graft site
  12. Encourage the patient to express feelings about changes in body image
  13. Administer antibiotics, as prescribed
  14. Assess the graft site for infection, hematoma, and fluid accumulation under the graft
  15. Keep the donor site dry and open to air

16. Prevent scratching
17. Apply heat lamp to the donor site
18. Keep the graft and donor sites free from pressure
19. Apply sterile saline or antibiotic solution to the graft site, as ordered

D. Possible surgical complications
   1. Infection of the graft and donor sites
   2. Graft rejection or failure
   3. Hematoma under the graft
   4. Fluid accumulation under the graft

E. Postoperative teaching goals (instructions to the patient and family)
   1. Keep follow-up appointments
   2. Exercise regularly
   3. Stop smoking
   4. Maintain a normal weight
   5. Know the action, side effects, and scheduling of medications
   6. Recognize the signs and symptoms of infection
   7. Continue physical therapy
   8. Apply lubricating lotion to the graft site
   9. Protect the graft site from direct sunlight
   10. Avoid trauma to the graft site
   11. Avoid extreme temperatures
   12. Demonstrate cosmetic camouflage techniques
   13. Complete daily dressing changes

VIII. Contact dermatitis

A. Definition — inflammatory response of the skin after contact with a specific antigen

B. Possible etiology
   1. Mechanical, biological, and chemical irritants
   2. Cosmetics and hair dyes
   3. Detergents, cleaning agents, and soaps
   4. Insecticides
   5. Poison ivy
   6. Wool

C. Pathophysiology
   1. Contact with an antigen triggers a localized inflammatory response
   2. Inflammatory response produces skin changes

D. Possible clinical manifestations
   1. Pruritus and burning
   2. Erythema at point of contact
   3. Localized edema
   4. Vesicles and papules
   5. LICHENIFICATION

6. Pigmentation changes
7. Eczema
8. Scaling

E. Possible diagnostic test findings
    1. Skin test (patch): positive to specific antigen
    2. Visual examination: area of dermatitis correlates with area of antigen contact

F. Medical management
    1. Position: elevation of extremity
    2. Activity: as tolerated
    3. Monitoring: VS and neurovascular checks
    4. Treatments: cool, wet dressings with aluminum acetate solution (Burow's solution) tepid baths, and bed cradle
    5. Antibiotic: ampicillin (Omnipen)
    6. Antipruritic: diphenhydramine hydrochloride (Benadryl)
    7. Corticosteroid: hydrocortisone (Cort-Dome)
    8. Antihistamine: diphenhydramine hydrochloride (Benadryl)
    9. Antianxiety agent: diazepam (Valium)

G. Nursing interventions and responsibilities
    1. Assess neurovascular status
    2. Maintain elevation of affected extremity
    3. Monitor and record VS and neurovascular checks
    4. Administer medications, as prescribed
    5. Encourage the patient to express feelings about changes in physical appearance
    6. Provide tepid baths, bed cradle, and cool, wet dressings
    7. Avoid soaps
    8. Avoid using heating pads or blankets
    9. Avoid temperature extremes
   10. Prevent scratching and rubbing of affected area
   11. Maintain a cool environment
   12. Provide diversional activities

H. Teaching goals (instructions to the patient and family)
    1. Keep follow-up appointments
    2. Stop smoking
    3. Know the action, side effects, and scheduling of medications
    4. Recognize the signs and symptoms of infection
    5. Monitor self for infection
    6. Avoid causative agent
    7. Avoid skin dryness and heat
    8. Avoid using soaps and over-the-counter medications
    9. Protect affected area from trauma, excessive sunlight, wind, and temperature extremes
   10. Avoid scratching and rubbing affected areas

I. Possible medical complications: infection

J. Possible surgical interventions: none

IX. Psoriasis

A. Definition – chronic, noninfectious skin inflammation that occurs in patches

B. Possible etiology
   1. Stress
   2. Epidermal trauma
   3. Streptococcal infection
   4. Changes in climate
   5. Genetics
   6. Anxiety
   7. Alcoholism
   8. Rheumatoid arthritis
   9. Drug induced: lithium, propranolol
   10. Hormones
   11. Obesity

C. Pathophysiology
   1. Loss of normal regulatory mechanisms of cell division leads to rapid multiplication of epidermal cells that interferes with formation of normal protective layer of skin
   2. Papules coalesce to form plaques

D. Possible clinical manifestations
   1. Pruritus
   2. Shedding, scaling plaques
   3. Yellow discoloration and thickening of nails
   4. Erythema
   5. Papules on sacrum, nails, palms

E. Possible diagnostic test finding: plaques, on visual examination

F. Medical management
   1. Monitoring: VS and neurovascular checks
   2. Treatments: bed cradle, daily soaks, and tepid, wet compresses
   3. Corticosteroids: triamcinolone acetonide (Kenalog) covered with occlusive dressing, betamethasone valerate (Valisone)
   4. Antipsoriatics: anthralin (Anthra-Derm), coal tar (Estar), followed by exposure to UV light, etretinate (Tegison)
   5. Antimetabolite: methotrexate (Amethopterin)
   6. Photochemotherapy (PUVA therapy): methoxsalen (Oxsoralen) followed by exposure to black light
   7. Keratolytics: benzoyl peroxide (Benzagel), salicylic acid (Keratex, Salacid)

8. Anti-microbial: sulfasalazine (Azulfidine)
9. Diet: high-protein, high-calorie, frequent feedings

G. Nursing interventions and responsibilities
1. Assess neurovascular status
2. Monitor and record VS and neurovascular checks
3. Administer medications, as prescribed
4. Encourage the patient to express feelings about changes in body image
5. Administer UV light and PUVA therapy
6. Apply occlusive dressings
7. Prevent scratching
8. Help the patient to remove scales during soaks
9. Provide information about the National Psoriasis Foundation
10. Maintain the patient's diet

H. Teaching goals (instructions to the patient and family)
1. Keep follow-up appointments
2. Stop smoking
3. Maintain a normal weight
4. Know the action, side effects, and scheduling of medications
5. Identify ways to reduce stress
6. Recognize the signs and symptoms of infection
7. Wear light cotton clothing over affected areas
8. Avoid over-the-counter medications
9. Demonstrate dressing changes
10. Complete skin care daily
11. Protect affected areas from trauma

I. Possible medical complications
1. Depression
2. Infection
3. Rheumatoid arthritis

J. Possible surgical interventions: none

X. Herpes zoster (shingles)

A. Definition — acute viral infection of nerve structure caused by varicella zoster

B. Possible etiology
1. Cytotoxic drug-induced immunosuppression
2. Hodgkin's disease
3. Exposure to varicella zoster
4. Debilitating disease

C. Pathophysiology
1. Activation of dormant varicella zoster virus causes an inflammatory reaction

   2. Affected areas include spinal and cranial sensory ganglia and posterior gray matter of the spinal cord

D. Possible clinical manifestations
   1. Neuralgia
   2. Malaise
   3. Pruritus
   4. Burning
   5. Unilaterally clustered skin vesicles along peripheral sensory nerves on trunk, thorax, or face
   6. Erythema
   7. Fever
   8. Anorexia
   9. Headache
   10. Parasthesia
   11. Edematous skin

E. Possible diagnostic test findings
   1. Antinuclear antibody (ANA): positive
   2. Skin cultures and stains: identification of organism
   3. Visual examination: vesicles along peripheral sensory nerves

F. Medical management
   1. Activity: as tolerated
   2. Monitoring: VS, seventh cranial nerve function, and neurovascular checks
   3. Treatments: air mattress, acetic acid compresses, tepid baths, and bed cradle
   4. Analgesics: acetaminophen (Tylenol), oxycodone hydrochloride (Tylox)
   5. Antianxiety agents: diazepam (Valium), hydroxyzine (Vistaril)
   6. Antipruritic: diphenhydramine hydrochloride (Benadryl)
   7. Corticosteroids: hydrocortisone (Cortef), triamcinolone acetonide (Kenalog)
   8. Nerve block using lidocaine (Xylocaine)
   9. Antiviral agents: acyclovir (Zovirax), vidarabine monohydrate (Vira-A), interferon (Roferon-A)
   10. Laboratory studies: culture and sensitivity

G. Nursing interventions and responsibilities
   1. Assess pain
   2. Monitor and record VS, laboratory results, and seventh cranial nerve function
   3. Administer medications, as directed
   4. Encourage the patient to express feelings about changes in physical appearance and recurrent nature of the illness
   5. Provide acetic acid compresses, tepid baths, bed cradle, and air mattress
   6. Prevent scratching and rubbing of affected areas

7. Allay the patient's anxiety

H. Teaching goals (instructions to the patient and family)
1. Keep follow-up appointments
2. Stop smoking
3. Know the action, side effects, and scheduling of medications
4. Recognize the signs and symptoms of infection and hearing loss
5. Monitor self for infection
6. Avoid wool and synthetic clothing
7. Wear lightweight, loose cotton clothing
8. Keep blisters intact
9. Avoid scratching and rubbing affected areas

I. Possible medical complications
1. Infection
2. Postherapeutic neuralgia
3. Ophthalmic herpes zoster
4. Facial paralysis
5. Vertigo
6. Tinnitus
7. Hearing loss
8. Visceral dissemination

J. Possible surgical interventions: none

XI. Burns

A. Definition – destruction of epidermis, dermis, and subcutaneous layers of skin

B. Possible etiology
1. Radiation: X-ray, sun, nuclear reactors
2. Mechanical: friction
3. Chemical: acids, alkalies, vesicants
4. Electrical: lightning, electrical wires
5. Thermal: flame, frostbite, scald

C. Pathophysiology
1. Cell destruction causes loss of intracellular fluid and electrolytes
2. Amount of cell destruction is directly related to extent (area) and degree (depth) of burn
3. First-degree (superficial partial thickness) involves epidermal layer
4. Second-degree (dermal partial thickness) involves epidermal and dermal layers
5. Third-degree (full thickness) involves epidermal, dermal, subcutaneous layers, and nerve endings

D. Possible clinical manifestations
1. First-degree

      a. Erythema
      b. Edema
      c. Pain
      d. Blanching
  2. Second-degree
      a. Pain
      b. Oozing, fluid-filled vesicles
      c. Erythema
      d. Shiny, wet subcutaneous layer after vesicles rupture
  3. Third-degree
      a. Eschar
      b. Edema
      c. Little or no pain

E. Possible diagnostic test findings
  1. Blood chemistry: increased potassium; decreased sodium, albumin, complement fixation, immunoglobulins
  2. Arterial blood gases (ABGs): metabolic acidosis
  3. 24-hour urine collection: decreased creatinine clearance, negative nitrogen balance
  4. Hematology: increased Hgb, Hct; decreased fibrinogen, platelets, WBCs
  5. Urine chemistry: hematuria, myoglobinuria
  6. Visual examination: extent of burn determined by Rule of Nines, Lund and Browder chart

F. Medical management
  1. Withhold oral food and fluids until allowed by the physician
  2. Diet: high in protein, fat, calories, carbohydrates; small, frequent feedings
  3. I.V. therapy: hydration and electrolyte replacement using Evan, Brooke, Parkland, or Massachusetts General Hospital protocols; heparin lock
  4. Oxygen therapy
  5. Intubation and mechanical ventilation
  6. Gastrointestinal decompression: nasogastric (NG) tube, Miller-Abbott tube
  7. Position: semi-Fowler's
  8. Activity: bed rest
  9. Monitoring: VS, UO, electrocardiogram (ECG), hemodynamic variables, I/O, neurovital signs, neurovascular checks, and stool for occult blood
  10. Laboratory studies: potassium, sodium, glucose, osmolality, creatinine, BUN, Hgb, Hct, platelets, WBCs, ABGs, culture and sensitivity
  11. Nutritional support: total parental nutrition (TPN), NG feedings
  12. Treatments: Foley catheter, postural drainage, chest physiotherapy (CPT), incentive spirometry, bed cradle, intermittent positive pressure breathing (IPPB), suction, Jobst clothing, and Hubbard tank bath

13. Precaution: protective
14. Transfusion therapy: fresh frozen plasma (FFP), platelets, packed RBCs, plasma
15. Antibiotic: gentamicin sulfate (Garamycin)
16. Anti-infectives: mafenide (Sulfamylon), silver sulfadiazine (Silvadene), silver nitrate, povidone-iodine (Betadine)
17. Antianxiety: diazepam (Valium)
18. Antitetanus: tetanus toxoid
19. Analgesic: morphine sulfate (Roxanol)
20. Antacids: magnesium and aluminum hydroxide (Maalox), aluminum hydroxide gel (ALternaGEL)
21. Histamine antagonists: cimetidine (Tagamet), ranitidine (Zantac)
22. Vitamins: phytonadione (AquaMEPHYTON), cyanocobalamin (vitamin B_{12})
23. Colloids: 5% albumin (Albuminar)
24. Diuretics: mannitol (Osmitrol)
25. Sedatives: phenobarbital (Luminal)
26. Cardiac glycosides: digoxin (Lanoxin)
27. Escharotomy
28. Biologic dressings
29. Early excisional therapy
30. Specialized bed: Air Fluidized (Clinitron, Skytron, Fluid Air)
31. Pulse oximetry
32. Mucosal barrier fortifier: sucralfate (Carafate)

G. Nursing interventions and responsibilities
   1. Maintain the patient's diet; withhold food and fluids, as ordered
   2. Administer I.V. fluids
   3. Administer oxygen
   4. Provide suction, TCDB, IPPB, CPT, and postural drainage
   5. Assess respiratory status and fluid balance
   6. Assess pain
   7. Maintain position, patency, and low suction of NG tube
   8. Keep the patient in semi-Fowler's position
   9. Monitor and record VS, UO, I/O, laboratory studies, hemodynamic variables, neurovital signs, stool for occult blood, specific gravity, calorie count, daily weight, neurovascular checks, and pulse oximetry
   10. Provide tracheostomy care or endotube care
   11. Administer TPN
   12. Administer medications, as prescribed
   13. Encourage the patient to express feelings about disfigurement, immobility from scarring, and a fear of dying
   14. Allay the patient's anxiety
   15. Provide treatments: ROM exercises, tanking, bed cradle, splints, and Jobst clothing
   16. Alternate periods of rest with activity

17. Elevate affected extremities
18. Maintain a warm environment during acute period
19. Maintain protective precautions
20. Provide skin and mouth care
21. Assess bowel sounds

H. Teaching goals (instructions to the patient and family)
1. Keep follow-up appointments
2. Exercise regularly
3. Stop smoking
4. Maintain a normal weight
5. Know the action, side effects, and scheduling of medications
6. Identify ways to reduce stress
7. Recognize the signs and symptoms of infection
8. Alternate periods of rest with activity
9. Monitor self for infection
10. Follow dietary recommendations and restrictions
11. Complete skin care daily
12. Demonstrate dressing changes
13. Avoid trauma to affected area
14. Avoid wearing restrictive clothing
15. Avoid using fabric softeners, harsh detergents, and soaps
16. Lubricate healing skin with cocoa butter
17. Maintain a cool environment
18. Protect the affected area from sunlight
19. Use splints and Jobst clothing

I. Possible medical complications
1. Paralytic ileus
2. Curling's ulcer
3. Acute renal failure
4. Pneumonia
5. Congestive heart failure
6. Septicemia
7. Pulmonary edema
8. Hypovolemic shock

J. Possible surgical interventions: skin grafting (see page 299)

XII. Skin cancer

A. Definition
1. Malignant primary tumor of the epidermal layer of the skin
2. Three types of skin cancer
   a. Basal cell epithelioma
   b. Melanoma
   c. Squamous cell carcinoma

B. Possible etiology
 1. Heredity
 2. Chemical irritants
 3. Ultraviolet rays
 4. Radiation
 5. Friction or chronic irritation
 6. Immunosuppressive drugs
 7. Precancerous lesions: leukoplakia, nevi, senile keratoses
 8. Infrared heat or light

C. Pathophysiology
 1. Unregulated cell growth and uncontrolled cell division result in the development of a neoplasm
 2. Basal cell epithelioma: basal cell keratinization causes tumor growth in basal layer of the epidermis
 3. Melanoma: tumor arises from melanocytes of the epidermis
 4. Squamous cell carcinoma: tumor arises from keratinocytes

D. Possible clinical manifestations
 1. Basal cell epithelioma: waxy nodule with telangiectasis
 2. Melanoma: irregular, circular bordered lesion with hues of tan, black, or blue
 3. Squamous cell carcinoma: small, red, nodular lesion that begins as an erythematous macule or plaque with indistinct margins
 4. Pruritus
 5. Local soreness
 6. Change in color, size, or shape of preexisting lesion
 7. Oozing, bleeding, crusting lesion

E. Possible diagnostic test findings (skin biopsy): cytology positive for cancer cells

F. Medical management
 1. I.V. therapy: heparin lock
 2. Monitoring: VS
 3. Radiation therapy
 4. Cryosurgery with liquid nitrogen
 5. Chemosurgery with zinc chloride
 6. Curettage and electrodesiccation
 7. Immunotherapy for melanoma: bacille Calmette-Guérin (BCG) vaccine
 8. Alkalating agents: carmustine (BiCNU), dacarbazine (DTIC-Dome)
 9. Antineoplastics: hydroxyurea (Hydrea), vincristine sulfate (Oncovin)
 10. Antimetabolites: fluorouracil (Adrucil)
 11. Antiemetic: nabilone (Cesamet)

G. Nursing interventions and responsibilities
 1. Monitor and record VS
 2. Administer medications, as prescribed

3. Encourage the patient to express feelings about changes in body image and a fear of dying
4. Provide postchemotherapeutic and postradiation nursing care
   a. Provide skin, mouth, and perineal care
   b. Encourage dietary intake
   c. Administer antiemetics and antidiarrheals, as prescribed
   d. Monitor for bleeding, infection, and electrolyte imbalance
   e. Provide rest periods
5. Assess lesions
6. Provide information about the Skin Cancer Foundation

H. Teaching goals (instructions to the patient and family)
   1. Keep follow-up appointments
   2. Know the action, side effects, and scheduling of medications
   3. Recognize the signs and symptoms of infection
   4. Avoid exposure to people with infections
   5. Alternate periods of rest with activity
   6. Monitor self for infection
   7. Seek help from community agencies and resources
   8. Avoid contact with chemical irritants
   9. Use sun-screening lotions and layered clothing when outdoors
   10. Monitor self for lesions that do not heal or that change characteristics
   11. Have moles removed that are subject to chronic irritation

I. Possible medical complications: metastasis (melanoma)

J. Possible surgical interventions
   1. Surgical excision of tumor
   2. Melanoma: bone marrow transplant (see page 322)

Points to remember

Infection is a common complication of integumentary disorders.

The patient's embarrassment from skin changes can cause social isolation.

Many risk factors associated with integumentary disorders are modifiable.

The nurse should assess a skin graft site for infection, hematoma, and fluid accumulation; the donor site should be kept dry and open to the air.

Burns that destroy cells can cause intracellular fluid loss and electrolyte imbalances.

A patient with skin cancer should use sunscreen lotions and wear protective clothing outdoors.

Glossary

The following terms are defined in Appendix A, page 354.

lichenification

nevi

pruritus

trophic

vesicle

Study questions

To evaluate your understanding of this chapter, answer the following questions in the space provided; then compare your responses with the correct answers in Appendix B, page 363.

1. What are the responsibilities of a nurse caring for a patient undergoing skin tests? _____

   _____

2. Which key nursing assessment should be performed after a skin graft?

   _____

   _____

3. Which medications might the physician prescribe for a patient with contact dermatitis? _____

   _____

4. Which clinical manifestations would a patient with psoriasis exhibit?

   _____

   _____

5. Where do the vesicles typically appear in herpes zoster? _____

   _____

   _____

6. What are the clinical manifestations of a second-degree burn? _____

   _____

   _____

7. What are the three types of skin cancer? _____

   _____

   _____

CHAPTER 9

Hematologic and Lymphatic Systems

Learning objectives

Check off the following items once you've mastered them:

☐ Describe the psychosocial impact of a hematologic or lymphatic system disorder.

☐ Differentiate between modifiable and nonmodifiable risk factors in the development of a hematologic or lymphatic system disorder.

☐ List three probable and three possible nursing diagnoses for the patient with a hematologic or lymphatic system disorder.

☐ Identify the nursing interventions and responsibilities for a patient with a hematologic or lymphatic system disorder.

☐ Write three goals for teaching a patient with a hematologic or lymphatic system disorder.

I. Anatomy and physiology

A. Lymphatic vessels
   1. Consist of capillary-like structures that are permeable to large molecules
   2. Prevent edema by moving fluid and proteins from interstitial spaces to venous circulation
   3. Reabsorb fats from the small intestine

B. Lymph nodes
   1. Tissue that filters out bacteria and other foreign cells
   2. Regional grouping of lymph nodes: cervicofacial, supraclavicular, axillary, epitrochlear, inguinal, and femoral

C. Lymph
   1. Fluid found in interstitial spaces
   2. Composition of lymph: water and end products of cell metabolism

D. Spleen
   1. Is the largest lymphatic organ
   2. Filters blood
   3. Traps formed particles
   4. Destroys bacteria
   5. Serves as blood reservoir
   6. Forms lymphocytes and monocytes

E. Erythrocytes: red blood cells (RBCs)
   1. RBCs are formed in the bone marrow
   2. RBCs contain hemoglobin (Hgb)
   3. Oxygen binds with Hgb to form oxyhemoglobin

F. Thrombocytes (platelets)
   1. Formed in the bone marrow
   2. Function in the coagulation of blood

G. Leukocytes: white blood cells (WBCs)
   1. WBCs are formed in the bone marrow and lymphatic tissue
   2. WBCs include granulocytes and agranulocytes
   3. Provide immunity and protection from infection by phagocytosis

H. Plasma
   1. Liquid portion of the blood
   2. Composition of plasma: water, protein (albumin and globulin), glucose, and electrolytes

I. ABO blood groups
   1. System of antigens located on the surface of RBCs that determines blood type
   2. Blood types: A antigen, B antigen, AB antigens, O (zero) antigens
   3. Universal donor: blood type O

    4. Universal recipient: blood type AB

J. Coagulation
    1. Blood clotting
    2. Series of reactions involving the conversion of prothrombin to thrombin to fibrinogen to fibrin to form a clot

K. Bone marrow
    1. Two types exist: red and yellow
    2. Hematopoeisis is carried out by red marrow
    3. Hematopoeisis produces erythrocytes, leukocytes, and thrombocytes
    4. Red bone marrow is a source of lymphocytes and macrophages
    5. Yellow bone marrow is red bone marrow that has changed to fat

L. Liver
    1. Is the largest organ in the body
    2. Produces bile (main function), which emulsifies fats and stimulates peristalsis
    3. Conveys bile to the duodenum at the sphincter of Oddi through the common bile duct
    4. Metabolizes carbohydrates, fats, and proteins
    5. Synthesizes coagulation factors VII, IX, X, and prothrombin
    6. Stores vitamins A, D, B_{12}, and iron
    7. Detoxifies chemicals
    8. Excretes bilirubin
    9. Receives dual blood supply from portal vein and hepatic artery
   10. Produces and stores glycogen
   11. Promotes erythropoiesis when bone marrow production is insufficient

II. Physical assessment findings

A. Subjective data that often accompany hematolymphatic disorders
    1. Enlarged glands
    2. Pain
    3. Fatigue and weakness
    4. Bleeding
    5. Pallor
    6. Lassitude
    7. Shortness of breath
    8. Fainting
    9. Vertigo
   10. Jaundice
   11. Night sweats
   12. Fever
   13. Weight loss
   14. Tachycardia
   15. Activity intolerance
   16. Frequent infections

17. Melena
18. Headache

B. Objective data to evaluate in hematolymphatic disorders
   1. Lymph node enlargement
   2. Anemia
   3. ECCHYMOSIS
   4. Skin: pallor, cyanosis, jaundice, PETECHIAE
   5. Gingivitis
   6. Ophthalmoscopic exam: bleeding fundi
   7. Sclera: jaundice, capillary hemorrhage
   8. Hepatomegaly
   9. Sternal tenderness
   10. Splenomegaly
   11. Myocardial hypertrophy
   12. EPISTAXIS
   13. Dyspnea on exertion

III. Diagnostic tests and procedures

A. Blood chemistry
   1. Definition and purpose
      a. Laboratory test of a blood sample
      b. Analysis for potassium, calcium, blood urea nitrogen (BUN), creatinine, protein, albumin, and bilirubin
   2. Nursing interventions and responsibilities
      a. Withhold food and fluids, as directed, before the procedure
      b. Check the site for bleeding after the procedure

B. Hematologic studies
   1. Definition and purpose
      a. Laboratory test of a blood sample
      b. Analysis for WBCs, RBCs, platelets, prothrombin time (PT), partial thromboplastin time (PTT), erythrocyte sedimentation rate (ESR), Hgb, and hematocrit (Hct)
   2. Nursing interventions and responsibilities
      a. Note current drug therapy before the procedure
      b. Check the site for bleeding after the procedure

C. Lymphangiography
   1. Definition and purpose
      a. Procedure involving an injection of radiopaque dye through a catheter
      b. Radiographic picture of lymphatic system and dissection of lymph vessel
   2. Nursing interventions and responsibilities before the procedure
      a. Note the patient's allergies to iodine, seafood, and radiopaque dyes

     b. Inform the patient of possible throat irritation and flushing of the face after injection of the dye

     c. Obtain written, informed consent

     d. Withhold food and fluids, as directed

  3. Nursing interventions and responsibilities after the procedure

     a. Assess vital signs (VS) and peripheral pulses

     b. Check catheter insertion site for bleeding

     c. Force fluids

     d. Advise the patient that skin, stool, and urine will have a blue discoloration

D. Bone marrow examination (aspiration or biopsy)

  1. Definition and purpose

     a. Procedure involving the percutaneous removal of bone marrow

     b. Examination of erythrocytes, leukocytes, and thrombocytes

  2. Nursing interventions and responsibilities before the procedure

     a. Obtain written, informed consent

     b. Determine the patient's ability to lie still during aspiration

  3. Nursing interventions and responsibilities after the procedure

     a. Maintain pressure dressing

     b. Check the aspiration site for bleeding and infection

E. Schilling test

  1. Definition and purpose

     a. Procedure involving administration of oral radioactive cyanocobalamin and intramuscular cyanocobalamin

     b. Microscopic examination of a 24-hour urine sample for cyanocobalamin (vitamin B_{12})

  2. Nursing interventions and responsibilities before the procedure

     a. Withhold food and fluids after midnight

     b. Obtain written, informed consent

  3. Nursing interventions and responsibilities after the procedure

     a. Instruct the patient to save all voided urine for 24 hours

     b. Keep urine at room temperature

F. Gastric analysis

  1. Definition and purpose

     a. Procedure involving the aspiration of stomach contents through a nasogastric (NG) tube

     b. Fasting analysis of gastric secretions to measure acidity and diagnose pernicious anemia

  2. Nursing interventions and responsibilities before the procedure

     a. Withhold food and fluids

     b. Instruct the patient not to smoke for 8 to 12 hours before the test

     c. Withhold medications that can affect gastric secretions

  3. Nursing interventions and responsibilities after the procedure

     a. Obtain vital signs

      b. Assess for reactions to gastric acid stimulant, if used

G. Urine urobilinogen
   1. Definition and purpose
      a. Laboratory test of a 2-hour or a 24-hour urine sample
      b. Microscopic examination to diagnose hemolytic jaundice
   2. Nursing interventions and responsibilities
      a. Use bottle with a preservative and refrigerate specimen
      b. Note salicylate use
      c. Start urine collection in the afternoon when food is being digested for a 2-hour specimen
      d. Begin the 24-hour collection after the first voided specimen in the morning

H. Erythrocyte life span determination
   1. Definition and purpose
      a. Procedure involving reinjection of the patient's blood that has been tagged with chromium 51
      b. Measurement of the life span of circulating RBCs
   2. Nursing interventions and responsibilities
      a. Inform the patient that frequent blood samples will be drawn over a 2-week period
      b. Check the venipuncture site for bleeding
      c. Apply a pressure dressing after the procedure

I. Bence Jones protein assay
   1. Definition and purpose
      a. Procedure involving a 24-hour urine sample
      b. Microscopic examination for the Bence Jones protein to diagnose multiple myeloma
   2. Nursing interventions and responsibilities
      a. Withhold all medications for 48 hours before the test
      b. Instruct the patient to void and note the time (collection of urine starts with the next voiding)
      c. Place urine container on ice
      d. Measure each voided urine
      e. Instruct the patient to void at the end of the 24-hour period
      f. Note any medications that might interfere with the test

J. Romberg test
   1. Definition and purpose
      a. Physical test
      b. Examination to assess loss of balance in pernicious anemia
   2. Nursing interventions and responsibilities
      a. Explain the procedure
      b. Monitor for imbalance
      c. Prevent the patient from falling

K. Erythrocyte fragility test
  1. Definition and purpose
     a. Laboratory test of a blood sample
     b. Analysis to measure the rate at which RBCs burst in varied hypotonic solutions
  2. Nursing interventions and responsibilities
     a. Explain the procedure
     b. Send the specimen to the laboratory

L. Rumpel-Leede capillary fragility tourniquet test
  1. Definition and purpose
     a. Crude physical test
     b. Examination of vascular resistance, platelet number, and function
  2. Nursing interventions and responsibilities: Explain that a blood pressure cuff will be placed on the arm for 5 minutes, followed by counting of petechiae

M. Bone scan
  1. Definition and purpose
     a. Procedure using an I.V. injection of radioisotope
     b. Visual imaging of bone metabolism
  2. Nursing interventions and responsibilities before the procedure: determine the patient's ability to lie still

IV. Psychosocial impact of hematologic and lymphatic disorders

A. Developmental impact
  1. Fear of dying
  2. Decreased self-esteem
  3. Fear of rejection

B. Economic impact
  1. Disruption or loss of employment
  2. Cost of hospitalization
  3. Cost of medications

C. Occupational and recreational impact
  1. Restrictions in work activity
  2. Changes in leisure activity

D. Social impact
  1. Changes in role performance
  2. Social isolation

V. Risk factors for developing hematologic and lymphatic disorders

A. Modifiable risk factors
  1. Exposure to chemical and environmental pollutants
  2. Sexual activity patterns

   3. History of aspirin use
   4. Alcohol consumption
   5. Drug toxicity
   6. Diet
   7. Exposure to occupational radiation or radiation therapy

B. Nonmodifiable risk factors
   1. Ethnic background
   2. Aging
   3. Malabsorption syndromes
   4. History of liver disease
   5. History of malignancy

VI. Nursing diagnostic categories for the patient with a hematologic and lymphatic disorder

A. Probable nursing diagnostic categories
   1. Activity intolerance
   2. Ineffective breathing pattern
   3. Pain
   4. Impaired gas exchange

B. Possible nursing diagnostic categories
   1. Potential for infection
   2. Altered nutrition: less than body requirements
   3. Altered oral mucous membranes
   4. Body image disturbance
   5. Self-esteem disturbance
   6. Anxiety
   7. Social isolation
   8. Impaired skin integrity

VII. Splenectomy

A. Definition — surgical removal of the spleen

B. Preoperative nursing interventions and responsibilities
   1. Complete patient and family preoperative teaching
      a. Determine the patient's understanding of the procedure
      b. Describe the operating room (OR), postanesthesia care unit (PACU), and preoperative and postoperative routines
      c. Demonstrate postoperative turning, coughing, and deep breathing (TCDB), splinting, leg exercises, and range-of-motion (ROM) exercises
      d. Explain the postoperative need for drainage tubes, surgical dressings, oxygen therapy, I.V. therapy, and pain control
   2. Complete a preoperative checklist
   3. Administer preoperative medications, as prescribed

4. Allay the patient's and family's anxiety about surgery
5. Document the patient's history and physical assessment data base
6. Monitor PT, PTT, and platelet count
7. Administer vitamin K
8. Verify inoculation with polyvalent pneumococcal vaccine 2 weeks before procedure
9. Administer antibiotics, as prescribed

C. Postoperative nursing interventions and responsibilities
1. Assess cardiac, respiratory, and neurologic status
2. Assess pain and administer postoperative analgesics, as prescribed
3. Assess for return of peristalsis; provide solid foods and liquids, as tolerated
4. Administer I.V. fluids, total parental nutrition (TPN), and transfusion therapy, as prescribed
5. Allay the patient's anxiety
6. Inspect the surgical dressing and change, as directed
7. Reinforce TCDB and splinting of incision
8. Keep the patient in semi-Fowler's position
9. Provide incentive spirometry
10. Increase activity as tolerated
11. Monitor and record VS, urinary output (UO), intake and output (I/O), laboratory studies, and pulse oximetry
12. Monitor and maintain position and patency of drainage tubes: wound drainage
13. Apply abdominal binder
14. Monitor for abdominal distention

D. Possible surgical complications
1. Pneumococcal pneumonia
2. Infection
3. Hemorrhage
4. Sepsis
5. Disseminated intravascular coagulation (DIC)
6. Atelectasis
7. Subphrenic abscess
8. Thrombophlebitis

E. Postoperative teaching goals (instructions to the patient and family)
1. Keep follow-up appointments
2. Exercise regularly
3. Stop smoking
4. Maintain a normal weight
5. Know the action, side effects, and scheduling of medications
6. Recognize the signs and symptoms of infection
7. Avoid exposure to people with infections
8. Complete incision care daily

9. State the need for prophylactic use of antibiotics
10. Avoid contact sports

VIII. Bone marrow transplant

A. Definition
   1. Bone marrow is aspirated from multiple sites along the iliac crest of the donor
   2. Donor bone marrow is infused intravenously into the recipient
B. Preoperative nursing interventions and responsibilities
   1. Complete patient and family preoperative teaching
      a. Determine the patient's understanding of the procedure
      b. Describe the OR, PACU, and preoperative and postoperative routines
      c. Demonstrate postoperative TCDB, splinting, and leg and ROM exercises
      d. Explain the postoperative need for drainage tubes, surgical dressings, oxygen therapy, I.V. therapy, and pain control
   2. Complete a preoperative checklist
   3. Administer preoperative medications, as prescribed
   4. Allay the patient's and family's anxiety about surgery
   5. Document the patient's history and physical assessment data base
   6. Verify bone marrow compatibility
   7. Administer chemotherapy for 3 days before the transplant
   8. Maintain the radiation treatment schedule
   9. Maintain protective isolation or the use of a laminar air flow room
   10. Monitor for infection
C. Postoperative nursing interventions and responsibilities
   1. Assess cardiac and respiratory status
   2. Assess for return of peristalsis; provide solid foods and liquids, as tolerated
   3. Administer I.V. fluids
   4. Allay the patient's anxiety
   5. Inspect the surgical dressing and change, as directed
   6. Keep the patient in semi-Fowler's position
   7. Maintain activity, as tolerated
   8. Monitor and record VS; UO; I/O; central venous pressure (CVP); laboratory studies; urine, stool, and emesis for occult blood; daily weight; specific gravity; urine glucose, ketones, and protein; and pulse oximetry
   9. Precautions: protective
   10. Encourage the patient to express feelings about a fear of dying
   11. Administer antibiotics, as prescribed
   12. Administer antidiarrheals, as prescribed
   13. Monitor for infection
   14. Provide mouth and skin care

15. Inspect for bruising and petechiae

D. Possible surgical complications
    1. Marrow graft rejection
    2. Graft versus host disease
    3. Cataracts
    4. Stomatitis
    5. Hemorrhage

E. Postoperative teaching goals (instructions to the patient and family)
    1. Keep follow-up appointments
    2. Know the action, side effects, and scheduling of medications
    3. Recognize the signs and symptoms of infection and bleeding
    4. Complete skin care daily
    5. Identify changes in vision

IX. Agranulocytosis (granulocytopenia)

A. Definition—profound decrease in the number of granulocytes

B. Possible etiology
    1. Idiopathic
    2. Exposure to chemicals
    3. Drug induced: chloramphenicol (Chloromycetin), chlorpromazine (Thorazine), phenytoin (Dilantin)
    4. Chemotherapy
    5. Radiation
    6. Radioisotopes
    7. Hemodialysis
    8. Viral infection

C. Pathophysiology
    1. Number of granulocytes is reduced because of increased utilization, lack of maturation, or shortened life span
    2. The reduced number of granulocytes diminishes resistance to disease

D. Possible clinical manifestations
    1. Fatigue
    2. Malaise
    3. Elevated temperature
    4. Chills
    5. Sore throat
    6. Multiple infections
    7. Weakness
    8. Dysphagia
    9. Enlarged cervical lymph nodes
    10. Tachycardia
    11. Ulcerations of oral mucosa and throat

E. Possible diagnostic test findings
   1. Hematology: decreased WBCs, granulocytes; increased ESR
   2. Bone marrow biopsy: absence of polymorphonuclear leukocytes
   3. Culture and sensitivity: positive identification of organisms

F. Medical management
   1. Diet: high-protein, high-vitamin, high-calorie, bland, and soft
   2. I.V. therapy: heparin lock
   3. Position: semi-Fowler's
   4. Activity: bed rest and active and passive ROM exercises
   5. Monitoring: VS, UO, and I/O
   6. Laboratory studies: WBCs, granulocytes, and urine and blood for culture and sensitivity
   7. Treatments: saline gargles
   8. Precautions: protective
   9. Transfusion therapy: packed WBCs and whole blood
  10. Antibiotics: ticarcillan (Ticar), tobramycin sulfate (Nebcin)
  11. Antipyretic: acetaminophen (Tylenol)
  12. Sedative: phenobarbital (Luminal)
  13. Stool softener: docusate sodium (Colace)
  14. Analgesic: ibuprofen (Motrin)

G. Nursing interventions and responsibilities
   1. Maintain the patient's diet
   2. Force fluids
   3. Provide TCDB
   4. Assess respiratory status
   5. Keep the patient in semi-Fowler's position
   6. Monitor and record: VS, UO, I/O, laboratory studies, and stool count
   7. Administer medications, as prescribed
   8. Encourage the patient to express feelings about imposed isolation
   9. Maintain bed rest
  10. Provide tepid baths and saline gargles
  11. Maintain protective precautions
  12. Administer transfusion therapy, as prescribed
  13. Provide gentle mouth and skin care
  14. Monitor for infection
  15. Avoid enemas and rectal temperatures

H. Teaching goals (instructions to the patient and family)
   1. Keep follow-up appointments
   2. Know the action, side effects, and scheduling of medications
   3. Recognize the signs and symptoms of infection
   4. Avoid exposure to people with infections
   5. Alternate rest periods with activity
   6. Monitor self for infection
   7. Follow dietary recommendations and restrictions

8. Complete gentle skin and mouth care daily
9. Avoid using over-the-counter medications
10. Prevent constipation

I. Possible medical complications
   1. Sepsis
   2. Rectal abscess
   3. Pneumonia
   4. Hemorrhagic necrosis of mucous membranes
   5. Parenchymal liver damage

J. Possible surgical interventions: splenectomy (see page 320)

X. Leukemia

A. Definition
   1. Uncontrolled proliferation of WBC precursors that fail to mature
   2. Three types
      a. Acute myelogenous (AML)
      b. Chronic lymphocytic (CLL)
      c. Chronic myelocytic (CML)

B. Possible etiology
   1. Unknown
   2. Genetics
   3. Virus
   4. Exposure to chemicals
   5. Radiation
   6. Altered immune system
   7. Chemotherapy
   8. Polycythemia vera

C. Pathophysiology
   1. Normal hemopoietic cells are replaced by leukemic cells in bone marrow
   2. Immature forms of WBCs circulate in the blood, infiltrating the liver, spleen, and lymph nodes

D. Possible clinical manifestations
   1. Petechiae
   2. Ecchymosis
   3. Frequent infections
   4. Elevated temperature
   5. Enlarged lymph nodes, spleen, and liver
   6. Joint, abdominal, and bone pain
   7. Gingivitis
   8. Night sweats
   9. Stomatitis
   10. Prolonged menses

11. Hematemesis
12. Melena
13. Jaundice
14. Tachycardia
15. Hypotension

E. Possible diagnostic test findings
   1. Hematology: decreased Hct, Hgb, RBCs, platelets; increased ESR, immature WBCs, bleeding time
   2. Bone marrow biopsy: large number of immature leukocytes

F. Medical management
   1. Diet: high-protein, high-vitamin and mineral, high-calorie, low-roughage, bland and soft in small, frequent feedings
   2. I.V. therapy: hydration and heparin lock
   3. Oxygen therapy
   4. Position: semi-Fowler's
   5. Activity: bed rest and active and passive ROM and isometric exercises
   6. Monitoring: VS, UO, and I/O
   7. Laboratory studies: Hgb, Hct, WBCs, platelets, BUN, creatinine, and surveillance cultures
   8. Nutritional support: TPN
   9. Radiation therapy
  10. Chemotherapy
  11. Treatments: sitz baths, bed cradle, and tepid baths
  12. Precautions: protective or laminar air flow room
  13. Transfusion therapy: platelets, packed RBCs, and whole blood
  14. Antibiotics: doxorubicin (Adriamycin), plicamycin (Mithracin)
  15. Antipyretic: acetaminophen (Tylenol)
  16. Stool softener: docusate sodium (Colace)
  17. Analgesic: ibuprofen (Motrin)
  18. Antigout: allopurinol (Zyloprim)
  19. Tranquilizer: diazepam (Valium)
  20. Systemic alkalinizer: sodium bicarbonate
  21. Antimetabolites: fluorouracil (Adrucil), methotrexate sodium (Mexate)
  22. Alkylating agents: busulfan (Myleran), chlorambucil (Leukeran)
  23. Antineoplastics: vinblastine (Velban), vincristine sulfate (Oncovin)
  24. Enzymes: L-asparaginase (Elspar)
  25. Estrogens: diethylstilbestrol (DES)
  26. Progestins: medroxyprogesterone (Provera)
  27. IgG antibody: immune globulin I.V. (Gammagard)
  28. Antiemetic: nabilone (Cesamet)

G. Nursing interventions and responsibilities
   1. Maintain the patient's diet
   2. Force fluids
   3. Administer I.V. fluids

4. Administer oxygen
5. Provide TCDB
6. Assess cardiovascular, neurologic, respiratory, and renal status and fluid balance
7. Keep the patient in semi-Fowler's position
8. Monitor and record VS, UO, I/O, laboratory studies, daily weight, and urine, stool, and emesis for occult blood
9. Administer TPN
10. Administer transfusion therapy, as prescribed
11. Administer medications, as prescribed
12. Encourage the patient to express feelings about changes in body image and a fear of dying
13. Maintain bed rest
14. Provide treatments: sitz baths, bed cradle, and tepid baths
15. Allay the patient's anxiety
16. Monitor for bleeding and infection
17. Maintain protective precautions
18. Provide gentle mouth and skin care
19. Avoid giving the patient intramuscular injections, enemas, and rectal temperatures
20. Avoid using straight razors on the patient
21. Provide postchemotherapeutic care
    a. Provide skin, mouth, and perineal care
    b. Encourage dietary intake
    c. Administer antiemetics and antidiarrheals, as prescribed
    d. Monitor for bleeding, infection, and electrolyte imbalance
    e. Provide rest periods
22. Provide information about the American Cancer Society

H. Teaching goals (instructions to the patient and family)
1. Keep follow-up appointments
2. Maintain a normal weight
3. Know the action, side effects, and scheduling of medications
4. Recognize the signs and symptoms of occult blood and infection
5. Avoid exposure to people with infections
6. Alternate rest periods with activity
7. Monitor self for infection
8. Follow dietary recommendations and restrictions
9. Seek help from community agencies and resources
10. Complete skin and mouth care daily
11. Prevent constipation
12. Use an electric razor
13. Avoid using over-the-counter medications
14. Monitor stool for occult blood
15. Increase fluid intake

I. Possible medical complications
 1. Gross systemic hemorrhage
 2. Acute renal failure
 3. Cerebrovascular accident (CVA)
 4. Thrombocytopenia
 5. Perirectal abscess
 6. Gastrointestinal bleeding
 7. Fungal and bacterial infection
 8. Meningitis

J. Possible surgical interventions: bone marrow transplant (see page 322)

XI. Lymphomas

A. Definition
 1. Hodgkin's disease: proliferation of malignant Reed-Sternberg cells within lymph nodes
 2. Non-Hodgkin's lymphoma: malignant tumors of lymph nodes and lymphatic tissues that cannot be classified as Hodgkin's disease
 3. Classes of non-Hodgkin's lymphoma: B-lymphocyte malignancies, T-lymphocyte malignancies, and histiocyte malignancies

B. Possible etiology
 1. Unknown
 2. Viral
 3. Genetic (Hodgkin's disease)
 4. Environmental (Hodgkin's disease)
 5. Immunologic

C. Pathophysiology
 1. Reed-Sternberg cells proliferate in a single lymph node and travel contiguously through the lymphathic system to other lymphatic nodes and organs (Hodgkin's disease)
 2. Immune system cell tumors occur throughout lymph nodes and lymphatic organs in unpredictable patterns (non-Hodgkin's lymphoma)

D. Possible clinical manifestations
 1. Enlarged, nontender, firm, and movable lymph nodes in lower cervical regions (Hodgkin's disease)
 2. Recurrent, intermittent fever
 3. Night sweats
 4. Weight loss
 5. Malaise
 6. Lethargy
 7. Severe pruritus
 8. Dyspnea (Hodgkin's disease)
 9. Anorexia
 10. Bone pain (Hodgkin's disease)

11. Cough
12. Recurrent infection
13. Hepatomegaly
14. Splenomegaly
15. Dysphagia (Hodgkin's disease)
16. Edema and cyanosis of face and neck (Hodgkin's disease)
17. Prominent, painless, generalized LYMPHADENOPATHY (non-Hodgkin's lymphoma)

E. Possible diagnostic test findings
   1. Bone marrow aspiration and biopsy: small, diffuse lymphocytic or large, follicular-type cells (non-Hodgkin's lymphoma)
   2. Hematology: decreased Hgb, Hct, platelets (non-Hodgkin's and Hodgkin's); increased ESR (Hodgkin's and non-Hodgkin's lymphoma); increased leukocytes, gammaglobulin (Hodgkin's)
   3. Lymphangiogram: positive lymph node involvement (Hodgkin's disease)
   4. Lymph node biopsy: positive for Reed-Sternberg cells (Hodgkin's disease)
   5. Chest X-ray: lymphadenopathy (Hodgkin's disease)
   6. Blood chemistry: increased alkaline phosphatase, copper (Hodgkin's disease)
   7. Stage I: asymptomatic: malignant cells found in a single lymph node
   8. Stage II: symptomatic; malignant cells found in two or three adjacent lymph nodes on the same side of the diaphragm
   9. Stage III: symptomatic; malignant cells widely disseminated to lymph nodes on both sides of the diaphragm and to organs
   10. Stage IV: symptomatic; malignant cells found in one or more extralymphatic organs or tissues with or without lymphatic involvement

F. Medical management
   1. Diet: high-protein, high-calorie, high-vitamin and mineral, high-iron, high-calcium, bland, and soft
   2. I.V. therapy: heparin lock
   3. Oxygen therapy
   4. Position: semi-Fowler's
   5. Acitvity: bed rest and active and passive ROM exercises
   6. Monitoring: VS, UO, and I/O
   7. Laboratory studies: Hgb, Hct, WBCs, and platelets
   8. Radiation therapy
   9. Precautions: protective
   10. Transfusion therapy: packed RBCs
   11. MOPP chemotherapy protocol: mechlorethamine (Mustargen), vincristine suslfate (Oncovin), procarbazine (Matulane), prednisone (Deltasone)

12. ABVD chemotherapy protocol: doxorubicin (Adriamycin), bleomycin (Blenoxane), vinblastine (Velban), dacarbazine (DTIC-Dome) for Hodgkin's disease
13. Analgesic: meperidine hydrochloride (Demerol)
14. Sedative: phenobarbital (Luminal)
15. Stool softener: docusate sodium (Colace)
16. Antipruritic: diphenhydramine (Benadryl)
17. CVP chemotherapy protocol (non-Hodgkin's lymphoma): cyclophosphamide (Cytoxan), vincristine sulfate (Oncovin), prednisone (Deltasone)
18. CHOP chemotherapy protocol (non-Hodgkin's lymphoma): cyclophosphamide (Cytoxan), doxorubicin (Adriamycin), vincristine sulfate (Oncovin), prednisone (Deltasone)
19. Antiemetic: nabilone (Cesamet)

G. Nursing interventions and responsibilities
1. Maintain the patient's diet
2. Force fluids
3. Administer I.V. fluids
4. Administer oxygen
5. Provide TCDB
6. Assess respiratory, cardiovascular, and neurologic status and fluid balance
7. Keep the patient in semi-Fowler's position
8. Monitor and record VS, UO, I/O, laboratory studies, and specific gravity
9. Administer medications, as prescribed
10. Encourage the patient to express feelings about changes in body image and a fear of dying
11. Maintain bed rest
12. Give frequent baths with mild soap
13. Provide mouth and skin care
14. Administer transfusion therapy, as prescribed
15. Allay the patient's anxiety
16. Avoid giving aspirin to the patient
17. Avoid using straight razors on the patient
18. Provide postchemotherapeutic and postradiation nursing care
    a. Provide skin, mouth, and perineal care
    b. Encourage dietary intake
    c. Administer antiemetics and antidiarrheals, as prescribed
    d. Monitor for bleeding, infection, and electrolyte imbalance
    e. Provide rest periods
19. Monitor for jaundice and infection
20. Maintain protective precautions
21. Provide information about the American Cancer Society

H. Teaching goals (instructions to the patient and family)
   1. Keep follow-up appointments
   2. Exercise regularly
   3. Maintain a normal weight
   4. Know the action, side effects, and scheduling of medications
   5. Recognize the signs and symptoms of infection and motor and sensory deficits
   6. Avoid exposure to people with infections
   7. Alternate rest periods with activity
   8. Monitor self for infection
   9. Follow dietary recommendations and restrictions
   10. Promote a safe environment
   11. Complete skin and mouth care daily
   12. Increase fluid intake
   13. Use electric razors
   14. Avoid using over-the-counter medications
   15. Avoid taking aspirin

I. Possible medical complications
   1. Metastasis (Hodgkin's disease)
   2. Hypersplenism
   3. Pleural effusion (Hodgkin's disease)
   4. Herpes zoster (Hodgkin's disease)
   5. Depression
   6. Pancytopenia (Hodgkin's disease)
   7. Pneumonitis (Hodgkin's disease)
   8. Paraplegia
   9. Pericarditis (Hodgkin's disease)
   10. Nephritis (Hodgkin's disease)
   11. Hypothyroidism (Hodgkin's disease)
   12. Neuralgia (Hodgkin's disease)
   13. Obstructive jaundice (Hodgkin's disease)
   14. Infections: viral, bacterial, fungal (non-Hodgkin's lymphoma)
   15. Intestinal obstruction (non-Hodgkin's lymphoma)
   16. Leukemia (non-Hodgkin's lymphoma)
   17. Superior vena cava obstruction (non-Hodgkin's lymphoma)

J. Possible surgical interventions: splenectomy (see page 320)

XII. Acquired immunodeficiency syndrome (AIDS)

A. Definition
   1. Defect in T-cell mediated immunity that allows the development of fatal opportunistic infections
   2. Caused by human immunodeficiency virus (HIV)

3. An illness characterized by laboratory evidence of HIV infection coexisting with one or more indicator diseases, such as herpes simplex virus, cytomegalovirus, mycobacteria, candidal infection, *Pneumocystis carinii*, Kaposi's sarcoma, wasting syndrome, and dementia

B. Possible etiology
1. Exposure to blood containing HIV: transfusions, contaminated needles, handling of blood, in utero
2. Exposure to semen containing HIV: sexual intercourse, handling of semen

C. Pathophysiology
1. HIV is transmitted by contact with infected blood or body fluids
   a. HIV-infected lymphocytes are carried in semen and blood
   b. Infected lymphocytes in semen are transferred through minute breaks in the skin and mucosa
   c. Infected lymphocytes in blood are transferred via transfusion, fetal circulation, and minute breaks in the skin and mucosa
2. HIV, a retrovirus, selectively infects human cells containing CD_4 antigen on their surface, the majority of which are T_4 lymphocytes
3. HIV virus reproduces within the T_4 lymphocytes and destroys them
4. The destruction of the T_4 lymphocytes diminishes resistance to disease

D. Possible clinical manifestations
1. Fatigue, weakness, anorexia, weight loss, recurrent diarrhea, fever, lymphadenopathy, pallor, night sweats, malnutrition
2. Disorientation, confusion, dementia
3. Opportunistic infections

E. Possible diagnostic test findings
1. Hematology: decreased WBCs, RBCs, platelets
2. Blood chemistry: increased transaminase, alkaline phosphatase, gamma globulin; decreased albumin
3. Enzyme linked immunosorbent assay (ELISA): positive HIV antibody titer
4. Western blot: positive

F. Medical management
1. Diet: high-calorie, high-protein in small, frequent feedings
2. I.V. therapy: hydration, electrolyte replacement, and heparin lock
3. Oxygen therapy
4. Position: semi-Fowler's
5. Activity: as tolerated, active and pasive ROM exercises
6. Monitoring: VS, UO, I/O, and neurovital signs
7. Laboratory studies: WBCs, RBCs, platelets, and albumin
8. Nutritional support: TPN
9. Treatments: chest physiotherapy (CPT), postural drainage, and incentive spirometry

10. Precautions: protective; blood and body fluid
11. Transfusion therapy: fresh frozen plasma (FFP), platelets, and packed RBCs
12. Antibiotics: aerosolized pentamidine (NebuPent), trimethoprim and sulfamethoxazole (Bactrim)
13. Antiviral: dapsone, didansine (Videx), ganciclovir (Cytovene), zidovudine (Retrovir, AZT), acyclovir (Zovirax), pentamidine (Pentam)
14. Plasmapheresis
15. Interferon
16. Interleukin II
17. Specialized bed: active or static, low air loss (Kin Air, Biodyne)
18. Antifungal: fluconazole (Diflucan), amphotericin B (Fungizone)
19. Pulse oximetry
20. Antiemetic: nabilone (Cesamet)

G. Nursing interventions and responsibilities
1. Maintain the patient's diet
2. Force fluids
3. Administer I.V. fluids
4. Administer oxygen
5. Provide incentive spirometry and TCDB
6. Assess respiratory and neurologic status and fluid balance
7. Keep the patient in semi-Fowler's position
8. Monitor and record VS, UO, I/O, laboratory studies, daily weight, specific gravity, and pulse oximetry
9. Administer TPN
10. Administer medications, as prescribed
11. Encourage the patient to express feelings about changes in body image, a fear of dying, and social isolation
12. Maintain activity, as tolerated
13. Allay the patient's anxiety
14. Provide rest periods
15. Provide skin and mouth care
16. Maintain protective blood and body fluid precautions
17. Monitor for opportunistic infections
18. Caution the patient to avoid anal sex
19. Caution an I.V. drug user to clean drug paraphernalia with bleach
20 Make referrals to community agencies for support

H. Teaching goals (instructions to the patient and family)
1. Keep follow-up appointments
2. Stop smoking
3. Maintain a normal weight
4. Know the action, side effects, and scheduling of medications
5. Recognize the signs and symptoms of infection
6. Avoid exposure to people with infections
7. Alternate rest periods with activity

8. Monitor self for infection
9. Follow dietary recommendations and restrictions
10. Seek help from community agencies and resources
11. Complete skin and foot care daily
12. Refrain from donating blood
13. Avoid using alcohol and recreational drugs
14. Use condoms during sexual intercourse

I. Possible medical complications
   1. *Pneumocystis carinii* pneumonia
   2. Cryptococcal meningitis
   3. Burkitt's lymphoma
   4. Encephalopathy
   5. Depression
   6. Herpes simplex virus
   7. Cytomegalovirus infection
   8. Epstein-Barr virus
   9. Oral and esophageal candidiasis
   10. Kaposi's sarcoma
   11. Toxoplasmosis
   12. *Mycobacterium avium* intracellular infection
   13. Neuropathies
   14. Myopathies

J. Possible surgical interventions: bone marrow transplant (see page 322)

XIII. Iron deficiency anemia

A. Definition—chronic, slowly progressive decrease in circulating RBCs

B. Possible etiology
   1. Acute and chronic bleeding
   2. Inadequate intake of iron-rich foods
   3. Gastrectomy
   4. Malabsorption syndrome
   5. Vitamin B_6 deficiency
   6. Pregnancy
   7. Menstruation
   8. Alcohol abuse
   9. Drug induced

C. Pathophysiology
   1. Iron deficiency is caused by inadequate absorption or excessive loss of iron
   2. Decreased iron affects formation of Hgb and RBCs
   3. Decreased Hgb and RBCs reduce the capacity of the blood to transport oxygen to cells

D. Possible clinical manifestations
   1. Palpitations
   2. Dizziness
   3. Sensitivity to cold
   4. Stomatitis
   5. Dyspnea
   6. Weakness and fatigue
   7. Pale, dry mucous membranes
   8. Papillae atrophy of the tongue
   9. Cheilosis
  10. Pallor
  11. Koilonychia

E. Possible diagnostic test findings
   1. Hematology: decreased Hgb, Hct, iron, ferritin, reticulocytes, red cell indices, transferrin saturation; absent hemosiderin; increased iron-binding capacity
   2. Peripheral blood smear: microcytic and hypochromic RBCs

F. Medical management
   1. Diet: high-iron, high-roughage, high-protein, high-vitamin with increased fluids
   2. Oxygen therapy
   3. Position: semi-Fowler's
   4. Activity: bed rest
   5. Monitoring: VS, UO, and I/O
   6. Laboratory studies: arterial blood gases (ABGs), Hgb, Hct, iron, iron-binding capacity
   7. Transfusion therapy: packed RBCs
   8. Antianemics: ferrous sulfate (Feosol), iron dextran (Imferon)
   9. Vitamins: pyridoxine hydrochloride (vitamin B_6), ascorbic acid (vitamin C)

G. Nursing interventions and responsibilities
   1. Maintain the patient's diet with increased fluids
   2. Force fluids
   3. Administer oxygen
   4. Assess cardiovascular and respiratory status
   5. Keep the patient in semi-Fowler's position
   6. Monitor and record VS, UO, I/O, and laboratory studies
   7. Administer medications, as prescribed
   8. Allay the patient's anxiety
   9. Monitor stool, urine, and emesis for occult blood
  10. Provide rest periods
  11. Provide mouth, skin, and foot care
  12. Protect the patient from falls
  13. Keep the patient warm

H. Teaching goals (instructions to the patient and family)
1. Keep follow-up appointments
2. Stop smoking
3. Maintain a normal weight
4. Know the action, side effects, and scheduling of medications
5. Recognize the signs and symptoms of bleeding
6. Avoid exposure to people with infection
7. Alternate rest periods with activity
8. Monitor self for infection
9. Follow dietary recommendations and restrictions
10. Promote a safe environment
11. Complete skin, mouth, and foot care daily
12. Monitor stools for occult blood
13. Avoid using hot pads and hot water bottles

I. Possible medical complications
1. Plummer-Vinson syndrome
2. Angina pectoris
3. Congestive heart failure (CHF)

J. Possible surgical interventions: none

XIV. Pernicious anemia

A. Definition – chronic, progressive macrocytic anemia caused by a deficiency of intrinsic factor

B. Possible etiology
1. Deficiency of intrinsic factor
2. Gastric mucosal atrophy
3. Genetics
4. Prolonged iron deficiency
5. Autoimmune disease
6. Lack of administration of vitamin B_{12} after small bowel resection or total gastrectomy
7. Malabsorption
8. Bacterial or parasitic infections

C. Pathophysiology
1. Without intrinsic factor, dietary vitamin B_{12} cannot be absorbed by the ileum
2. Normal DNA synthesis is inhibited, resulting in defective maturation of cells

D. Possible clinical manifestations
1. Weakness
2. Pallor
3. Dyspnea
4. Palpitations

5. Fatigue
6. Sore mouth
7. Glossitis
8. Weight loss and anorexia
9. Dyspepsia
10. Constipation or diarrhea
11. Mild jaundice of sclera
12. Tingling and paresthesia of hands and feet
13. Paralysis
14. Depression
15. Delirium
16. Gait disturbances
17. Tachycardia

E. Possible diagnostic test findings
   1. Schilling test: positive
   2. Romberg test: positive
   3. Gastric analysis: hypochlorohydria
   4. Peripheral blood smear: oval, macrocytic, hyperchromic erythrocytes
   5. Bone marrow: increased megaloblasts; few maturing erythrocytes; defective leukocyte maturation
   6. Blood chemistry: increased bilirubin, lactic dehydrogenase (LDH)
   7. Hematology: decreased Hct, Hgb
   8. Upper GI series: atrophy of gastric mucosa

F. Medical management
   1. Diet: high in iron and protein, with increased intake of vitamin B_{12} and folic acid; restrict highly seasoned, coarse, or extremely hot foods
   2. Position: semi-Fowler's
   3. Activity: as tolerated
   4. Monitoring: VS and neurovital signs
   5. Laboratory studies: Hgb, Hct and bilirubin
   6. Treatments: bed cradle
   7. Transfusion therapy: packed RBCs
   8. Antianemics: ferrous sulfate (Feosol), iron dextran (Imferon)
   9. Vitamins: pyridoxine hydrochloride (vitamin B_6), ascorbic acid (vitamin C), cyanocobalamin (vitamin B_{12}), folic acid (Folvite)

G. Nursing interventions and responsibilities
   1. Maintain the patient's diet
   2. Assess neurologic and respiratory status
   3. Keep the patient in semi-Fowler's position
   4. Monitor and record VS, laboratory studies, and neurovital signs
   5. Administer medications, as prescribed
   6. Allay the patient's anxiety
   7. Maintain activity, as tolerated
   8. Provide treatments: bed cradle

9. Monitor and record amount, consistency, and color of stools
10. Provide mouth care before and after meals
11. Use soft toothbrushes
12. Maintain warm environment
13. Provide foot and skin care
14. Prevent the patient from falling

H. Teaching goals (instructions to the patient and family)
1. Keep follow-up appointments
2. Stop smoking
3. Maintain a normal weight
4. Know the action, side effects, and scheduling of medications
5. Recognize the signs and symptoms of skin breakdown
6. Alternate rest periods with activity
7. Follow dietary recommendations and restrictions
8. Promote a safe environment
9. Complete skin, mouth, and foot care daily
10. Alter activities of daily living (ADLs) to compensate for paresthesia
11. Comply with lifelong, monthly injections of vitamin B_{12}
12. Avoid using heating pads and electric blankets

I. Possible medical complications
1. Chronic renal failure
2. Arrhythmias
3. Gastric cancer
4. Gastrointestinal bleeding
5. CHF
6. Angina
7. Neurogenic bladder
8. CVA

J. Possible surgical interventions: none

XV. Aplastic anemia (pancytopenia)

A. Definition — failure of bone marrow to produce adequate amounts of erythrocytes, leukocytes, and platelets

B. Possible etiology
1. Idiopathic
2. Exposure to chemicals
3. Drug induced: chloramphenicol (Chloromycetin), phenylbutazone (Butazolidin), phenytoin (Dilantin)
4. Chemotherapy
5. Radiation
6. Viral hepatitis

C. Pathophysiology
   1. Bone marrow suppression, destruction, or aplasia results in failure of bone marrow to produce an adequate number of stem cells
   2. Without an adequate number of stem cells, sufficient amounts of erythrocytes, leukocytes, and platelets cannot be produced
   3. Pancytopenia includes leukopenia, thrombocytopenia, and anemia

D. Possible clinical manifestations
   1. Fatigue
   2. Dyspnea
   3. Multiple infections
   4. Elevated temperature
   5. Headache
   6. Weakness
   7. Anorexia
   8. Gingivitis
   9. Epistaxis
   10. Purpura
   11. Petechiae
   12. Ecchymosis
   13. Pallor
   14. Palpitations
   15. Tachycardia
   16. Tachypnea
   17. Melena

E. Possible diagnostic test findings
   1. Peripheral blood smear: pancytopenia
   2. Hematology: decreased granulocytes, thrombocytes, RBCs
   3. Fecal occult blood: positive
   4. Urine chemistry: hematuria
   5. Bone marrow biopsy: fatty marrow with reduction of stem cells

F. Medical management
   1. Diet: high-protein, high-calorie, high-vitamin
   2. I.V. therapy: hydration; heparin lock
   3. Oxygen therapy
   4. Position: semi-Fowler's
   5. Activity: as tolerated
   6. Monitoring: VS, UO, and I/O
   7. Laboratory studies: RBCs, WBCs, platelets, and stool for occult blood
   8. Treatments: tepid sponge baths, cooling blankets
   9. Precautions: protective
   10. Transfusion therapy: platelets, packed RBCs
   11. Antibiotics: penicillin G potassium (Pentids), ticarcillin sodium (Ticar), tobramycin sulfate (Nebcin)
   12. Analgesics: ibuprofen (Motrin), acetaminophen (Tylenol)

13. Antithymocyte globulin (ATG or RATG)
14. Androgenic steroids: fluoxymesterone (Halotestin), oxymetholone (Anadrol)
15. Recombinant human granulocyte-macrophage colony stimulating factor (GMCSF)

G. Nursing interventions and responsibilities
1. Maintain the patient's diet
2. Force fluids
3. Administer I.V. fluids
4. Administer oxygen
5. Provide TCDB
6. Assess cardiovascular and respiratory status and fluid balance
7. Keep the patient in semi-Fowler's position
8. Monitor and record VS; UO; I/O; laboratory studies; stool, urine, and emesis for occult blood; and specific gravity
9. Administer transfusion therapy, as prescribed
10. Administer medications, as prescribed
11. Allay the patient's anxiety
12. Alternate rest periods with activity
13. Provide cooling blankets and tepid sponge baths
14. Maintain protective precautions
15. Provide mouth care before and after meals
16. Provide skin care
17. Protect the patient from falls
18. Avoid giving the patient intramuscular injections
19. Avoid using hard toothbrushes and straight razors on the patient
20. Monitor for infection, bleeding, and bruising

H. Teaching goals (instructions to the patient and family)
1. Keep follow-up appointments
2. Stop smoking
3. Maintain a normal weight
4. Know the action, side effects, and scheduling of medications
5. Recognize the signs and symptoms of bleeding and infection
6. Avoid contact sports
7. Avoid exposure to people with infections
8. Alternate rest periods with activity
9. Monitor self for infection
10. Follow dietary recommendations and restrictions
11. Promote a safe environment
12. Complete gentle skin and mouth care daily
13. Wear a medical identification bracelet
14. Avoid using over-the-counter medications
15. Monitor stool for occult blood
16. Use an electric razor
17. Avoid taking aspirin

I. Possible medical complications
1. Hemorrhage
2. Infection
3. Septicemia
4. CVA
5. Gastrointestinal bleeding

J. Possible surgical interventions
1. Bone marrow transplant (see page 322)
2. Splenectomy (see page 320)

XVI. Idiopathic thrombocytopenia purpura (ITP)

A. Definition—increased premature destruction of platelets

B. Possible etiology
1. Unknown
2. Autoimmune disease
3. Viral infection

C. Pathophysiology
1. Antibody-coated platelets are removed from circulation by reticuloendothelial cells of the spleen and liver
2. Decreased number of circulating platelets cause bleeding

D. Possible clinical manifestations
1. Petechiae
2. Ecchymosis
3. Epistaxis
4. Gingivitis
5. Visual disturbances
6. Dizziness
7. Menorrhagia
8. Hematomas
9. Increased bleeding after dental extraction
10. Gastrointestinal bleeding

E. Possible diagnostic test findings
1. Hematology: decreased Hgb, Hct, platelets; PT, PTT normal; prolonged bleeding time
2. Urine chemistry: hematuria
3. Fecal occult blood: positive
4. Blood chemistry: increased immunoglobins (IgG), complement fixation
5. Bone marrow biopsy: increased and abnormal megakaryocytes
6. Rumpel-Leede capillary fragility tourniquet test: positive with increased capillary fragility

F. Medical management
1. Diet: soft and bland

2. I.V. therapy: heparin lock
3. Activity: bed rest
4. Monitoring: VS, UO, daily weight, and stool for occult blood
5. Laboratory studies: Hgb, Hct, and platelets
6. Precautions: protective
7. Transfusion therapy: FFP, platelets, packed RBCs, and plasma
8. IgG antibody: immune globulin I.V. (Gammagard)
9. Stool softener: docusate sodium (Colace)
10. Immunosuppressants: azathioprine (Imuran), cyclophosphamide (Cytoxan), vincristine sulfate (Oncovin)
11. Anabolic steroid: danazol (Cyclomen)
12. Corticosteroid: prednisone (Deltasone)

G. Nursing interventions and responsibilities
1. Maintain the patient's diet
2. Force fluids
3. Administer I.V. fluids and transfusion therapy
4. Assess for bruising, bleeding, and infection
5. Monitor and record VS; UO; I/O; laboratory studies; daily weight; stool, urine, and emesis for occult blood; neurovital signs; pad count; and blood loss
6. Administer medications, as prescribed
7. Allay the patient's anxiety
8. Provide gentle mouth care
9. Protect the patient from falls
10. Avoid giving the patient intramuscular injections, aspirin, enemas, and rectal temperatures
11. Avoid using straight razors, tape, and tourniquets on the patient
12. Alternate rest periods with activity
13. Rotate extremities for blood pressure monitoring

H. Teaching goals (instructions to the patient and family)
1. Keep follow-up appointments
2. Know the action, side effects, and scheduling of medications
3. Recognize the signs and symptoms of bleeding and infection
4. Avoid contact sports
5. Avoid exposure to people with infections
6. Alternate rest periods with activity
7. Monitor self for infection
8. Promote a safe environment
9. Complete skin care daily
10. Wear a medical identification bracelet
11. Use electric razors and soft toothbrushes
12. Avoid sneezing, coughing, nose blowing, straining at stool, and heavy lifting
13. Avoid using over-the-counter medications

I. Possible medical complications
   1. Hypersplenism
   2. CVA
   3. Shock
   4. Hemothorax
   6. Peripheral paralysis and paresthesia
   7. Bleeding into diaphragm

J. Possible surgical interventions: splenectomy (see page 320)

XVII. Polycythemia vera

A. Definition — myeloproliferative disorder that results in the increased production of erythrocytes, hemoglobin, myelocytes, and thrombocytes

B. Possible etiology
   1. Unknown
   2. Hypernephroma
   3. Hepatoma
   4. Uterine fibroids
   5. Pheochromocytoma
   6. Lung tumors
   7. Adrenal cancer
   8. Cerebral hemangioblastoma

C. Pathophysiology
   1. Hyperplasia of bone marrow results in increased production of erythrocytes, hemoglobin, granulocytes, and platelets
   2. Overproduction results in increased blood viscosity, increased total blood volume, and severe congestion of all tissues and organs

D. Possible clinical manifestations
   1. Ruddy complexion
   2. Dusky mucosa
   3. Vertigo
   4. Headaches
   5. Dyspnea and orthopnea
   6. Tachycardia
   7. Ecchymosis
   8. Hepatomegaly and splenomegaly
   9. Increased gastric secretions
   10. Weakness and fatigue
   11. Pruritus
   12. Epistaxis
   13. Gastrointestinal bleeding
   14. Angina

E. Possible diagnostic test findings
   1. Blood chemistry: increased uric acid, unconjugated bilirubin, vitamin B_{12}, alkaline phosphatase, serum aspartate aminotransferase (AST, formerly serum glutamic oxaloacetic transaminase [SGOT]), serum alanine aminotransferase (ALT, formerly serum glutamic pyruvic transaminase [SGPT]), LDH
   2. Hematology: increased erythrocytes, leukocytes, platelets, Hct, Hgb
   3. Bone marrow biopsy: increased number of immature cell forms, decreased iron in marrow
   4. Urine chemistry: hematuria
   5. Stool specimen: positive for blood
   6. ABGs: normal PaO_2

F. Medical management
   1. Diet: soft, low-iron
   2. I.V. therapy: heparin lock
   3. Activity: as tolerated
   4. Monitoring: VS, UO, CVP, I/O, and neurovital signs
   5. Laboratory studies: Hgb, Hct, WBCs, RBCs, platelets, and unconjugated bilirubin
   6. Treatments: tepid sponge baths
   7. Analgesic: acetaminophen (Tylenol)
   8. Antacids: magnesium and aluminum hydroxide (Maalox), aluminum hydroxide gel (ALternaGEL)
   9. Histamine antagonists: cimetidine (Tagamet), ranitidine (Zantac)
   10. Antihistamine: diphenhydramine hydrochloride (Benadryl)
   11. Antigout: colchicine (Colsalide), allopurinal (Zyloprim)
   12. Radioactive phosphorus (P_{32})
   13. Phlebotomy
   14. Myelosuppressants: busulfan (Myleran), chlorambucil (Leukeran), cyclophosphamide (Cytoxan)
   15. Muscosal barrier fortifier: sucralfate (Carafate)

G. Nursing interventions and responsibilities
   1. Maintain the patient's diet
   2. Force fluids
   3. Assess cardiovascular and respiratory status
   4. Keep the patient in semi-Fowler's position
   5. Monitor and record VS, UO, I/O, laboratory studies, CVP, neurovital signs, and fecal occult blood
   6. Administer medications, as prescribed
   7. Allay the patient's anxiety
   8. Protect the patient from falls
   9. Provide treatments: tepid baths and ROM exercises
   10. Provide postchemotherapeutic and postradiation nursing care
       a. Provide skin, mouth, and perineal care
       b. Encourage dietary intake

   c. Administer antiemetics and antidiarrheals, as prescribed
   d. Monitor for bleeding, infection, and electrolyte imbalance
   e. Provide rest periods

H. Teaching goals (instructions to the patient and family)
   1. Keep follow-up appointments
   2. Stop smoking
   3. Know the action, side effects, and scheduling of medications
   4. Recognize the signs and symptoms of infection, CHF, and thrombophlebitis
   5. Avoid exposure to people with infections
   6. Alternate rest periods with activity
   7. Monitor self for infection
   8. Follow dietary recommendations and restrictions
   9. Promote a safe environment
   10. Complete skin care daily
   11. Avoid taking hot showers

I. Possible medical complications
   1. Hypertension
   2. CHF
   3. CVA
   4. Myocardial infarction (MI)
   5. Deep vein thrombosis
   6. Hemorrhage
   7. Peptic ulcer
   8. Gout
   9. Acute leukemia

J. Possible surgical interventions: none

XVIII. Disseminated intravascular coagulation

A. Definition — body's response to injury or disease in which microthrombi obstruct blood supply of organs and hemorrhage occurs throughout the body

B. Possible etiology
   1. Unknown
   2. Frequent, rapid transfusions
   3. Gram-negative sepsis
   4. Neoplastic disease
   5. Massive burns
   6. Massive trauma
   7. Anaphylaxis
   8. Chronic disease

C. Pathophysiology
   1. Underlying disease causes release of thromboplastic substances that promote the deposition of fibrin throughout the microcirculation
   2. Red blood cells are trapped in fibrin strands and are hemolyzed
   3. Platelets, prothrombin, and other clotting factors are destroyed, leading to bleeding
   4. Excessive clotting activates the fibrinolytic system that inhibits platelet function, causing further bleeding
   5. Acute activation of clotting mechanism results in consumption of plasma-clotting factors that the liver cannot replenish quickly enough
   6. Activation of the thrombin and fibrinolytic system results in simultaneous bleeding and thrombosis

D. Possible clinical manifestations
   1. Petechiae
   2. Ecchymosis
   3. Prolonged bleeding after venipuncture
   4. Hemorrhage
   5. Oliguria
   6. Anxiety
   7. Restlessness
   8. Purpura
   9. Acrocyanosis
   10. Joint pain
   11. Dyspnea
   12. Hemoptysis
   13. Rales

E. Possible diagnostic test findings
   1. Hematology: decreased platelets, RBCs, fibrinogen, factor assay (II, V, VII); increased fibrin split products, thrombin, PT, PTT; positive protamine sulfate test
   2. Urine chemistry: hematuria
   3. ABGs: metabolic acidosis
   4. Ophthalmoscopic exam: retinal hemorrhage
   5. Fecal occult blood: positive

F. Medical management
   1. Diet: withhold food and fluids
   2. I.V. therapy: hydration, electrolyte replacement, and heparin lock
   3. Oxygen therapy
   4. Intubation and mechanical ventilation
   5. Gastrointestinal decompression: NG tube
   6. Position: semi-Fowler's
   7. Activity: bed rest and active and passive ROM exercises
   8. Monitoring: VS, UO, I/O, ECG, and hemodynamic variables

    9. Laboratory studies: PT, PTT, platelets, fibrinogen, and fibrin split products
  10. Nutritional support: TPN
  11. Treatments: indwelling urinary (Foley) catheter
  12. Transfusion therapy: platelets, packed RBCs, FFP, whole blood, volume expanders, and cryoprecipitates
  13. Glucocorticoids: prednisone (Deltasone), hydrocortisone (Cortef)
  14. Analgesics: ibuprofen (Motrin), acetaminophen (Tylenol)
  15. Antacids: magnesium and aluminum hydroxide (Maalox), aluminum hydroxide gel (Gelusil)
  16. Stool softener: docusate sodium (Colace)
  17. Anticoagulant: heparin sodium (Lipo-Hepin)
  18. Hemodialysis
  19. Precautions: seizure
  20. Pulse oximetry

G. Nursing interventions and responsibilities
    1. Withhold food and fluids
    2. Administer I.V. fluids
    3. Administer oxygen
    4. Provide suction and TCDB
    5. Assess cardiovascular and respiratory status and fluid balance
    6. Maintain position, patency, and low suction of NG tube
    7. Irrigate NG tube gently and do not reposition it
    8. Keep the patient in semi-Fowler's position
    9. Monitor and record VS, UO, I/O, laboratory studies, hemodynamic variables, neurovital signs, fecal occult blood, and pulse oximetry
  10. Administer TPN
  11. Administer medications, as prescribed
  12. Allay the patient's anxiety
  13. Maintain bed rest
  14. Provide gentle mouth and skin care
  15. Avoid giving the patient intramuscular injections, enemas, and rectal temperatures
  16. Avoid using straight razors and tape on the patient
  17. Rotate extremities for blood pressure monitoring
  18. Maintain seizure precautions
  19. Administer transfusion therapy, as prescribed
  20. Maintain endotracheal tube to mechanical ventilator

H. Teaching goals (instructions to the patient and family)
    1. Keep follow-up appointments
    2. Stop smoking
    3. Know the action, side effects, and scheduling of medications
    4. Recognize the signs and symptoms of occult bleeding
    5. Alternate rest periods with activity
    6. Promote a safe environment

    7. Complete gentle skin and mouth care daily
    8. Wear a medical identification bracelet
    9. Avoid straining at stool
  10. Avoid using over-the-counter medications
  11. Monitor stool for occult blood
  12. Use an electric razor
  13. Avoid using aspirin and enemas

I. Possible medical complications
    1. Acute renal failure
    2. Shock
    3. CVA
    4. Convulsions
    5. Hemothorax
    6. Hemorrhage
    7. Coma

J. Possible surgical interventions: none

XIX. Multiple myeloma

A. Definition — abnormal proliferation of plasma cells in the bone marrow

B. Possible etiology
    1. Unknown
    2. Genetic
    3. Environmental

C. Pathophysiology
    1. Single tumor in bone marrow disseminates into lymph nodes, liver, spleen, kidneys, and bone
    2. Plasma cell tumors produce abnormal amounts of immunoglobulins
    3. Tumor cells trigger osteoblastic activity, leading to bone destruction throughout the body

D. Possible clinical manifestations
    1. Headaches
    2. Constant, severe bone pain
    3. Pathologic fractures
    4. Skeletal deformities of sternum and ribs
    5. Renal calculi
    6. Multiple infections
    7. Hepatomegaly
    8. Splenomegaly
    9. Loss of height
  10. Hemorrhage

E. Possible diagnostic test findings
1. X-ray: diffuse, round, "punched out" bone lesions; osteoporosis, osteolytic lesions of the skull, widespread demineralization
2. Bone scan: increased uptake
3. Bone marrow biopsy: increased number of immature plasma cells
4. Hematology: decreased Hct, WBCs, platelets; increased ESR
5. Blood chemistry: increased calcium, uric acid, BUN, creatinine, globulins, protein; decreased albumin-globulin (A-G) ratio
6. Urine chemistry: increased calcium, uric acid
7. Immunoelectrophoresis: monoclonal spike
8. Bence Jones protein assay: positive

F. Medical management
1. Diet: high-protein, high-carbohydrate, high-vitamin and mineral in small, frequent feedings
2. I.V. therapy: hydration, electrolyte replacement, and heparin lock
3. Activity: as tolerated
4. Monitoring: VS, UO, I/O, and neurovital signs
5. Laboratory studies: Hct, calcium, BUN, creatinine, uric acid, WBCs, protein, platelets, and surveillance cultures
6. Radiation therapy
7. Chemotherapy
8. Precautions: seizure
9. Transfusion therapy: packed RBCs
10. Antibiotics: doxorubicin (Adriamycin), plicamycin (Mithracin)
11. Antigout: allopurinol (Zyloprim)
12. Muscle relaxant: diazepam (Valium)
13. Alkylating agents: melphalan (Alkeran), cyclophosphamide (Cytoxan)
14. Antineoplastics: vinblastine (Velban), vincristine sulfate (Oncovin)
15. Analgesics: meperidine hydrochloride (Demerol)
16. Diuretic: furosemide (Lasix)
17. Glucocorticoid: prednisone (Deltasone)
18. Antacids: magnesium and aluminum hydroxide (Maalox), aluminum hydroxide gel (Gelusil)
19. Androgen: fluoxymesterone (Halotestin)
20. Orthopedic devices: braces, splints, casts
21. Peritoneal and hemodialysis
22. Phosphates: K-Phos
23. Antiemetic: nabilone (Cesamet)

G. Nursing interventions and responsibilities
1. Maintain the patient's diet
2. Force fluids
3. Administer I.V. fluids
4. Provide TCDB
5. Assess renal, cardiovascular, and respiratory status and fluid balance

    6. Monitor and record VS, UO, I/O, laboratory studies, specific gravity, daily weight, urine and stool for occult blood, and neurovital signs
    7. Administer transfusion therapy, as prescribed
    8. Administer medications, as prescribed
    9. Allay the patient's anxiety
  10. Maintain seizure precautions
  11. Provide skin and mouth care
  12. Alternate rest periods with activity
  13. Monitor for infection and bruising
  14. Prevent the patient from falling
  15. Provide postchemotherapeutic and postradiation nursing care
    a. Provide skin, mouth, and perineal care
    b. Encourage dietary intake
    c. Administer antiemetics and antidiarrheals, as prescribed
    d. Monitor for bleeding, infection, and electrolyte imbalance
    e. Provide rest periods
  16. Assess bone pain
  17. Move the patient gently
  18. Apply and maintain braces, splints, casts
  19. Provide information about the American Cancer Society

H. Teaching goals (instructions to the patient and family)
    1. Keep follow-up appointments
    2. Exercise regularly, with particular attention to muscle-strengthening exercises; alternate rest periods with activity
    3. Maintain a normal weight
    4. Know the action, side effects, and scheduling of medications
    5. Recognize the signs and symptoms of renal calculi, infection, fractures, and seizures
    6. Avoid lifting, constipation, over-the-counter medications, and exposure to people with infections
    7. Monitor self for infection and stools for occult blood
    8. Follow dietary recommendations and restrictions
    9. Complete skin and mouth care daily
  10. Use braces, splints, casts

I. Possible medical complications
    1. Paraplegia
    2. Acute renal failure
    3. Hemorrhage
    4. Infection
    5. Urolithiasis
    6. Pathologic fractures
    7. Seizures
    8. Gout

J. Possible surgical interventions: none

Points to remember

After bone marrow transplantation, the patient should be placed in protective isolation.

AIDS results from a defect in T-cell mediated immunity that allows development of opportunistic infections.

A patient with pernicious anemia has a positive Schilling test and hypochlorohydria.

The nurse should avoid intramuscular injections, enemas, and rectal temperatures when caring for a patient with DIC.

Glossary

The following terms are defined in Appendix A, page 354.

ecchymosis

epistaxis

lymphadenopathy

petechiae

Study questions

To evaluate your understanding of this chapter, answer the following questions in the space provided; then compare your responses with the correct answers in Appendix B, pages 363 and 364.

1. Which nursing interventions are appropriate after a lymphangiogram?

   _____

   _____

2. What key information should the nurse teach a patient who has had a splenectomy? _____

   _____

3. How is donor bone marrow transplanted? _____

   _____

   _____

4. What is agranulocytosis? _____

   _____

5. What would a bone marrow biopsy reveal about a patient with leukemia?

   _____

   _____

6. What are the chemotherapy protocols for Hodgkin's disease? _____

   _____

   _____

7. Which clinical manifestations describe the early, or acute, stage of AIDS?

   _____

   _____

8. What is the recommended diet for a patient with iron deficiency anemia?

   _____

   _____

Study questions *(continued)*

9. What is the pathophysiology of ITP? _____

_____

10. What would blood chemistry tests reveal about a patient with polycythemia vera? _____

_____

11. How does DIC develop? _____

_____

12. What type of diet would the physician prescribe for a patient with multiple myeloma? _____

_____

Appendices

A: Glossary

Anuria – absence of urine output

Ascites – fluid in the peritoneal cavity

Ataxia – lack of muscular coordination

Bruit – sound of abnormal blood flow heard on auscultation

Crackles – abnormal inspiratory or expiratory lung sound, usually associated with the presence of fluid

Crepitation – grating sound produced by bone rubbing against bone

Decerebration – abnormal extension and internal rotation of arms and legs

Dysphagia – difficulty in swallowing

Dyspnea – difficult, labored breathing

Ecchymosis – bruise

Epistaxis – bleeding from the nose

Hematemesis – vomiting of blood

Hematuria – blood in the urine

Hemoptysis – expectoration of bloody sputum

Hirsutism – excessive hair growth or unusual distribution of hair

Intermittent claudication – calf pain caused by walking and relieved by rest

Jugular venous distention – distended neck veins that may indicate increased central venous pressure

Lichenification – thickening and hardening of the epidermis

Lymphadenopathy – enlargement of the lymph nodes

Melena—black, tarry stools

Mineralocorticoid—substance, such as aldosterone, produced by the adrenal cortex that regulates electrolyte and water balance

Neurovital signs—neurologic assessment of pupils, motor and verbal response, level of consciousness, vital signs, pulse pressure, mean arterial pressure, and intracranial pressure

Nevi—mole or birthmark

Oliguria—urine output of less than 30 ml/hour

Orthopnea—respiratory distress that is relieved by sitting upright

Pannus—granular tissue that covers and invades articular cartilage

Papilledema—swelling of the optic nerve head

Paroxysmal nocturnal dyspnea—respiratory distress that occurs after lying in a recumbent position for several hours

Petechiae—multiple, small, hemorrhagic areas on the skin

Point of maximal impulse (PMI)—point on the anterior chest wall located at the midclavicular line at the fifth intercostal space, that the tip of the left ventricle hits during ventricular systole; using light palpation, the nurse can feel a tap with each heartbeat

Polydipsia—excessive thirst

Polyphagia—excessive eating

Polyuria—excessive urination

Pruritus—itching

Ptosis—drooping of the eyelid

Pyuria—pus in the urine

Renal colic—flank pain that radiates to the groin

Rhonchi — abnormal inspiratory or expiratory lung sound, usually associated with airway constriction

Steatorrhea — fatty stools

Subluxation — partial dislocation of a joint

Sympathectomy — surgical removal of ganglia to improve blood flow to the skin (usually performed on the lumbar ganglia)

Tachypnea — abnormally fast rate of breathing

Thenar — musculature at the thumb's base

Tophi — urate crystals deposited in areas of diminished blood flow, such as joints and ear lobes

Trophic — integumentary changes (such as hair loss or skin thickening and drying) caused by prolonged tissue ischemia and malnutrition

Vasopressin — antidiuretic hormone

Vesicle — fluid-filled sac

B: Answers to Study Questions

CHAPTER 1

1. Cardiac output equals stroke volume times heart rate: $CO = SV \times HR$.

2. After cardiac catheterization, the nurse should monitor the patient's vital signs (VS) and peripheral pulses, check the insertion site for bleeding, maintain a pressure dressing, promote bed rest, force fluids unless contraindicated, and allay the patient's anxiety.

3. The modifiable risk factors for developing cardiovascular disorders include smoking, hypertension, hypercholesterolemia, obesity, physical inactivity, and emotional stress.

4. After cardiac surgery, medications given to the patient might include antiarrhythmics, anticoagulants, vasopressors, beta adrenergics, diuretics, and cardiac glycosides.

5. After vascular grafting, the key assessment is peripheral circulation, which includes checking temperature, color, pulses, and sensations distal to the graft site.

6. A patient with hypertension should consume a low-sodium, low-calorie, low-cholesterol, low-fat diet with limited intake of alcohol and caffeine.

7. An ECG for a patient with coronary artery disease will show ST depression and T wave inversion.

8. A patient with angina might describe the pain as substernal and crushing, or compressing. The pain might radiate to the arms and last for 3 to 5 minutes after exertion, emotional excitement, or exposure to cold.

9. In a patient experiencing an acute MI, blood chemistry results include increased CPK, LDH, AST, lipids; positive CPK-MB fraction; and flipped LDH-1 and LDH-2 isoenzymes.

10. In left-sided heart failure, decreased myocardial contractility or increased myocardial workload results in increased left ventricular pressure, increased left atrial pressure, and decreased CO. As a result of the increased pressure in the pulmonary capillaries, oxygenation decreases and respiratory signs of fluid overload appear.

11. The clinical manifestations of acute pulmonary edema include dyspnea; paroxysmal cough; blood-tinged, frothy sputum; orthopnea; tachypnea; agitation; restlessness; intense fear; chest pain; syncope; tachycardia; cold, clammy skin; and gallop rhythms, S_3 and S_4.

12. A patient in cardiogenic shock would have metabolic acidosis.

13. A chest X-ray for a patient with mitral stenosis would reveal pulmonary congestion and enlargement of the left atrium and right ventricle.

14. Aortic stenosis refers to a narrowing of the aortic valve; aortic insufficiency refers to incomplete closure of the aortic valve.

15. Three clinical manifestations of PVD are trophic changes, diminished or absent pulses, and temperature changes in the extremities.

CHAPTER 2

1. An EMG is a noninvasive test that graphically records the electrical activity of a muscle at rest and during contraction.

2. After a total hip replacement, the patient's hips should be kept in abduction. Hip flexion should be limited to 90 degrees when the patient is sitting or being turned to the side, as ordered.

3. The patient with an external fixation needs to recognize the signs and symptoms of soft tissue and bone infection.

4. After an amputation, the stump should be rewrapped before the patient is assisted out of bed.

5. After a laminectomy, the patient should be turned by the logrolling technique.

6. A patient with a spinal fusion should sleep on the side with the hips and knees flexed. A firm mattress is recommended.

7. Patients commonly describe the pain of rheumatoid arthritis as morning stiffness and the pain of osteoarthritis as joint stiffness. The discomfort of osteoarthritis lessens with rest and worsens in damp, cold weather.

8. Medications for treating gouty arthritis include uricosuric agents, xanthine-oxidase inhibitors, antigout agents, analgesics, and NSAIDs.

9. Osteomyelitis, an infection causing bone destruction, results from organisms reaching the bone through an open wound or the bloodstream. As the infection progresses, bone fragments die. During healing, new bone cells form over the sequestum. The result is nonunion.

10. Fractures are a possible complication of osteoporosis.

11. Osteosarcoma is a malignant bone tumor that invades the ends of long bones.

12. A patient with carpal tunnel syndrome should avoid manual activities requiring dorsiflexion and volar flexion of the wrist.

13. Clinical manifestations of lumbar HNP include acute lower back pain radiating across the buttock and down the leg; weakness, numbness, and tingling in the foot and leg; pain when walking; and straightening of the normal lumbar curve with scoliosis away from the affected side. Clinical manifestations of cervical HNP include neck pain that radiates down the arm to the hand; neck stiffness; weakness, numbness, and tingling in the hand; weakness in the affected upper extremities; and atrophy of the biceps and triceps.

14. The three types of fractured hips are intracapsular, extracapsular, and intertrochanteric.

15. A key manifestation of SLE is a butterfly rash on the face.

CHAPTER 3

1. After an LP, the nurse should keep the patient flat in bed for 24 hours, administer prescribed analgesics, check the insertion site for bleeding, monitor the patient's neurovital signs, and force fluids.

2. Two key postoperative nursing interventions after a craniotomy are to check the patient for signs of increased intracranial pressure and to maintain seizure precautions.

3. In MS, scattered demyelinization occurs in the brain and the spinal cord. Degeneration of the myelin sheath results in patches of sclerotic tissue and in impaired conduction of motor nerve impulses.

4. In Guillain-Barré syndrome, paralysis begins in the legs and ascends the body.

5. When a patient has a seizure, the nurse should observe and record: aura incontinence, initial movement, respiratory pattern, duration of the seizure, loss of consciousness, and pupillary changes.

6. Head injury is classified by the type of fracture, hemorrhage, or trauma to the brain.

7. Clinical manifestations of a CVA include syncope, paresthesia, headache, aphasia, seizures, paralysis, labile emotional responses, and change in level of consciousness.

8. The clinical manifestations for a patient with a cerebellar tumor include poor coordination and impaired equilibrium.

9. Two key nursing interventions for a patient with a spinal cord injury are to assess for autonomic dysreflexia and to check for spinal shock.

CHAPTER 4

1. Before an endoscopy, the nurse should withhold food and fluids; obtain written, informed consent; obtain baseline vital signs; and administer sedatives, as prescribed. After the procedure, the nurse should assess the patient's gag and cough reflexes; withhold food and fluids until the gag reflex returns; and assess the patient's vasovagal response.

2. After pancreatic surgery, the patient should learn to monitor urine glucose and ketones and to recognize the signs of hyperglycemia.

3. Three types of portal systemic shunts are portacaval, splenorenal, and mesocaval.

4. Dumping syndrome is a possible complication of a partial gastrectomy.

5. In an abdominoperineal resection, the distal sigmoid colon, rectum, and anus are removed. A permanent colostomy is then created.

6. A patient with a hiatal hernia should be instructed to follow dietary recommendations and restrictions; eat small, frequent meals; avoid carbonated beverages and alcohol; and maintain an upright position for 2 hours after eating.

7. The patient with a gastric ulcer should eliminate caffeine, alcohol, and spicy or fried foods.

8. The fecal occult blood test would be positive for a patient with gastric cancer.

9. Ulcerative colitis is an inflammation of the large bowel; Crohn's disease is a chronic inflammatory disease of the small intestine. Usually, Crohn's disease affects the terminal ileum and ascending colon. It progresses slowly with exacerbations and remissions.

10. A patient with diverticulosis should avoid corn, nuts, and fruits and vegetables with seeds.

11. The clinical manifestations of an intestinal obstruction include nausea, singultus, constipation, cramping pain, abdominal distention, elevated temperature, diminished or absent bowel sounds, weight loss, and vomiting of fecal material.

12. Heat should not be applied to the abdomen of a patient with peritonitis.

13. A patient with hemorrhoids should follow a high-fiber, low-roughage diet and should increase fluid intake.

14. Colorectal cancer commonly metastasizes to the liver.

15. A patient with cholecystitis is placed on a low-fat, high-carbohydrate, high-protein, high-fiber, and low-calorie diet, with small, frequent feedings. Intake of gas-forming foods is restricted.

16. Blood chemistry tests for a patient with hepatic cirrhosis would show increased AST, ALT, LDH, alkaline phosphatase, ammonia, bilirubin, and BSP and decreased albumin.

17. Type A hepatitis virus is transmitted through oral ingestion of fecal-contaminated food and liquids, such as water and milk.

CHAPTER 5

1. For 3 days before a urine VMA test, the patient should avoid vanilla, coffee, tea, citrus fruits, bananas, nuts, and chocolate.

2. Endocrine disorders may lead to decreased self-esteem, changes in body image, and embarrassment from changes in body function and structure.

3. After an adrenalectomy, the patient should be taught that hormonal replacement will be lifelong.

4. Complications of a hypophysectomy include diabetes insipidus, increased ICP, hemorrhage, adrenal crisis, thyroid storm, meningitis, and diplopia.

5. After a parathyroidectomy, the patient should have a diet high in calcium and vitamin D, with calcium and vitamin D supplements.

6. Signs and symptoms of thyroid storm include tachycardia, delirium, agitation, coma, hyperpyrexia, dehydration, arrhythmias, and diarrhea.

7. The clinical manifestations of hypothyroidism include fatigue, weight gain, dry flaky skin, edema, intolerance to cold, coarse hair, alopecia, thick tongue, swollen lips, mental sluggishness, menstrual disorders, constipation, hypersensitivity to drugs (narcotics, barbiturates, and anesthetics), anorexia, decreased diaphoresis, and hypothermia.

8. For a patient with thyroid cancer, blood chemistry tests would reveal increased calcitonin, serotonin, and prostaglandins.

9. Medications for a simple goiter include iodine preparations and thyroid hormone replacements.

10. In hyperparathyroidism, excessive PTH secretion leads to bone demineralization and hypocalcemia.

11. For a patient with hypoparathyroidism, the key nursing intervention is to maintain seizure precautions.

12. Diagnostic tests for Cushing's syndrome include dexamethasone suppression test, X-rays, angiography, CT scan, urine chemistry, blood chemistry, ultrasonography, hematology, and GTT.

13. The urine chemistry test for Addison's disease would show decreased 17-KS and 17-OH-CS.

14. In pheochromocytoma, a tumor in the adrenal medulla secretes large amounts of catecholamines. The increased catecholamines cause hypertension, an increased BMR, and hyperglycemia.

15. The acid-base imbalance seen with hyperaldosteronism is metabolic alkalosis.

16. Two key clinical manifestations of diabetes insipidus are polyuria (greater than 5 liters/day) and polydipsia (4 to 40 liters/day).

17. Acromegaly is the hypersecretion of growth hormone by the anterior pituitary gland.

CHAPTER 6

1. A patient with a kidney transplant should be placed in protective isolation.

2. A patient's nephrostomy tube should not be irrigated or manipulated.

3. Four types of urinary diversions are ureterosigmoidostomy, nephrostomy, ileal conduit, and cutaneous ureterostomy.

4. In a patient with glomerulonephritis, a urine chemistry test would reveal increased RBCs, WBCs, protein, casts, and specific gravity. A blood chemistry test for the same patient would reveal increased BUN and creatinine but decreased protein, creatinine clearance, C-reactive protein, and albumin.

5. Pyelonephritis warrants a soft, high-calorie, low-protein diet.

6. A diet high in calcium, vitamin D, milk, protein, oxalate, and alkali is associated with urolithiasis.

7. The diet therapy for acute renal failure is low-protein, increased carbohydrate, moderate-calorie with potassium, sodium, and phosphorus intake regulated according to serum levels.

8. Diagnostic tests for bladder cancer include cystoscopy, IVP, KUB, cytologic exam, urine chemistry, and hematology.

9. Key manifestations of BPH are urinary frequency, urgency, or hesitancy; burning on urination; and decreased force and amount of stream.

CHAPTER 7

1. After bronchoscopy, nursing interventions include assessing the patient's cough and gag reflex, assessing the patient's sputum, determining the patient's respiratory status, withholding the patient's food and fluids until the gag reflex returns, and checking the patient's vasovagal response.

2. A total laryngectomy involves the surgical removal of the larynx, hyoid bone, and tracheal rings; the closure of the pharynx; and the formation of a permanent tracheostomy.

3. A key postoperative assessment for a radical neck dissection is determining the patient's gag and cough reflex plus the patient's ability to swallow.

4. Following a pneumonectomy, the patient should be placed on the back or the side of the surgery.

5. Possible surgical complications of an embolectomy include hemorrhage, embolus, and thrombus.

6. A vena caval filter is used to partially occlude the inferior vena cava and, thus, prevent pulmonary emboli.

7. Possible clinical manifestations of pneumonia include cough, malaise, chills, shortness of breath, dyspnea, elevated temperature, rales, rhonchi, pleural friction rub, pleuritic pain, and sputum production.

8. The four diseases associated with COPD include bronchiectasis, asthma, bronchitis, and emphysema.

9. In ARDS, the ABGs would reveal respiratory acidosis.

10. TB is transmitted through droplets produced during coughing.

11. The key clinical manifestation present in a pneumothorax is diminished or absent breath sounds unilaterally.

12. The patient with a pulmonary embolism should be instructed to avoid smoking, stress, prolonged sitting and standing, constrictive clothing, leg crossing, and oral contraceptives.

13. The four histologic types of lung cancer are epidermoid, adenocarcinoma, large cell anaplastic, and small cell anaplastic.

14. Antineoplastics used to treat laryngeal cancer might include methotrexate, vincristine sulfate, bleomycin sulfate, and cisplatin.

CHAPTER 8

1. Nursing interventions for a patient undergoing skin tests include keeping the test area dry; recording the site, date, and time of the test; checking the test site for erythema, papules, vesicles, edema, and induration; and recording the date and time for the follow-up site reading.

2. The key assessment after a skin graft is to inspect the recipient site for infection, hematoma, and fluid accumulation under the graft.

3. Medications for contact dermatitis include antibiotics, antipruritics, corticosteroids, antihistamines, and antianxiety agents.

4. Clinical manifestations of psoriasis include pruritus; shedding, scaling plaques; yellow discoloration and thickening of the nails; erythema; and papules on sacrum, nails, and palms.

5. The vesicles of herpes zoster appear unilaterally clustered along peripheral sensory nerves on the trunk, thorax, and face.

6. The clinical manifestations of second degree burns reveal pain; oozing, fluid-filled vesicles; erythema; and a shiny, wet subcutaneous layer after vesicles rupture.

7. Three types of skin cancer are basal cell epithelioma, melanoma, and squamous cell carcinoma.

CHAPTER 9

1. After a lymphangiogram, the nurse should assess the patient's VS and peripheral pulses; inspect the catheter insertion site for bleeding; force fluids; and advise the patient that skin, stool, and urine will have a blue discoloration.

2. After a splenectomy, the patient should be taught about the need for prophylactic antibiotics.

3. Donor bone marrow is transplanted through an I.V. infusion into the recipient.

4. Agranulocytosis refers to a profound decrease in the number of granulocytes.

5. In leukemia, a bone marrow biopsy would reveal a large number of immature leukocytes.

6. Two chemotherapy protocols for Hodgkin's disease are MOPP and ABVD.

7. In the early, or acute, stage of AIDS, clinical manifestations include fatigue, weakness, anorexia, weight loss, recurrent diarrhea, fever, lymphadenopathy, pallor, night sweats, and malnutrition.

8. Diet therapy for iron deficiency anemia would include a high intake of iron, roughage, protein, and vitamins. Fluids should also be increased.

9. In ITP, antibody-coated platelets are removed from circulation by the reticuloendothelial cells of the spleen and liver. The decrease in the number of circulating platelets causes bleeding.

10. For a patient with polycythemia vera, blood chemistry tests would reveal increased uric acid, unconjugated bilirubin, vitamin B_{12}, alkaline phosphatase, AST, ALT, and LDH.

11. DIC is the a body's response to an injury or disease in which microthrombi obstruct the blood supply to organs and hemorrhage occurs throughout the body. Activation of the thrombin and fibrinolytic system results in simultaneous bleeding and thrombosis.

12. The diet therapy for multiple myeloma includes a high intake of protein, carbohydrate, vitamins, and minerals in small, frequent feedings.

C: NANDA Taxonomy of Nursing Diagnoses

This list represents the North American Nursing Diagnosis Association (NANDA) approved nursing diagnoses for clinical use and testing (1992).

PATTERN 1: Exchanging

1.1.2.1 Altered nutrition: More than body requirements

1.1.2.2 Altered nutrition: Less than body requirements

1.1.2.3 Altered nutrition: Potential for more than body requirements

1.2.1.1 High risk for infection

1.2.2.1 High risk for altered body temperature

1.2.2.2 Hypothermia

1.2.2.3 Hyperthermia

1.2.2.4 Ineffective thermoregulation

1.2.3.1 Dysreflexia

*1.3.1.1 Constipation

1.3.1.1.1 Perceived constipation

1.3.1.1.2 Colonic constipation

*1.3.1.2 Diarrhea

*1.3.1.3 Bowel incontinence

1.3.2 Altered urinary elimination

1.3.2.1.1 Stress incontinence

1.3.2.1.2 Reflex incontinence

1.3.2.1.3 Urge incontinence

1.3.2.1.4 Functional incontinence

1.3.2.1.5 Total incontinence

1.3.2.2 Urinary retention

*1.4.1.1 Altered (specify type) tissue perfusion (renal, cerebral, cardiopulmonary, gastrointestinal, peripheral)

1.4.1.2.1 Fluid volume excess

1.4.1.2.2.1 Fluid volume deficit

1.4.1.2.2.2 High risk for fluid volume deficit

*1.4.2.1 Decreased cardiac output

1.5.1.1 Impaired gas exchange

1.5.1.2 Ineffective airway clearance

1.5.1.3 Ineffective breathing pattern

#1.5.1.3.1 Inability to sustain spontaneous ventilation

#1.5.1.3.2 Dysfunctional ventilatory weaning reponse (DVWR)

1.6.1 High risk for injury

1.6.1.1 High risk for suffocation

1.6.1.2 High risk for poisoning

1.6.1.3 High risk for trauma

1.6.1.4 High risk for aspiration

1.6.1.5 High risk for disuse syndrome

1.6.2 Altered protection

1.6.2.1 Impaired tissue integrity

(continued)

New diagnostic categories approved in 1992.
* Categories with modified label terminology.

NANDA Taxonomy of Nursing Diagnoses (continued)

*1.6.2.1.1 Altered oral mucous membrane

1.6.2.1.2.1 Impaired skin integrity

1.6.2.1.2.2 High risk for impaired skin integrity

PATTERN 2: Communicating

2.1.1.1 Impaired verbal communication

PATTERN 3: Relating

3.1.1 Impaired social interaction

3.1.2 Social isolation

*3.2.1 Altered role performance

3.2.1.1.1 Altered parenting

3.2.1.1.2 High risk for altered parenting

3.2.1.2.1 Sexual dysfunction

3.2.2 Altered family processes

#3.2.2.1 Caregiver role strain

#3.2.2.2 High risk for caregiver role strain

3.2.3.1 Parental role conflict

3.3 Altered sexuality patterns

PATTERN 4: Valuing

4.1.1 Spiritual distress (distress of the human spirit)

PATTERN 5: Choosing

5.1.1.1 Ineffective individual coping

5.1.1.1.1 Impaired adjustment

5.1.1.1.2 Defensive coping

5.1.1.1.3 Ineffective denial

5.1.2.1.1 Ineffective family coping: Disabling

5.1.2.1.2 Ineffective family coping: Compromised

5.1.2.2 Family coping: Potential for growth

#5.2.1 Ineffective management of therapeutic regimen (Individuals)

5.2.1.1 Noncompliance (specify)

5.3.1.1 Decisional conflict (specify)

5.4 Health-seeking behavior (specify)

PATTERN 6: Moving

6.1.1.1 Impaired physical mobility

#6.1.1.1.1 High risk for peripheral neurovascular dysfunction

6.1.1.2 Activity intolerance

6.1.1.2.1 Fatigue

6.1.1.3 High risk for activity intolerance

6.2.1 Sleep pattern disturbance

6.3.1.1 Diversional activity deficit

6.4.1.1 Impaired home maintenance management

6.4.2 Altered health maintenance

*6.5.1 Feeding self-care deficit

6.5.1.1 Impaired swallowing

6.5.1.2 Ineffective breast-feeding

#6.5.1.2.1 Interrupted breast-feeding

6.5.1.3 Effective breast-feeding

New diagnostic categories approved in 1992.
* Categories with modified label terminology.

NANDA Taxonomy of Nursing Diagnoses *(continued)*

#6.5.1.4 Ineffective infant feeding pattern

*6.5.2 Bathing or hygiene self-care deficit

*6.5.3 Dressing or grooming self-care deficit

*6.5.4 Toileting self-care deficit

6.6 Altered growth and development

#6.7 Relocation stress syndrome

PATTERN 7: Perceiving

*7.1.1 Body image disturbance

*7.1.2 Self-esteem disturbance

7.1.2.1 Chronic low self-esteem

7.1.2.2 Situational low self-esteem

*7.1.3 Personal identity disturbance

7.2 Sensory or perceptual alterations (specify) (visual, auditory, kinesthetic, gustatory, tactile, olfactory)

7.2.1.1 Unilateral neglect

7.3.1 Hopelessness

7.3.2 Powerlessness

PATTERN 8: Knowing

8.1.1 Knowledge deficit (specify)

8.3 Altered thought processes

PATTERN 9: Feeling

*9.1.1 Pain

9.1.1.1 Chronic pain

9.2.1.1 Dysfunctional grieving

9.2.1.2 Anticipatory grieving

9.2.2 High risk for violence: Self-directed or directed at others

#9.2.2.1 High risk for self-mutilation

9.2.3 Post-trauma response

9.2.3.1 Rape-trauma syndrome

9.2.3.1.1 Rape-trauma syndrome: Compound reaction

9.2.3.1.2 Rape-trauma syndrome: Silent reaction

9.3.1 Anxiety

9.3.2 Fear

New diagnostic categories approved in 1992.
* Categories with modified label terminology.

Source: North American Nursing Diagnosis Association (1992). *NANDA Nursing Diagnoses: Definitions and Classification 1992-1993.* Philadelphia: NANDA.

D: Common Laboratory Test Values

Hematologic tests

Erythrocyte sedimentation rate
0 to 20 mm/hour; rates gradually increase with age

Hematocrit
- Adult males: 42% to 52%
- Adult females: 38% to 46%

Hemoglobin
- Adult males: 14 to 18 g/dl
- Adult females: 12 to 16 g/dl

Iron and total iron-binding capacity (TIBC)

	Men	Women
Serum iron	70 to 150 μg/dl	80 to 150 μg/dl
TIBC	300 to 400 μg/dl	300 to 450 μg/dl
Saturation	20% to 50%	20% to 50%

Red blood cell count
- Adult males: 4.5 to 6.2 million/μl of venous blood
- Adult females: 4.2 to 5.4 million/μl of venous blood

Reticulocyte count
0.5% to 2% of total RBC count

White blood cell count
4,100 to 10,900/μl

White blood cell differential
Adult values—
- Neutrophils: 47.6% to 76.8%
- Lymphocytes: 16.2% to 43%
- Monocytes: 0.6% to 9.6%
- Eosinophils: 0.3% to 7%
- Basophils: 0.3% to 2%

Coagulation tests

Activated partial thromboplastin time (APTT)
25 to 36 seconds

Bleeding time
- Template: 2 to 8 minutes
- Ivy: 1 to 7 minutes
- Duke: 1 to 3 minutes

Platelet count
130,000 to 370,000/mm³

Prothrombin time
- Males: 9.6 to 11.8 seconds
- Females: 9.5 to 11.3 seconds

Whole blood clotting time
5 to 15 minutes

Arterial blood gases

PaO_2
75 to 100 mm Hg

$PaCO_2$
35 to 45 mm Hg

pH
7.35 to 7.42

O_2 Sat
94% to 100%

HCO_3-
22 to 26 mEq/liter

O_2Ct
15% to 23%

Total carbon dioxide content
22 to 34 mEq/liter

Serum electrolytes

Calcium
4.5 to 5.5 mEq/liter (Atomic absorption: 8.9 to 10.1 mg/dl)

Common Laboratory Test Values *(continued)*

Chloride
100 to 108 mEq/liter

Magnesium
1.5 to 2.5 mEq/liter (atomic absorption: 1.7 to 2.1 mg/dl)

Phosphates
1.8 to 2.6 mEq/liter (atomic absorption: 2.5 to 4.5 mg/dl)

Potassium
3.8 to 5.5 mEq/liter

Sodium
135 to 145 mEq/liter

Serum enzymes

Acid phosphatase
- 0 to 1.1 Bodansky units/ml
- 1 to 4 King-Armstrong units/ml
- 0.13 to 0.63 BLB units/ml

Alanine aminotransferase (ALT)
- Adult males: 10 to 32 units/liter
- Adult females: 9 to 24 units/liter

Alkaline phosphatase
- 1.5 to 4 Bodansky units/dl
- 4 to 13.5 King-Armstrong units/dl
- Chemical inhibition method: Men, 90 to 239 units/dl; Women < age 45, 76 to 196 units/liter; women > age 45, 87 to 250 units/liter

Amylase
60 to 180 Somogyi units/dl

Angiotensin converting enzyme
18 to 67 U/liter (adults)

Aspartate aminotransferase (AST)
8 to 20 units/liter

Creatine phosphokinase
- Total: Men, 23 to 99 units/liter; women, 15 to 57 units/liter
- CPK-BB: none
- CPK-MB: 0 to 7 IU/liter
- CPK-MM: 5 to 70 IU/liter

Hydroxybutyric dehydrogenase (HBD)
- Serum HBD: 114 to 290 units/ml
- LDH/HBD ratio: 1.2 to 1.6:1

Lactic dehydrogenase (LDH)
- Total: 48 to 115 IU/liter
- LDH_1: 18.1% to 29% of total
- LDH_2: 29.4% to 37.5% of total
- LDH_3: 18.8% to 26% of total
- LDH_4: 9.2% to 16.5% of total
- LDH_5: 5.3% to 13.4% of total

Serum hormones

Aldosterone
1 to 21 ng/dl

Antidiuretic hormone
1 to 5 pg/ml

Chorionic gonadotropin
< 3 mIU/ml

Cortisol (plasma)
7 to 28 µg/dl in the morning to 2 to 18 µg/dl in the afternoon

Estrogens
- Premenopausal women: 24 to 68 pg/ml on days 1 to 10, 50 to 186 pg/ml on days 11 to 20, and 73 to 149 pg/ml on days 21 to 28
- Men: 12 to 34 pg/ml

Free thyroxine (FT₄)
0.8 to 3.3 ng/dl

(continued)

Common Laboratory Test Values (continued)

Free triiodothyronine
0.2 to 0.6 ng/dl

Growth hormone
● Men: 1 to 5 ng/ml
● Women: 0 to 10 ng/ml

Insulin
0 to 25 μU/ml

Parathyroid hormone
210 to 310 pg/ml

Prolactin
0 to 23 ng/dl in nonlactating females

Thyroxine (T₄)
5 to 13.5 μg/dl

Triiodothyronine
90 to 239 ng/dl

Serum lipids and lipoproteins

Lipoprotein-cholesterol fractionation
● HDL: 29 to 77 mg/dl
● LDL: 62 to 185 mg/dl

Total cholesterol
● Ideal: <200 mg/dl
● Borderline high: 200 to 239 mg/dl
● High: >240 mg/dl

Triglycerides
● Ages 0 to 29: 10 to 140 mg/dl
● Ages 30 to 39: 10 to 150 mg/dl
● Ages 40 to 49: 10 to 160 mg/dl
● Ages 50 to 59: 10 to 190 mg/dl

Serum proteins and pigments

Bilirubin, serum
Adult: direct, <0.5 mg/dl; indirect, ≤1.1 mg/dl

Blood urea nitrogen (BUN)
8 to 20 mg/dl

Creatinine
● Males: 0.8 to 1.2 mg/dl
● Females: 0.6 to 0.9 mg/dl

Proteins
● Total serum protein: 6.6 to 7.9 g/dl (100%)
● Albumin: 3.3 to 4.5 g/dl (53%)
● Alpha₁ globulin: 0.1 to 0.4 g/dl (14%)
● Alpha₂ globulin: 0.5 to 1 g/dl (14%)
● Beta globulin: 0.7 to 1.2 g/dl (12%)
● Gamma globulin: 0.5 to 1.6 g/dl (20%)

Uric acid
● Men: 4.3 to 8 mg/dl
● Women: 2.3 to 6 mg/dl

Serum carbohydrates

Fasting plasma glucose
70 to 100 mg/dl

Lactic acid
0.93 to 1.65 mEq/liter

Oral glucose tolerance test (OGTT)
Peak at 160 to 180 mg/dl, 30 to 60 minutes after challenge dose

Two-hour postprandial plasma glucose
<145 mg/dl

Urinalysis

Routine urinalysis
● *Appearance:* clear
● *Casts:* none, except occasional hyaline casts
● *Color:* straw
● *Crystals:* present
● *Epithelial cells:* none

Common Laboratory Test Values (continued)

- *Odor:* slightly aromatic
- *pH:* 4.5 to 8.0
- *Specific gravity:* 1.025 to 1.030
- *Sugars:* none
- *Red blood cells:* 0 to 3 per high-power field
- *White blood cells:* 0 to 4 per high-power field
- *Yeast cells:* none

Urine concentration test
- Specific gravtiy: 1.025 to 1.032
- Osmolality: > 800 mOsm/kg water

Urine dilution test
- Specific gravity: < 1.003
- Osmolality: < 100 mOsm/kg; 80% of water excreted in 4 hours

Urine chemistry tests

Amylase
10 to 80 amylase units/hour

17-ketosteroids (17-KS)
- Men: 6 to 21 mg/24 hours
- Women: 4 to 17 mg/24 hours

Creatinine clearance
- Men (age 20): 90 ml/minute/1.73 m²
- Women (age 20): 84 ml/minute/ 1.73 m²

Protein
< 150 mg/24 hours

Uric acid
250 to 750 mg/24 hours

Glucose oxidase
Negative

Ketones
Negative

Calcium
- Males: < 275 mg/24 hours
- Females: < 250 mg/24 hours

Phosphate
< 1,000 mg/24 hours

Sodium
30 to 280 mEq/24 hours

Chloride
110 to 250 mEq/24 hours

Cerebrospinal fluid

Glucose
50 to 80 mg/100 ml (two-thirds of blood glucose)

Pressure
50 to 180 mm H₂O

Protein
15 to 45 mg/dl

Stool tests

Lipids
Less than 20% of excreted solids, with excretion of less than 7 g/24 hours

Occult blood
2.5 mg/24 hours

Urobilinogen
50 to 300 mg/24 hours

Source: *Nurse's FactFinder.* Springhouse, Pa.: Springhouse Corp., 1991.

Selected References

Brunner, L.S., and Suddarth, D.S. *The Lippincott Manual of Nursing Practice,* 5th ed. Philadelphia: J.B. Lippincott Co., 1991.

Brunner, L.S., and Suddarth, D.S. *Textbook of Medical-Surgical Nursing,* 6th ed. Philadelphia: J.B. Lippincott Co., 1988.

Govoni, L., and Hayes, J.E. *Drugs and Nursing Implications,* 7th ed. East Norwalk, Conn.: Appleton and Lange, 1991.

Gruendemann, B.J., and Meeker, M.H. *Alexander's Care of the Patient in Surgery,* 9th ed. St. Louis: C.V. Mosby Co., 1991.

Holman, S.R. *Essentials of Nutrition for the Health Professions.* Philadelphia: J.B. Lippincott Co., 1987.

Ignatavicius, D. *Medical Surgical Nursing.* Philadelphia: W.B. Saunders, Co., 1991.

Kim, M.J., et al. *Pocket Guide to Nursing Diagnoses,* 4th ed. St. Louis: Mosby-Year Book, Inc., 1991.

Kneisl, C.R., and Ames, S.W. *Adult Health Nursing: A Biopsychosocial Approach.* Reading, Mass.: Addison-Wesley Publishing Co., 1986.

Luckmann, J., and Sorensen, K.C. *Medical-Surgical Nursing: A Psychophysiologic Approach,* 2nd ed. Philadelphia: W.B. Saunders Co., 1987.

Pagana, K.D., and Pagana, T.J. *Diagnostic Testing and Nursing Implications: A Case Study Approach,* 3rd ed. St. Louis: C.V. Mosby Co., 1990.

Patrick, M.L., et al. *Medical Surgical Nursing: Pathophysiological Concepts.* 2nd ed. Philadelphia: J.B. Lippincott Co., 1991.

Phipps, W.J., et al., eds. *Medical-Surgical Nursing: Concepts and Clinical Practice,* 4th ed. St. Louis: Mosby-Year Book, Inc., 1991.

Price, S.A., and Wilson, L.M. *Pathophysiology,* 4th ed. New York: McGraw-Hill Book Co., 1991.

Swearingen, P.L., ed. *Manual of Nursing Therapeutics: Applying Nursing Diagnoses to Medical Disorders,* 2nd ed. Menlo Park, Calif.: Addison-Wesley Publishing Co., 1990.

Thompson, J.M., et al. *Clinical Nursing.* St. Louis: C.V. Mosby Co., 1989.

Ulrich, S.P., et al. *Nursing Care Planning Guides: A Nursing Diagnosis Approach,* 2nd ed. Philadelphia: W.B. Saunders Co., 1990.

Index

Sulkowitch's test, 186
Sweat glands, 295
Sympathectomy, 38, 356
Synovectomy, 53
Synovium, 48
Systemic lupus erythematosus, 81-83

T
Tachypnea, 278
Tendons, 48
Thenar, 74, 356
Thoracentesis, 263
Thrombocytes, 314
Thrombophlebitis, 38-40
Thyroidectomy, 190-191
Thyroid gland, 180
Thyroid storm, 194
Tophi, 49, 356
Trachea, 261
Transplantation
    kidney, 233-235
    marrow, 322-323
Transverse carpal ligament, release of,
    57-58
Tuberculosis, pulmonary, 280-282
Tumor, brain, 118-120

U
Ulcer, gastric, 144-146
Ultrasonography, 7, 132, 184
Ureter, 227
Ureterosigmoidostomy, 238-239
Ureterostomy, cutaneous, 238-239
Urethra, 227
Urine
    diagnostic tests of, 183-184, 228-229,
        318
    formation of, 227
Urolithiasis, 245-247
Urologic system. *See* Renal and urologic
    system.

V
Vagotomy, 137
Valve replacement, 9
Valvular annuloplasty, 9
Valvuloplasty, 9
Vasopressin, 180, 356
Vena caval filter, 272-273
Venogram, 7
Vesicle, 297, 356

W-X-Y-Z
Wedge resection, 269-271
White blood cells, 314
Wood's light, 297
X-ray
    bone and joint, 51
    chest, 6, 262
    kidneys, ureters, bladder (KUB), 229
    skull, 92-93